Twelve Therapists

How They Live and Actualize Themselves

Arthur Burton & Associates

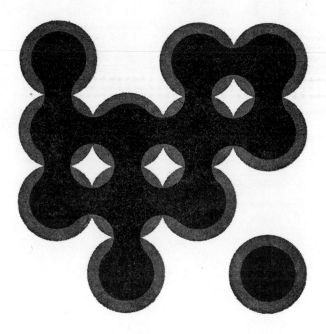

TWELVE
THERAPISTS

Jossey-Bass Inc., Publishers
San Francisco • Washington • London • 1972

921
B95t

TWELVE THERAPISTS
How They Live and Actualize Themselves
    by Arthur Burton and Associates

Copyright © 1972 by Jossey-Bass, Inc., Publishers

Published and copyrighted in Great Britain by
Jossey-Bass, Inc., Publishers
3, Henrietta Street
London W.C.2

Library of Congress Catalogue Card Number LC 72-83966

International Standard Book Number ISBN 0-87589-139-X

Manufactured in the United States of America

JACKET DESIGN BY WILLI BAUM

FIRST EDITION

Code 7224

The Jossey-Bass Behavioral Science Series

General Editors

WILLIAM E. HENRY
University of Chicago

NEVITT SANFORD
Wright Institute, Berkeley

To James A. Kennedy, M.D.
The physician as humanist

Preface

The objectivity required of science when applied to the field of psychotherapy has at times obscured the human events played out on the healing scene. Never are these more crystalline than in the perpetuated belief that the doctor has the precision of his instruments. A century of psychotherapy has revealed that this assumption is false—that indeed the psychotherapist brings as much art as science to his work. Should he refuse artistic creativity and improvisation, he fails in his primary mission of healing.

It is ironic that although Freud revealed the innermost secrets of his psyche to a world often hostile to them, in the practice of psychoanalysis a pattern of aloofness was carried far beyond any conceptual credence or necessity. In this developing pattern the person of the analyst was incredibly protected. I believe that a stimulus for the creation of *Twelve Therapists* was the experience during my training analysis of accidentally seeing my analyst urinating at a nearby hotel where I had stopped for a strengthening coffee. I almost believed at the time that he did not pee—and that he did not need to! Today, this incident is the subject of some personal humor when I tell my classes about it.

The courageous psychotherapists who elected to participate in *Twelve Therapists* reveal themselves as quite human indeed. We might even say that they are full of problems we do not expect to find in psychotherapists. But the point is that to meliorate the distinctive problems of living, one has also to be human, and that means to have problems like everyone else. The distinction between client and therapist comes only in that the therapist works his problems through, recovers thereby a consistent and fulfilling philosophy of existence, and then offers it to others in a spirit of comradeship. We might say he shares his problems rather than broods on them.

In a radical way I suggest that anyone contemplating becoming a client first ask his doctor about his (the doctor's) life. If the doctor refuses or is hurt or defensive about the question, the client-to-be should perhaps go to someone else. This suggestion does not mean that a proper sense of timing for disclosure is not required by therapists; but with many disclosure never comes at all.

I want to salute the grand people who offered their lives for public inspection in this book and did it with an eagerness which also characterizes their entire treatment work. (Others invited were not so fortunate with themselves.) Their willingness implies that these very special therapists can laugh at themselves, their mistakes, their weaknesses, but also their strengths. Psychotherapists need to laugh more.

Davis and Sacramento, California   ARTHUR BURTON
March 10, 1972

Contents

Contributors

ARTHUR BURTON, *psychotherapist in private practice, Sacramento and Davis, Calif.; professor of psychology, California State University, Sacramento*

RUDOLF EKSTEIN, *director, Childhood Psychosis Project, Reiss-Davis Child Study Center, Los Angeles; clinical professor of medical psychology, University of California, Los Angeles; senior faculty member, Los Angeles Psychoanalytic Society and Institute and Southern California Society and Institute*

ALBERT ELLIS, *director, Institute for Advanced Study in Rational Psychotherapy, New York*

O. SPURGEON ENGLISH, *professor of psychiatry, Temple University School of Medicine; member, Philadelphia Psychoanalytic Society*

REUBEN FINE, *director, Center for Creative Living, New York; visiting professor, Adelphi University*

JUAN J. LOPEZ-IBOR, *professor of psychiatry and medical psychology, University of Madrid; past president, World Congress of Psychiatry*

WERNER M. MENDEL, *professor of psychiatry, University of Southern California School of Medicine; member, Los Angeles Psychoanalytic Institute*

ERVING POLSTER, *chairman and founding member, postgraduate training faculty, Gestalt Institute of Cleveland*

CARL R. ROGERS, *resident fellow, Center for Studies of the Person, La Jolla, Calif.*

BERNARD STEINZOR, *psychotherapist in private practice, New York; lecturer, Union Theological Seminary*

HELM STIERLIN, *acting chief, Adult Psychiatry Branch, National Institute of Mental Health, Bethesda, Md.; member, Washington-Baltimore Psychoanalytic Institute*

JOHN WARKENTIN, *member, Atlanta Psychiatric Clinic; past editor,* Voices

Twelve Therapists

How They Live and Actualize Themselves

Healing as a Life Style

Arthur Burton

One inspiration for this book was the growing awareness that the psychotherapist as a person was somehow being left out of contemporary psychotherapy. Recent developments in psychotherapy have all focused on the client, often to the exclusion of the therapist. In part this focus may be due to the times, which downgrade wisdom, information, and authority and is perhaps best socially reflected in the encounter group movement. Here all healing and to-be-healed members are believed to be equal. Classical psychoanalysis certainly exaggerated the contribution of the psychoanalyst, and the pendulum is now on the return sweep of accommodation. But my growing concern has been the recognition that the inner structure of the therapist has very much to do with the kind of psychotherapy he does and may indeed be the critical element in the therapeutic equation. As long as we could fool ourselves with a dubious scientific objectivity, as long as we could apply a strictly medical model, then the question of the healer's

1

personality and needs was a quiet or unformulated one. It was not the
egalitarian view of psychotherapy as an equal partnership (seen perhaps in most extreme form in Steinzor) which changed the situation
so much as a dawning recognition that psychotherapy succeeds best
when the therapist himself participates deeply in the process as a human being. When some of his own growth needs are met, the therapy
prospers; when they are not, the therapy languishes.

Therapist satisfaction has long been a gritty or closed issue. We
are constantly concerned with satisfying clients, if only because when
too many of them fail to keep their appointments we consider ourselves
a failure, and we also lose income. I would argue that the treatment
satisfactions of the therapist are as important, if not more important,
than the client's, for the simple reason that the unconscious takes over
in extreme therapist dissatisfaction and punishes or even eliminates the
client. But the question of what gives therapists satisfaction is un-
answered; up to now we dared not even ask the question. This book
responds to this need on the deepest levels using an autobiographical
mode. It dares to ask such questions as "Who is the therapist and
what is his inner person? What gave him form and substance, and
what is the milieu in which he operates?" We have assumed that all
therapists healed equally, particularly if they had the same training.
Nothing is further from the truth. Therapists, even more than do other
professionals, evidence unequal zeal, skill, and humanity in applying
their theories. Since the self is what he works with, it makes a difference whether the therapist is given to depressions, hypomania, or
schizoid behavior, let alone the normative personality question of being
a feeling, intuiting introvert—to use Jung's typology for the healer.

Creative artists reveal the widest intellectual and feeling phenomena—sometimes at the borderlands of normality—and healing is
above all a creative act. Whatever is charismatic in the therapist and
helps attract clients to him is not necessarily the scientific ideal and an
assurance of high-quality practice. Our profession willy-nilly obscures
the guidelines by which clients can judge competence once the wildest
extremes are ruled out. It therefore becomes important to match in
some way the life of the healer with the life of the client, just as in a
marriage some minimal conjunction of personality trends is necessary.
This approach puts a sophisticated matter in a gross way, but that is
perhaps appropriate. The "presentation of self" in one's treatment

office often covers all the anguish one feels inside, and if therapy is defined as shared feeling, then the client has a right to the anguish he never gets. Any therapist who consistently refuses to disclose himself is precisely fearful of that hiatus between his office persona and his real self. In this book, perhaps for the first time, the personal anguish, despair, hatred, joys, and attainments of gifted therapists are offered to the public at large. It is not masochism of any kind but the ego strength to look at what heals in the self which allows our biographees to disclose themselves in this way.

Why have we so carefully shielded our person from the client? Why has it been so difficult to share our humanity and to see clients as persons as well as transferences? Freud was ever-ready to use himself and his life experiences as an experimental laboratory, and some of his clients must surely have read *The Interpretation of Dreams* and the *Three Contributions to a Theory on Sex*. His inner life was in one way or another on public display. Jung similarly used aspects of his life to assist the therapy of a client. I suspect that therapists do a lot more of this than anyone ever really knows, but we have lost a certain openness in treatment which is the proper foundation of a generic psychotherapy.

In this age of Everyman autobiography, the paucity of such productions by psychotherapists is almost a source of embarrassment. This is why Mowrer's autobiographical denudation of self came first as a blow to the solar plexus. Certainly, as English points out, autobiographical material is not well received by either colleagues or clients, and this poor reception has perhaps been one major deterrent to publication. But I insist that the dangers are strictly overrated and will, as was found with the first psychotherapeutic tape recording, reveal themselves to be more figment than reality. Anyone who has unmasked in an encounter group, and felt afraid because of it, knows that the dangers to the self were badly overestimated. What colleagues think about us, particularly those we work with closely, is something to ponder about; but they also have the same access to autobiographical truth as we do, and if they cannot tolerate truth, they had better look to their foundations and what they are professing. The governing condition is that the science of psychotherapy now mandates the willingness to be open in this way—to share fully in what we ask the client himself to do. This mandate is in a sense the preamble to this book.

My function in this chapter is to attempt to collate the variegated autobiographical material into some kind of pattern. What generally can we say about these personalities and the way they have directed their lives? What draws them to make a positive thing out of suffering and to offer nurture to the unnurturable? Why do they come fully alive while healing and why are they bound to it? In this I draw upon my own three decades as a therapist as well as the work that has been done elsewhere on creative artists and scientists and psychotherapists by Eiduson, Henry, Stein, Holt, Roe, and others. What follows, then, is not so much a product of clinical or even literary research as a set of provisional character hypotheses on how people find personal and professional meaning in psychotherapy—indeed, how they manage to do it at all. While I have long pondered on these questions, even written some on them and examined a number of autobiographies seeking answers, I consider what follows heuristic and subject to the findings of designs involving larger samples. But lives have a way of refusing scientific controls, and a beginning must be made.

Some attributes of psychotherapy apply regardless of where or by whom it is practiced. Even though they are more properly related to classical forms of treatment, these aspects or functions are generic and apply to all healing situations where growth, fulfillment, or even cure is a goal. Exemplary are: (1) that reason is applied to an anti-reasoning process; (2) that verbal symbols become the method of molar transformation; (3) that pleasure and sex are the vehicle of the healing work; (4) that a form of "morality" is employed to counter superego "shoulds" which constitute the illness; (5) that love and mutual negation are the cement of the process; (6) that loneliness in one person is used to cure loneliness in the other; (7) that an intellectual process becomes both the quest for and answer to a less than satisfactory existence; (8) that to become less "crazy" the process first calls for becoming more so. All of these are part and parcel of the discussion to follow.

Rational Man

Some explanation is needed about why, in its evolution as a healing discipline, psychotherapy strangely found itself in the corner of medicine, the science of the healing of the pathology of the body. Considering the social or behavioral science model of treatment, or perhaps the pastoral or friendship model, it might appear that psychotherapy would have developed more brilliantly or more happily in any field *but* medicine. I do not necessarily concur in this point of view even though I know that the nonmedical therapist invariably suffers from fewer handicaps in his psychotherapeutic work than does his medical counterpart. But, to face facts, many nonmedical healing systems have come and gone and none has withstood the test of time as has medicine. Virchow, Pasteur, Roentgen, Fleming, and others made basic discoveries about man which transcend time and place. They are not matched even by Sigmund Freud. Even Scientology, that burgeoning international treatment organization of Ron Hubbard, survives because for most of its way it translates psychoanalytic discoveries into popular face validity but now has to proclaim itself a religion to exist.

The history of science is the chronicle of those campaigns which unseated the divine revelation as the fountainhead of knowledge and placed it squarely on the pivot of human and repeatable observation. Man became his own master by searching his own soul. The divine and the devil being of a piece, science brought with it a limitation not only of the God-given but of the hidden machinations of the devil as well. Mental disease had always been a province of the latter, in whatever form he wished to appear, and do not discount the people who still believe this in some form. The rational and the irrational have interminably locked horns historically, and rationality, we must say, exists only because such a dialogue was possible. I have noted with some astonishment that clients are now bringing astrological interpretations to their therapy, perhaps hoping in this way for understanding which the rational aspects of therapy cannot provide. Man lives by the rational at the same time he intimately adopts the irrational. Rationality becomes that organizational process by which social and creative discoveries are made, but as applied to any single person it rapidly falls into a dilution. Not even the most rigorous physicist lives by rationality at home, and the fact that he lights up a cigarette reveals that his inner hungers displace his rational cognitions of the statistical dangers of smoking. Logical positivism, that most exquisite philosophical statement of scientific postulation and method, was spawned in the same womb as was psychoanalysis. No one worth his salt then escaped Hegel, not to speak of the lights of Descartes. It is thus no happenstance that Freud was first a neuropathologist, and then a practicing physician, before he became a psychoanalyst and that from this basic fount of medicine came something as medically remote as psychoanalysis.

The fact is that making diagnoses—and healing—calls first for the use of logical and inductive processes; otherwise one is apt to be overwhelmed by the complexity of the disease phenomena. In the psychic arena the pathology—and the pathogen—is in its most extreme form; that is, it rarely has specific form and promises not to have any. Freedom without structure is no freedom at all, and fulfillment without conflict is not fulfilling. Psychopathology is dis-order, for which a limited order is the necessary anodyne. Rational processes, if they do little else, bring order to the wild anarchy of nature and in this way limit biological destruction. The sick are precisely those whose death science postpones.

To personify the situation a little, there are men who live by order and those who die by disorder. Scientists invariably turn out to be the former. The bringing of order (structure) to anarchy is one of the most creative acts open to sober men, and whether this action occurs on a molecular level or involves political systems is only incidental. These creations are the great achievements of a Linnaeus, Mendeleyev, Darwin; but also a Jefferson, Marx, and Sun Yat Sen.

Thus some of us are necessarily challenged by the wild anarchy of the beast within us, of imagination run riot, of the mind become uncivilized. Society, it should be noted, cannot countenance madness, which is why it provides for and fosters psychotherapy and a whole host of intramural services. The Russian situation shows that politics and psychiatric diagnosis are not so far apart as we once thought. Psychosis is felt dangerous to group survival and to civilization itself, and at best it is a return to feral man. Therapists, it seems, have a social mandate to put things mentally in order, to set things right, to provide harmony and joy. They want rationality to prevail and furthermore see this as the way to man's salvation. The intellect thereby becomes extolled—sometimes at the expense of the emotions—and art and science historically blend in this twentieth-century amalgam of psychotherapy.

In applying rationality to man's life the therapist is simply conforming to at least three millennia of Greco-Roman philosophical doctrine; but it should be noted that problem solving by rationality is by now deeply introjected and the motive itself has been lost. Rationality here is beyond reason, although it may masquerade as the apogee of reason, and in its own way it is as compelling as the priest who believes his mission is lodged in the godhead.

One pundit sees the future importance of rationality in the following way: "Clearly, a democracy in which Everyman is considered equal is the only political form in which such a universal consciousness is possible. In a secular meritocracy if you do not have a high I.Q. or a Ph.D. (or the money to protect yourself from thought police with Ph.D.s in the behavioral sciences) you are damned more effectively than you would be in the darkest ages of religion: because there is no god in whose sight all men are equal, and because there is no life after death, you are damned without hope of redemption."[1]

Every therapist keeps at least a few books visible to his clients, and some have walls lined with them. They are the cross or the Buddha of his spiritual office, and the books announce that Reason is practiced here. As we will see later, the therapist is attempting to rationalize his own historical person in this way.

Intelligence has been a most valuable social commodity and promises to become even more so in the days to come. The black never feels so desperate as when his I.Q. is believed not to be innately up to par. But reason is a massively derided and discounted phenomenon, particularly in America. It has never attained the dignity or position of, say, past aristocracy, the presiding churchman, the moneyed capitalist, or the sportsman, except possibly for extremely brief intervals. Intelligence has been kept isolated and individual, and the attempt of intelligence to band together has not been a shouting success. Yet, intelligence is a caste or ruling class which operates everywhere clandestinely in most powerful ways. The man who moves symbols moves mountains. Many moneyed men sooner or later want to give up their money because what they really want is the power of the word and symbol—that is, the spiritual and humanistic dimension in moving men.

The therapist is a man of the book, and as such he assumes the

[1] W. Thompson, *At the Edge of History.* Quoted in *The New York Times,* January 1, 1972.

power of reason and intelligence, the "wise old man archetype." Whether so many Jews become therapists because their historical definition is the "people of the book," or because Jews bring the "word" to whatever they do or are allowed to do, is a question I cannot answer. At any rate, such dynamisms arise reciprocally to feed a common personal and social need. Analytics as intelligence may yet turn out to be the most potent social force of all, and in the Age of Therapeutic Man the therapist may yet inherit the earth.

Joseph Knecht, in *Magister Ludi*,[2] has by great ardor and effort attained the supreme and exalted position of Grand Master of the Order, which brings with it a mystical and deep contemplation of man: his being, his happiness, and his future. He believes that the final bit of understanding which he lacks will be found in the "bead game" (whose nature Hesse never exactly specifies), in which there are implications of mathematics, ontology, epistemology, biology, and physics. Knecht believes that if only he can find the one key combination of monads all of man's problems will be once and for all solved. He has come closer than anyone ever has before and is momentarily on the point of the great discovery!

Now, if we for the moment place psychotherapy (in all its variant forms and in the widest sense) in the Knecht equation as the problem solving root power, then we have analogically the missing solution he sought. That is, we act as though not mathematics, not logic, not ontogeny, not molecular biology, not ethology, not religion but the therapeutic encounter is the missing radical. Is it? Millions of people believe it, I perhaps among them, and the therapeutic process now becomes the bead game universally played. Therapists are people who particularly delight in solving the happiness equation and shuffle their kings, queens, bishops, and pawns endlessly, hoping for a final solution for their clients. They are the rational men, and Reuben Fine reveals that chess, love, and therapy are not so far apart as we might have them.

Love and Mutual Negativity

Most therapists believe that what binds them to their clients— and their clients to them—is love. (Fine manifests this position most

[2] H. Hesse, *Magister Ludi: The Glass Bead Game* (New York: Bantam, 1970).

sanguinely in his psychotherapy.) I have never met one who abjured the word. They further believe that they have a greater capacity for love than have other people. I submit that this view puts the cart before the horse. What truly binds client and therapist is mutual negativity which, however, wears the facade of love. The negative charge is more explosive than the positive—and thus has greater growth potential. I have always wondered why, if therapeutic growth is merely a process of love, it went so hostilely afoul so often, why it left both participants so dissatisfied so often at the end. And the track record for therapists' loving each other, or for loving their spouses, is not at all a beautiful thing. How can we give such great quanta of love to our clients and so little to other people? Not only are divorce, suicide, schizophrenia known to occur among us but often their incidence is higher than that for the general population. Are these not examples more of negativity than of love?

All observers of the neonate focus on the positive thrust of mother and child. Their expectation is that mother will love her child —and the child will return the love of mother. They invariably fail to note the many exceptions to this loving expectation. Basic human trust, a foundation for love, does not come about through imprinting but requires an evolvement and maturation of its own. For every single erogenous zone, and for every age-level mastery, there is a dynamic of thesis and antithesis.[3] Out of the reconciliation of opposites and inherent resistance comes mastery. What I mean is that no oral, anal, phallic, or oedipal phase of human life is ever transacted without its negative or aggressive aspect. And there is no age mastery in growth and development without a first refusal of that development—perhaps we might call it an antidevelopment. Regression is in a more precise sense refusal and aggression, and positiveness and growth can take place only in the reciprocating dialogue of resistance and thrust.

Growth being ambivalence, therapy is therefore also ambivalence. It is no happenstance that countertransference comes in for such momentous stress in psychoanalysis. Beginning analysts are mortally afraid of their countertransferences, and it takes years before countertransference security is gained. The opportunity to be mutually negative within the positive, loving framework of therapy duplicates an

[3] A. Freud, *Ego and the Mechanisms of Defense* (rev. ed.) (New York: International Universities Press, 1967).

ancient and residual family situation in which mutual negativity was left unresolved. Family love was therefore never totally complete. Furthermore, it was contingent upon the therapist-to-be to solve the family riddle and to make the family happy. He believed that without his ministrations the family might well go down the drain. Albert Ellis describes this responsibility most poignantly in his autobiography.

A child is in some strange way selected to provide happiness for all, and to him is given the role of healer. Obviously, a grown-up is better prepared to handle such a mandate than a child, so the child, in the face of the impossibility of the task, carries it over to adulthood. The demand becomes a latency and is repressed but remains as a draft on the currency of the personality. How else do we explain the total acceptance of unbridled venom from some clients, the terrible vicissitudes of doing psychotherapy with chronic regressed schizophrenics, the endless complaints and victimization of the neurotic, the narcissism and infantility of the character disorders? On the face of it, no therapist would rationally submit to psychotherapy for any of the rewards now extant.

Jews are known for not leaving their families, for "hanging in" no matter how inadequate and miserable the family, and they do not easily desert their familial responsibilities. They make do, work things through, and live fully to the level of their despair and misery. The Christian therapists in this book seem to have the same family dynamics since they also cannot easily leave the family field. How do we explain the fact that so little physical sexuality, so little long-term love, and so few marriages come out of therapy? Therapists actually require two families: one for living and loving out—wife and children—and the other, the therapeutic marriage, with mutual negativity, pseudo-intimacy, but no acted upon love and marriage. And never do the twain meet.

Loneliness

Therapists find their best consolation within their inner selves. This is the way it was with Sigmund Freud and C. G. Jung. Carl Rogers reiterates again and again how he preferred to read rather than seek the company of his fellow mill workers in his youth. It is not that therapists are uncomfortable with the social scene but that their inner life is so much richer than the often ritualized allegro which passes for social life. The words introvertive or schizoid do not describe this creative state of being—these are pejorative terms—for it is voluntarily elected, and some people require more incubation of their creativity than do others. This inner dialogue with the parts of self, or with the self temporally and spatially juxtaposed, satisfies the interpersonal Self-Other need but also provides an epiphenomenal feeling of being separated or special. We could call this quality of existence "passionate loneliness," and I believe that therapists do indeed feel more lonely than other people. All serious creative artists have this form of loneliness (and fight mightily against it) which revolves around feelings of the significance of their productions. Sartre had to give up many a session at the Cafe Flore to set down the written word!

Society abets the passionate loneliness of the therapist by conferring special privileges upon him, by raising him above the herd, and by mystifying his messages. And by so doing it makes him somewhat untouchable. Lest this make any therapist feel smug, society tends to do the same with garbage collectors and others who work with waste. A disturbing fact in general medicine today is the rise of malpractice suits, but what bothers physicians most is not the lawsuits but that the *populi* dares to challenge their untouchability. It is interesting that in any ordinary commercial transaction one has only to reveal that one is a therapist to have the entire basis of the transaction shift away from economics. Most people in the world have never met a therapist face to face, and doing so socially or economically changes the straightforwardness of the engagement. People are both attracted to and repelled by those who joust with the demon (or who handle dirt), and if this work is believed done by magic or quasimagic, the therapist cannot thereafter be treated as a mere mortal. The total effect of such social forces surrounding healing is to thrust the therapist deeper into himself, his family, and the therapeutic ghetto. By a simple transformation, passionate loneliness becomes pride, self-sufficiency, creativeness, arrogance, tenacity, and the like. But it also serves to draw the therapist deeper into the ambience of his clients. Only a man who has had tuberculosis knows what the healing entails on the quiet mountain. Only the passionately lonely can understand the despair and loneliness

of the client who wants intimate social participation but is invariably
left out. The therapist is, in a sense, in the same boat, but he knows the
joy of self-communion, embraces it fully, lives by it, and helps others
with it. For most therapists compassion for the healthy is normative,
but for the maimed, withdrawn, or underprivileged, it knows no
bounds.

Justice and Charity

Henry[4] cites the not-astonishing fact that 50 per cent of the
therapists in his large study sample were Jewish or of Jewish extraction.

> *There is indeed a marked tendency for practitioners in the
> mental health field to have Jewish cultural origins. Moreover, the
> prevailing stereotype of the Jewish psychotherapist is an apt descrip-
> tion of the sample as a whole and is not confined to psychoanalysis.
> Not only do a majority of mental health professionals in the sample
> claim a Jewish cultural affinity, but the proportion of practitioners hav-
> ing a Jewish affinity is twice as large as the proportion claiming an
> affinity with the second most popular tradition, Protestantism. As a
> result of this pattern, the mental health field is, in terms of professional
> composition, not only more Jewish than most other professional fields
> but also more culturally homogeneous than other fields. Thus cultural
> affinity may exercise a stronger influence on entry into the mental
> health professions than is true for most other professions.*

The interest in medicine on the part of the Jew has always
been strong and the new psychological medicine has an added attraction for him—in part because he was filling a vacuum and a role no
one else wanted but also because the demonic and irrational has a
special fascination for him. To provide hope where there is no hope is
precisely the function of the professional person of this ethnic group.
My prophecy is that the field will become even more heavily saturated
with Jews in the future, and the ratio of seven Jews to five non-Jews,
which occurred on a chance basis in this book, will in later editions
turn out to be nine out of twelve.

Of interest also perhaps is that most of the therapists in his

---

[4] W. E. Henry, J. H. Sims, S. L. Spray, *The Fifth Profession* (San
Francisco: Jossey-Bass, 1971).

study were only one or two generations removed from specific European origins. The residual world centers of influence of psychoanalysis and psychotherapy in England and the United States—the English-speaking countries—were formed because these are precisely the areas where nineteenth-century Jewish emigration from Russia, Poland, Austria, Hungary, Lithuania, found its greatest outlet.

The tenacity of Jewish existence over more than four millennia, and in the face of the most militant pressure for elimination or assimilation, is a startling thing and requires sociological explanation. Of course, there is no convincing documentation, but on a psychological basis we know that forces leading to extinction have their expression in a yet even greater will to live.[5] There is also the peculiar paradox that six million Jews were more or less docilely led to gas chambers by Hitler at the time that the will to survive in them was greater than ever. This docility has been blamed on the Hassidim and the imminence of the Messiah who the Torah promised would appear mysteriously one day. The psychological problem is that the will to live is also the will to die—in a careful balance.

The archetypal values of being a Jew, reinforced by ever-present survival needs, are part and parcel of what every Jewish boy has dinned into him. Only a rare few can escape their fate. One of these values is the love of wisdom and the love of learning. In Lvov or Kiev, the Jewish father was not expected to work and support his family. His work was to study the Talmud and become wise in Jewish ritual and law. The rabbi was not only a religious and spiritual man but the secular leader of the community. He served as judge and jury about most matters of daily living. He was the Wise Old Man backed by millennial tradition, contact with God, an overriding morality, and an ethic of health and happiness. Today Israel is rocked by the internecine struggle between the god-fearing of three thousand years ago and the secularists who want to be more in tune with the scientific world around them. The issue is not yet decided. I predict that the resolution, when it comes, will carry with it a Talmudic dynamic acceptable in

[5] Scholars studying this survival phenomenon attribute it to monotheism, the imminent coming of the Messiah, Mosaic Law and the Talmudic tradition, and to values surrounding learning and abstraction. None suffices.

some way to the modern world but also fully integrated with Jewish history. Of course, success for Jews also came to mean trading and acquisition of money, yet rarely was money itself the end. Gaining it meant shelter from anti-Semitism and more plausible social accommodation and assimilation, but in the long run it offered the opportunity to exercise justice and charity. The Hebrew words for these two virtues are interestingly the same. And Aris[6] quotes Sir Isaac Wolfson as follows: "My father said that there are two things I want to tell you that you must remember all your life. God gives to him who gives; and the man who transforms a miserable wretch into a contented mind merits a place on the right hand of God."

Humanistic psychotherapy is not so much a matter of eliminating uncomfortable symptoms as it is a penetration to the heart of the philosophy of existence. What the manifest symptoms mean to the psyche and what the client makes of them in his overall life constitute his disablement. The creative excitement in therapy, unknown to other professions, is derived from being present at the ontic birth of a new being—assisting in its re-formation, definition, and extrusion. I would say that no husband no matter how long he is married to his wife attains this specific form of therapeutic ecstasy in his marriage. Other forms of pleasure, yes, but not this, for if he has to reconstruct his wife, give her rebirth, he has a divorce on his hands. For a therapist whose existence has problematic aspects reflected in his unconscious, "charitably" helping a client work out his fate is tantamount to helping the therapist resolve his own. I do not speak here of a clinical neurosis in the therapist, which is an entirely different matter. What becomes resolved by the therapist in his psychotherapeutic work in unaware ways is his survival and the perpetuation of his ages-old values and of his identification as a Jew. Psychotherapy is one situation where the Jewish therapist is not only not discriminated against but is actively wooed because, being Jewish, he knows the cabbala well enough to work with the demonic.

One theory of the origins of Jewish professional affiliation is:

> *The Jews have produced many famous businessmen but they have also provided outstanding scientists, academics, and musicians. It*

[6] S. Aris, *But There Are No Jews in England* (New York: Stein and Day, 1971), p. 174.

*is not easy to analyse why Jews have made such an outstanding con-
tribution to mathematics, physics, chemistry and biology any more
than it is simple to untangle the reason why many should have succeeded so well in business. But I think part of the answer is to be
found in the* shtetl *where the study of the Torah was an inevitable,
unavoidable part of a Jewish boy's education. Not all of them, of
course, became rabbis, however much their parents might wish it. But
it did provide them with an intellectual training of a very special and
formidable kind. It was a rigorous, scholastic discipline very similar
to that which the medieval schoolmen, who were forever arguing about
how many angels sit on the point of a needle, endured.*[7]

Dimont[8] points out the influence of the study of the Talmud
in that peculiar mixture of logic, love, and faith which the historical
Yeshiva left on its many participants. "Anything in the Talmud came
to be regarded as Judaism itself; any deviation with a horror usually
reserved for apostates. It became a strait jacket constricting the universal ideas of the Jews. . . Here, in cheerless, bleak classrooms, the
pale ghetto students of the Talmud were taught subtle rules of law and
logic. At an early age they came into contact with the humanism of
Rashi and rationalism of Maimonedes. They learned to think in abstract terms, to apply obsolete laws to nonexistent situations, to deal
with the imagination in concrete terms."

Aris, a journalist by profession, omits psychiatry from the fields
focused on by Jews, perhaps because he subsumes psychiatry under
science. But the reason for the oversight may have another source: it
is both an obscure and a sensitive subject that Jews have become pre-
dominant in mental healing. It is no longer fashionable or feasible for
the masses of Jewish boys to succeed in business in the old way and
they have looked for new fields to conquer. Like other youths today,
the young Jew is redirected away from corporate business to humanitarian service. Becoming a psychoanalyst, psychiatrist, or clinical psychologist or psychiatric social worker now best meets a variety of Jewish personal and archetypal needs—that is, intellectual expression,
outlet for creative imagination, social power, economic security, personal identity, charity, Talmudic morality, and the like. This role

[7] Aris, p. 174.
[8] M. I. Dimont, *Jews, God and History.* (New York: Signet,
1962), pp. 180–181.

provides Jewish growth and survival at their best; through it the Jew
fights the dybbuk and socializes him for the common weal.

Moral Values

Despite a recent book[9] which indirectly impugns psychotherapy
as immoral and panders to popular belief, therapy is a highly moral
business. Rieff correctly and not surprisingly calls Freud a moralist.
Every therapist is a moralist whether or not he believes he is. Where
guilt and restitution are common features of the content; where love
and sex are the vehicles of neurosis and need to be aired; where the
couch is the symbol and actuality of cure, then therapy must by conventional definition be a moral process. Morality is concerned with
fulfillment and happiness, and immorality is the conflict about being
happy.

In no other profession I know of are pleasure and sexuality so
regularly a part of the transaction, yet in no other profession is there
so little absolute physical sexuality—in face of the grand opportunities
available—as in this one. Psychotherapy is a kind of pseudo-sexual
relationship, backed by true feelings of love, with concealed signals
that this is not to be consummated. It is not transference but transfer-
incest, and the taboo is as strong as actual incest. This does not mean
that both types do not occur. But I ask myself the following questions
in the everlasting face of temptation. Would I be willing to give up
healing this lovely client to go to bed with her (you cannot do both)?
Would I want her permanently in place of my wife?

In my experience very few therapists report changing clients
for wives. But why not? Are they not in a sense our products, and do
we not know their interior even better than we do our wives? Well, it
is a superego question, and in the two families which every therapist
has, only one is for real, and that reality is a "covenant made on the
mount." I have known therapists who have slept with clients, and
even one or two who married them. The sky did not fall in. But the
point is that any therapist *qua* therapist who uses his office for sexual
recruitment cannot really enjoy his sexuality or ever make something
permanent out of it. There is also a good probability that his love is

[9] M. Shepard, *The Love Treatment* (New York: Wyden, 1971).

neurotic or counterfeit love. More seriously yet, this action is prima facie evidence that his treatment work is inadequate and that he does not even know it is.

Therapists are perhaps more sensual people than others, and they are certainly titillated by the sexual secrets they hear. Fine uses the word *excited*, which I believe is perhaps too strong. But it is a fact that there are not many Casanovas in the psychoanalytic profession, except possibly in the public imagination. I have earlier written that becoming a therapist calls for a full development of the feminine side of the therapist's personality, and experience shows that those therapists who are overburdened by masculine needs do not remain long in direct treatment with clients. Intuition, sensitivity, affect, feeling, artistry, color, all highly relevant to the work of the therapist, are better realized as feminine qualities, and they are most certainly correlated with success and gratification in work as a therapist. This does not at all mean that masculinity has no place in psychotherapy, only that a primary focus on the phallus and its expression leaves something to be desired.

Mothers, Fathers, and Problem-Solving

Albert Ellis to the contrary, a therapist is made in childhood. The specific kind of therapy he does is determined by experiential factors, backed of course by the particular endowment he brings to his experience. Ellis may believe that rational-emotive therapy is his considered judgment of what is best for clients, and Rogers similarly the client-centered approach, but learning, style and temperamental and metaphysical factors also make these approaches the best for these two personalities. The study of the lives of therapists reveals that the great majority of them were early given the responsibility for the happiness of their families. Since every study shows that they mostly come from disrupted or disjointed families, often with the father physically or psychically absent, the therapists-to-be were delegated the task of assuring the fate and fulfillment of the family. They became, and are, the family nurturer. They had a very low threshold for family argument, family pain, and could not bind it. This is a sometimes subtle thing, but the important point is that all therapists recall something like this in their background. Growing up for our therapists was a

constant turmoil, a daily solving of living problems, as they attempted
to reconcile as many family members as possible. Ellis and Rogers
bring this out most poignantly. Do some of us then feel our mission
to be the healing of marriages or the divorcing of them? It really makes
no difference which, in the sense that we are out to bring individual
and collective happiness to families, and the consideration of which
persons or which family is perhaps secondary.

Our therapists are, by and large, highly critical of their mothers
and much more laudatory of their fathers. English says, for example,
of his father "that he was unusually endowed with confidence, optimism, overt humor and courage, did not tend to be distrustful of his
fellow man, and was forward looking and successful." Rogers also
quietly respects his father and made at least one close and lengthy
trip with him when he was in trouble. Mothers were furthermore seen
by many of our therapists as interfering with the father's success and,
directly or indirectly, estranging him from the family, sometimes putting the therapist-to-be in his place.

One would expect that the mothers of therapists would be
Florence Nightingale types, inspiring their sons to heal people at whatever cost to themselves. But nothing seems further from the truth. If
not merely a pallid or uninspired group of women, they actually neglected or were indifferent to the welfare of their therapist-to-be child
and their other children. Or, more properly, they manipulated the
therapist-to-be for their private benefits—for their own happiness. I
believe one reason therapists are so finicky about the conditions under
which they do psychotherapy—therapy can actually be done anywhere
—is that they are unconsciously attempting to reinstate the perfect
family milieu where healing and fulfillment can be maximized. Any
detraction from perfection comes through as an irritability, a not unknown trait in our profession.

The fact that most patients are women but most psychotherapists men creates an interesting heterosexual therapeutic situation.[10]

[10] The current membership of the American Psychoanalytic Association is composed of 88 per cent males and 12 per cent females; in
1970–1971, the American Psychiatric Association had 89 per cent males
and 11 per cent females; the Division of Psychotherapy of the American
Psychological Association indicates a fellowship of 86 or 87 per cent men

Is there a male/female need which is socially and personally met in this approved way? Is this a revenant of an unresolved oedipal situation which is perhaps now approaching universality in our society? We become transferential father figures to women, overlooking the fact that female clients become countertransferential mother figures to us. But it is the introjected idealized father who wants to relate to the female client, and thus to the countertransferential mother. In this way father and mother can be happily merged and a fulfilled family life prevail. The therapist satisfies his repetition compulsion of quieting the tension of his family and replacing it by something more ideal. One therapist says, "Patients have been and still are all important for without them I would go unchallenged and stale." Another insists that his clients and his friends are the same, and he regularly interchanges both. The rest of us anyway treat clients with a special reverence, which is strange in the face of past history of exorcism of the devil as therapy. Clients are not merely clients to us but the bedrock of our existence. Does this not indicate an unresolved past?

The rather strong fathers in the backgrounds of our therapists were a surprise. Fathers are such shadowy figures in modern developmental psychology that it is instructive that they stand forth so clearly here. I believe the therapist-to-be was, for one reason or another, not allowed to admire or emulate his father and was forced back on fantasy for the father-son relationship. Indeed, the father was quite often away on one basis or another. This secret fantasy carries over as background organization for "the third ear" and becomes the therapist's reserve against which the love and hate of the client are played out. At no other time in his life is the therapist so much a father, and a father to the treatment as well. The client who said to me that getting married would be like "marrying her beloved father, her therapist, and the man who first took her maidenhead" was valuing her therapist as a most important part of this holy trinity. The Jewish father, furthermore, is a strange phenomenon in that he is a regular tiger in the marketplace but frequently reduces to an amoeba at home. But in

and 13 or 14 per cent women. If case work, educational guidance, marital counseling, and the like were included as psychotherapy, the percentages for women would of course be higher.

therapy the Jewish father comes into his own and, perhaps for the first time, can relate to women with a feeling of parity and have the fatherhood status he missed so much in his own family.

Psychotic Analogue

The lives of therapists, from Freud and Jung and Sullivan onward, convince me that most therapists experience themselves as closer to the shoals of psychosis than do other people. Their reality is somewhat different from the ordinary; conscious, preconscious, and unconscious fuse for them into a greater integral harmony. Therapists who have psychotic episodes invariably come out of them with greater ego strength than they had before and then develop more intense rapport with their clients. They have a greater desire to cure and they want to share their psychotic-consciousness experience. Some people react similarly with psychedelic drugs, feeling a missionary zeal to spread the gospel. The opening of consciousness, the diminution of cultural pull, the immediate rapport with the unconscious, the feeling of awe and mysterium, the freeing of rigid Protestant reality, and similar apperceptions, lead the one who has been to the Promised Land to want to go there again—and to bring a companion. Only rarely is man permitted to see behind the persona facade he—and his family—have spent years in erecting, and only the rare experience— such as conversion or the death bed—mobilizes the true personality in a brilliant way. Psychosis is one such.

It is ridiculous to say that one has to become psychotic to become authentic. Even though something like this view is held by Laing, the practical wisdom of it in sufficient titres is still to be determined. Yet many of the most creative therapists have experienced either very brief psychotic interludes, or their marginal equivalents, and may even have a latent depression or schizophrenia as a personality base. Stierlin raises this interesting possibility for Binswanger and Jung, and certainly Sullivan has to be included in this pantheon. The psychotic experience clarifies purpose and meaning and points the way to the healing posture. The assuredness, even smugness, of the authentic therapist is that he has found the way—he has been close to psychosis and back, and nothing can shake his foundation. This experience he in turn passes on to his clients in the form of skill, safety, and confidence.

Ego Satiation

The autobiographies reveal that our therapists do not tolerate boredom well. Boredom and surfeit have been generally overlooked in psychology, which unfortunately focuses primarily on stimulus and motive. The drive is deified while its consummation and end response is relatively ignored. The gourmand is an artist but the glutton a disaster. Fromm[11] has recently suggested that current social irritability may result more from boredom than from specific deprivations produced by poverty, race, and so on. Some people bind boredom better than do others, and possibly there is a genetic basis to this tolerance. High achievement seems related not only to the availability of a high quantum of energy but also to the need not to be bored. In Victorian and Edwardian society being bored was considered an egregious social error, and those with leisure time sought gamely not to be bored. The specific drive to reduce boredom to its lowest common denominator is behind much of modern alienation. More marriages, and more careers, fail because of boredom than any other single psychological factor, and the oft-repeated "I'm dying of boredom" is not such a far-fetched cry today.

Therapists have low boredom thresholds and discover that contact with people reduces their ennui. The fact that they have become therapists rather than bankers, or the like, indicates that being with people who get to the heart of the matter reduces boredom even further. I have experienced very little boredom in my therapeutic work, and I do not know any therapist who is perpetually bored. There is sometimes a routine and uniformity in therapy, but there is also the opportunity to select interesting clients to begin with and to employ a diversity of dyadic and polyadic approaches and forms in healing them. Clients also try very hard not to bore their therapists; they know it goes hard with them if they do. If anyone becomes bored listening to sexual and similar titillating secrets reported by intelligent, beautiful,

[11] E. Fromm, Paper presented at the Fifth World Congress of Psychiatry, Mexico City, December 2, 1971.

well-dressed, affluent, and achieving clients, then they may have to look to their own personality for answers to their ennui. Psychotherapy is by definition excitement—the excitement that only people in the active business of living can bring to a situation. Being a part of that excitement is not only what fulfills the therapist but entertains him as well.

Thanatos Deferred

Psychotherapists by and large live closer to the dynamics of mood—depression and ecstasy—than do other people. This I believe is generally true for the Jewish ethnic group. Depression goes along with sensitivity, growth, and extraordinary achievement so that we need not be concerned about it. Depression, rather than neurosis as such, provides the empathic experience with the client and depression must be taken seriously, whereas neurosis can be gamed or malingered. Depression, as we know, is dynamically coupled with love, guilt, and aggression, and interestingly enough, these behaviors are the stuff of psychotherapy. But depression is also rehearsal or preparation for death. In one important sense, psychotherapy is the place where the idea of death is first seriously tried on. It appears true as well that Thanatos is more involved in the cause of neuroses than we have heretofore believed.[12] Ideas and fears of finiteness bring a lowered mood, and the process of biological death itself may have matched depressive overtones, for otherwise death would be an impossible social achievement.

Doing therapy is therefore jousting with Thanatos as well as Eros, bringing them both into a proper relationship, and making one serve the other. In order to accomplish these tasks the therapist must come to terms with his own finiteness and its anxiety. It helps if the ethnic background of the therapist provides him with a palette of sadness, depression, and the social proximity of death, as it does in the Jew and those similar to him.

The Antisystem

Modern organizations or organizational systems bring with them their own indigeneous entropy. The larger and more complex

[12] This idea was first broached to me by J. J. Lopez-Ibor. See "The Neurotic Society," *Totus Homo,* 1971, *3,* 47–52.

the systems become, the greater is the dehumanization factor. This is why modern economics now takes seriously the new anti-growth movement, and the hipster who refuses progress gets in the way of corporate society. Every top manager knows that expansion of his organization may not necessarily lead to human rewards even though the company's profits may go up. The Gross National Product is no longer a qualitative indicator of the social weal, of how well we are doing as people, and millionaires are, regretfully, apt candidates for suicide. It seems probable that the industry of the twenty-first century will project humanistic goals for itself rather than profit margins in the old ways. If it does not, it may indeed not survive as a system. Economics is now becoming political science, and money no longer follows its own trends but is manipulated by governments for political expediency. In this only mass man is involved for the individual becomes obscured by his organizational gross phenomena.

It seems to me that Szasz perceives the social compulsiveness of psychotherapy only in part fashion. Psychotherapists, in my experience, are invariably anti-system, belonging to their culture but still not belonging to it, meliorating for the individual as opposed to his civilization, liberal rather than conservative in outlook, and fully on the side of justice.

There are few unified systems in psychotherapy, which is perhaps why so many styles of therapy functionally operate side by side. And therapists have an inside view of the ravages of systems and organization and become hostile toward them. Seldom do therapists choose to sit at the head of corporate organization and very few are interested in running for political office. Therapists are basically sympathetic with Szasz and Leiter on the covert uses of psychiatry for social conformance, and most of us want to be assured of the voluntariness of a client before we take him on. We minimize organization in every way we can. This is humanism applied to technical melioration, and therapy in one way or another involves reducing the ravages of the system. Though psychotherapy as a profession is itself not free from a power structure, and certainly doctrine often becomes institutional, *in camera,* in the therapeutic hour itself, it fights for freedom, self-expression, and actually against itself. At what point such anti-system burrowing from within stops, or should stop, is a delicate question. But therapists become therapists because they know that monolithic culture militates against personal freedom, and they are fearful of what that which we call civilization can do to man's dignity and pleasure.

Overconscious Man

A pervasive theme in contemporary psychology reiterates that man uses only a fraction of his awareness and that psychoanalysis and psychotherapy have not led him to his full conscious capabilities. The LSD experience, plus the urgings of Aldous Huxley, Timothy Leary, and Alan Watts, among others, reinforced this idea in the popular mind. Catharsis and insight have at any rate always been basic psychoanalytic structures, and are in effect much older than Freud's treatment of them. Analysis is by definition the coming awareness of that of which one was unaware.

My view is that the task of psychotherapy is to make some over-conscious clients less painfully conscious, and that it is an error to correlate awareness with health in a univocal way. The ultimately self-conscious person is apt to become paralyzed by his inner vision and refuse to live in this real but absurd world of ours. This is after all what schizophrenia is all about—awareness gone riotous. The poetic vision must be coupled with the sweat of the brow to become actualized, and not much which is socially creative can be expected from the persistent hashish or heroin user. Subjectivity must power its motor only enough to make the motor run and reach some place. Otherwise, profundity goes awry. It is precisely those who move masses of energy who meditate best and meditation without energy is simply vegetation. To put stasis and force in balance, to return a certain naivete and naturalness to the person, to make him more animal and less saint, to make him less conscious of self and things are also goals of psychotherapy.

Ideal Client

Psychotherapists prefer certain kinds of clients. In one study[13] they said that "married females, twenty to forty years old, with some

[13] W. Schofield, *Psychotherapy: The Purchase of Friendship* (Englewood Cliffs, N.J.: Prentice-Hall, 1964).

college education, and having professional/managerial status made the most desirable clients." On a more abstract level, all of us are on the watch for the "ideal client," which is at the same time our ideal self, our ideal Other, and our ideal mothering person. I have often wondered how the people we treat differ from those we live with. My glimmering insight is that we can idealize clients but not our wives and children. There has always been something unreal about the therapeutic process, and the unreality lies in our ability to cut the therapeutic relationship from the whole cloth. By this I mean that certain images, icons, metaphors, and aspirations can be projected onto the therapeutic encounter that cannot be lived out at home. All persons on the couch are beautiful; but off of it, the snake begins to come into Eden. Steinzor says in this connection, "Such vicarious pleasures [psychotherapy] do much to help me accommodate to the lives I never can live. Yet these unsolicited, unintended gifts also provide the context for the continuous rearousal and reinterpretation of my anguish."

The reality of the therapist's family life is apparently so difficult or so pedestrian that it has to be buttressed by another: the family life with the client. Of course, most of the office life is ideational, but the images and feelings evoked are real and exist in their own right, and in gestalt therapy, for example, quite a bit of touching may go on. Therapy is therefore a life within a life; and in therapy, the expectations are invariably beyond what they can be in the life outside. My thesis must not be misunderstood. It is not a matter of a man using the therapeutic ambience to live a life he cannot live outside. What I am suggesting can only take place with those therapists who already have a fulfilled private life. Only then can they therapeutically take on the second family function.

I seem to be searching for those clients whom I call "Harvard types"—I actually do have some clients from Harvard—who can themselves become psychotherapists some day and therefore follow in the pathway of Sigmund Freud and C. G. Jung. They must be bright, verbal, cultured, ontic, and value beauty, justice, and growth. Their joys and suffering must transcend them, and in them I hopefully recognize the fate of psychotherapy. On their rationality and sensitivity I fully believe rests also the fate of the world. I look for my ideal in the person who just phoned, and, mirabile dictu, he comes often enough. Therapists are dreamers who do not easily give up their ideals.

Religious Identification

What is the significance of the perhaps not so startling finding that not one of our biographees mentions religion as an important force in becoming a therapist? Polster and Rogers came from homes in which religion and worship were taken seriously. The latter even formally enrolled in a theological seminary, and the former must certainly have countenanced becoming a rabbi at some time. Other early therapists' environments reveal fundamental identification with Christian and Judaic tenets, such that professional identification might have been expected to be closer to the priesthood. As a matter of fact, a repugnance is now expressed with institutional religion by precisely those therapists who ought all the more firmly to embrace it.

Henry[14] found a trend toward secularization in his therapist sample in the generations removed from primary European immigration, and this mirrors a growing secularization at large in the community. But psychotherapy is a business of the spirit, and the agnosticism and atheism of the profession is actually the dynamic which fuels the need for "soul." It is a religion of atheistic and agnostic clients coupled to atheistic and agnostic therapists; that is, nonreligion becomes itself the religion. But the agnosticism of the participants is not to be taken at face value, for underneath lies the religion of the Fathers. The dynamic of religion is faith; the dynamic of psychotherapy is faith as well. Wherein do the two faiths differ? Perhaps in theology the faith goes primarily outside the believer; in psychotherapy it becomes internalized in the self. But we must not abjure the evident truth that in order to attain such self-sufficiency we must first create a dependency which matches that of priest on God. Freud rejected formal religion because he considered it infantile and therefore neurotic. A visitor from Mars might say the same if he observed psychotherapy at first hand.

My perception of the outcomes of psychotherapy is that the client is left not only a wiser, quieter, and more dignified human being,

[14] Henry, Sims, Spray, 1971.

but a more spiritual one as well. Community, fraternity, mystery, ritual, beauty, symbolism, faith, worship, hope are all now part of his values. If he was formerly a church member he may return to it. (However, he need not do so in order to be fulfilled and to be religious.) But therapy does assuredly change the client in the direction of the therapist, who is today's manifestation of the archetypal religionist, in my opinion. That is to say, the therapist has totally defended himself against religion by assuming a profession which deals with souls but which has no blessings and full negation from the church. In the Middle Ages, therapists would have been burned at the stake as heretics. Today they are slowly taking over the church. The priest or minister who does not use psychological techniques somewhere and at some time is passe. A recent survey of Protestant ministers revealed that they want now to "counsel" and not to give sermons. Many are even going into independent private practice and thus leaving the church. The wildly successful evangelical preachers, say Billy Graham and Oral Roberts, could by a simple transformation become successful psychotherapists, and they are more indebted to Sigmund Freud than they know.

It is a mistake to phrase the religious aspects of psychotherapists only in terms of Judaic-Christian tenets, for the intellect brings in Buddha, Vishnu, Siva, Confucius, Lao-tzu, and others as well. Psychotherapy is the universal rather than doctrinaire aspect of religion— Jung knew this better than Freud; and from Rogers to Lopez-Ibor to Warkentin we offer our clients ages-old life principles in new forms which move them and have meaning in this century.

II

My Personal Growth

Carl R. Rogers

I assume the purpose of an autobiography is to reveal the person as
he is to himself and, either directly or indirectly, to reveal some of the
factors and forces which entered into the making of his personality and
his professional interests. So perhaps the first question to answer is
"Who am I?" Who is this person whose life history is to be explored?

I am a psychologist; a clinical psychologist I believe, a humanistically oriented psychologist certainly; a psychotherapist and facilitator, deeply interested in the dynamics of personality change; a
scientist, to the limit of my ability investigating such change; an educator, challenged by the possibility of facilitating learning; a philoso-

Written in 1965–1966 and updated in 1971 for this volume. Pub-
lished in its original form in E. G. Boring and G. Lindzey, *A History of
Psychology in Autobiography* (Vol. V) (New York: Appleton-Century-
Crofts, 1967). Permission to publish this version has been granted by The
Educational Division, Meredith Corp.

pher in a limited way, especially in relation to the philosophy of science and the philosophy and psychology of human values. As a person I see myself as fundamentally positive in my approach to life; somewhat of a lone wolf in my professional activities, socially rather shy but enjoying close relationships; capable of a deep sensitivity in human interaction though not always achieving this; often a poor judge of people, tending to overestimate them; possessed of a capacity for setting other people free, in a psychological sense; capable of a dogged determination in getting work done or in winning a fight; eager to have an influence on others but with very little desire to exercise power or authority over them.

These are some of the ways I would describe myself. Others, I am sure, often see me quite differently. How I became the person I am is something of which I am not at all sure. I believe the individual's memory to his own dynamics is often decidedly inadequate. So I shall try to give enough of the factual data for the reader to draw his own conclusions. Part of these data consists of the feelings and attitudes which I remember in various events and periods throughout my life. I will not hesitate to draw some of my own inferences from the data, with which the reader can compare his own.

Early Days

Though as a clinician I feel the individual reveals himself in the present, and that a true history of his psychogenesis is impossible, I will yield to the traditional mode and give my own memory and perception of my past, pegged to such objective facts as are available to me.

I was born January 8, 1902, in Oak Park, a Chicago suburb, the fourth of six children, five of whom were boys. My parents had both been reared on farms and were highly practical, down to earth individuals. In a day when college education was not widespread, my father had completed his engineering degree and even some graduate work at the University of Wisconsin, and my mother had also attended for two years. In spite of this they both tended to be rather anti-intellectual, with some of the contempt of the practical person toward the long-haired egghead. They both worked very hard and, more important than this, had a strong belief in the virtue of work. There was almost nothing that a little hard work wouldn't cure. My mother was a person with strong religious convictions whose views became increasingly fundamentalist as she matured. Two of her biblical phrases, often used in family prayers, stick in my mind and give the feeling of her religion: "Come out from among them and be ye separate"; "All our righteousness is as filthy rags in thy sight, oh Lord." (The first expressed her conviction of superiority, that we were of the "elect" and should not mingle with those who were not so favored; the second her conviction of inferiority, that at our best we were unspeakably sinful.) My father was involved too in the family prayers, church attendance, and the like, but in a less emotional way. They were both devoted and loving parents, giving a great deal of time and energy to creating a family life which would "hold" the children in the way in which they should go. They were masters of the art of subtle and loving control. I do not remember ever being given a direct command on an important subject, yet such was the unity of our family that it was understood by all that we did not dance, play cards, attend movies, smoke, drink, or show any sexual interest. For some reason swearing was not quite so strictly tabooed—perhaps because father would, on occasion, vent his anger in that way.

My father formed his own business—contractor and civil engineer—in partnership with an older man. Due to hard work (and doubtless good fortune) the business prospered and by the date of my birth the early "hard times" were past, and we were a middle-class or upper-middle-class family. Our home was one of good family times, occasional pleasant gatherings of young people (the friends of my oldest brother), and much family humor which very often had a cutting and biting edge to it. We teased each other unmercifully, and I did not realize until I was adult that this was not a necessary part of human relationships.

I learned to read long before I went to school—from my older sibs, I presume—and was reading heavy Bible story books before I went to first grade at age seven. The principal, being informed of this, took me to the second, third, and fourth grade rooms for a brief trial at their reading material. I could read any of it. Nothing was made, at school or at home, of this (as I now realize) rather unusual performance. I was placed in second grade, which pleased me because I was very fearful of the stern-looking first grade teacher. I soon had a crush on Miss Littler, my teacher. This was repeated in fifth grade when I was so devoted to Miss Kuntz that I stayed after school to help her with tasks around the schoolroom. This was flying in the face of the family expectation that children came *directly home* when school was out. It was perhaps my first minor personal independence.

I was a dreamy youngster all through these grammar school years, so lost in fantasy most of the time that my absentmindedness was legendary. I was teased a great deal about this and called "Professor Moony," an absent-minded comic strip character of the period. I was buried in books—stories of Indian and frontier life to the extent that I could lay hands on them, but *anything* was grist to my mill. If there was nothing else, I read the encyclopedia, or even the dictionary. I can still recall some of the attempts to gain sex information through these channels, only to come to a dead end at a crucial point.

I felt guilty about my reading, since it so often meant that I was not doing my "chores" or had blissfully forgotten all about the things I had been told to do. To "have your nose in a book," except perhaps in the evening, was not a good or practical or hardworking thing. (Years later, as a college professor, I can remember the vaguely guilty feelings which would arise when I sat down to read a book in the *morning!*)

I felt that my parents cared more for my next older brother than they did for me. This feeling must have been quite strong for I recall that I developed the theory that I had been adopted. (Many years later I learned how common this fantasy is.) As might be expected, there was much rivalry and hard feeling between me and this brother, Ross, who was three years older. There was also, however, much companionship since we went to school together and shared in many activities. My closest family link was with my next younger brother, Walter. He and John, my youngest brother, were less than two years apart in age and were respectively five and seven years younger than I. In spite of this age difference we were a very close trio. I had an attitude of real hero-worship toward my oldest brother, Lester, though the age difference was too great for us to have much companionship. I remember the pride I felt when it was reported in the newspapers that he had made the highest score of any recruit (on the old Army Alpha Intelligence Test) at Camp Grant in World War I.

I had almost no social life outside the family, but I have no

recollection of being disturbed by this. Our family life seemed sufficient. I recall just one fist fight while in elementary school. I was
frightened to death but did my best in what ended as pretty much of
a draw.

I recall one experience which seems to indicate that my parents
were concerned about my withdrawn, dreamy, and impractical nature.
At about the time of my twelfth birthday, while in seventh grade,
plans were made for me to take a long trip of two or three weeks
with my father, while he visited various construction jobs in the south
and east. Permission was obtained for me to leave school on the basis
that I would present a written report of my experience when I returned. Father and I visited New Orleans, Norfolk, Virginia, and
New York City, spending much time visiting construction projects. I
enjoyed myself, though I did not become enamored of engineering as
a result. It is only as I look back at this trip that I realize its unusual
nature. I do not recall that my brothers were taken on similar trips.
My best guess is that it was an attempt to help me become more interested in real life than fantasy and to help me become aware of the
fact that the world was one of work and that I should be thinking
about my future occupation. I am not sure that the trip accomplished
these aims, but it was an exciting and broadening experience. I came
back thrilled by the chanting Negro workers on the New Orleans
docks and with a passionate taste (acquired in Norfolk) for raw
oysters!

When I was twelve, my parents bought a large farm some
thirty miles west of Chicago, and after spending weekends and a summer there, a home was built and we moved to the country. There
were several reasons for this step. My father liked farming and made
a hobby of having the farm handled in the best scientific fashion.
Mother too liked gardening and cared little for the social life of the
suburb. The major reason, however, was that with six growing children, ranging at that time from age six to twenty, they were concerned
about the temptations and evils of suburban and city life and wished
to get the family away from these threats.

When we moved to the farm, I loved it. To play in the woods
(the "forest" to me) and to learn the birds and animals was bringing
my frontier stories to life. Many are the Indians I have crept up on,

all unsuspecting, in those wooded glades. What if they were only imaginary? My brothers and I thoroughly enjoyed the new setting.

I recall two events—the first very vividly—which occurred before I was fifteen, which turned me toward the world of science. To provide background for the first I should say that Gene Stratton-Porter was at that time writing her "Girl of the Limberlost" books, in which nature, but particularly the large night-flying moths, played an important part. I had of course read all these books. So I was in a responsive mood when I discovered in the woods close to home, against the dark-fissured bark of a black oak tree, two lonely luna moths, just emerged from their cocoons. These beautiful pale green creatures, large as a small bird, with long "swallowtail" wings spotted with purple, would have intrigued anyone. They fascinated me. I began my first "independent study project," as it would be termed today. I obtained books on moths. I found and raised their caterpillars. I hatched the eggs and raised caterpillars through their whole series of moults, into the cocoons, until the twelve-month cycle was complete and they emerged again as moths—Polyphemus, Cecropia, Prometheus, or one of the dozens of other varieties I came to know. I even "tied out" a female moth on the roof to attract males—a very successful experiment—and was continually busy getting leaves of the special sorts which the caterpillars demanded as food. In my own very small and specialized field I became something of a biologist.

A less sharply focused experience has to do with scientific agriculture. My father wanted his farm conducted in the most modern way and brought in agricultural scientists from the universities to instruct the farm foreman, herdsman, and others. He also acquired many books on the latest approaches to agriculture. I can remember reading these books—particularly the heavy scientific tome by Morison on *Feeds and Feeding*. The descriptions of all the scientific experiments on feeding, on milk and egg production, on the use of different fertilizers, different varieties of seed, of soil, and so on, gave me a thoroughgoing feeling for the essential elements of science. The design of a suitable experiment, the rationale of control groups, the control of all variables but one, the statistical analysis of the results—all of these concepts were unknowingly absorbed through my reading at the ages of thirteen to sixteen.

My experience in high school was very fragmented. I attended three different high schools and in each case had to travel from our farm home to attend high school—by horse and buggy, by train, by automobile, and combinations of these. I was expected to return home at once after school in order to do chores and work at home. Consequently, I made no lasting associations or friendships in any of these schools. I was a good student and never had any difficulty with the work. Neither did I have any problems in getting along with the other students so far as I can recall. It is simply that I knew them only in a very surface fashion and felt decidedly different and alone, but this was compensated for by the fact that my brother and I went together much of this time and there was always the family at home.

When I speak of working at home, both morning and night, while going to high school, I do not mean light work. I was up at five o'clock or earlier and milked a dozen cows morning and night while attending high school. I remember this particularly because the milking was evidently more than my muscles could stand and my hands and arms were continually "asleep" during the day. I could never get them quite free of the prickles. I recall that at one time I also took care of all of the pigs on the farm. During the summer months I rode a cultivator all day long, usually being assigned to the cornfield at the far end of the farm which was full of quack grass. It was a lesson in independence to be on my own, far away from anyone else. When the cultivator needed repair or adjustment, when the team was troublesome, or the soil or weather conditions were not right, I had to make the necessary decisions and take appropriate action on my own. It was a type of responsibility experienced by few young people today.

At school my best work was in English and science. I received straight A grades in almost all my courses. I remember best Miss Graham, a spinsterish teacher of English at Naperville High School. Though she was a strict disciplinarian and rarely if ever smiled, she had a true scholarly interest in her work. I somehow felt that she would understand what I wrote, so for themes in English I wrote personal accounts as well as rebellious papers on "Shakespeare as an overrated author."

I never had a real "date" in high school. In my junior year I was elected president of the class (presumably because I had good grades and did not belong to any of the cliques). The one social event of the year was a class dinner to which it was necessary to take a girl. I remember the agony I went through in inviting an auburn-haired lass whom I had admired from a distance. Fortunately for me, she accepted. If she had not, I don't know what I would have done.

There is one summer during this period which tells a great deal about me and about my upbringing. It was the summer between high school graduation and the beginning of college. I was seventeen. It was part of the family tradition that of course I would work during the summer. On this particular occasion my father arranged for me to work in one of a string of lumberyards throughout the Northwest, owned by three of my uncles. I was excited by the opportunity of going all by myself to a small town in North Dakota for the summer. I had been given a graduation present of fifty dollars and spent it on the beautifully printed, small leather-bound books which were all the rage at that time. I took my books with me and was given a room in the lumberyard itself where I lived and slept, being the only person on the premises. I worked hard from about eight o'clock in the morning until five o'clock, loading and unloading lumber, filling customers' orders, shoveling coal, unloading bricks, and the like. I ate at a boarding house and remember no contact beyond superficial conversation with any of the individuals at the boarding house. My relationship with the kindly boss of the lumberyard was similar. We worked together and I felt he was fair and friendly. He invited me twice to his house during the summer. Aside from that I remember no social life at all. I was not too lonely, however, because I spent the long evenings with my new books. During that period I read Carlyle, Victor Hugo, Dickens, Ruskin, Robert Louis Stevenson, Emerson, Scott, Poe, and many others. I found this most stimulating. I realize that I lived in a world of my own, created by these books.

College

At some point in my high school years I had chosen scientific agriculture as my field. I went to the University of Wisconsin in 1919. It was an appropriate place to go because it had a very good college of agriculture. This, however, was not my real reason for going to Wisconsin. It was simply assumed that every member of the family would go to Wisconsin since my parents and my two older brothers and sister had all studied there. I roomed with my brother Ross at the YMCA dormitory.

Following my own religious inclinations—built on the religious traditions at home—I became a member of a Sunday morning YMCA group composed of students of agriculture. Professor George Humphrey was the leader. I saw him then as a well-intentioned individual but somewhat weak. To this day I do not know whether he really understood what he was doing in leaving everything up to the group, but it was (I realize now) an excellent example of facilitative leadership. Left to our own decisions and choices, the group set up its own curriculum, organized all kinds of social and educational activities, conducted its business in first-class parliamentary fashion, discussed topics deeply, and became very close-knit. For the first time in my life outside of my family I found real closeness and intimacy. The friendship and companionship which developed in this group of about twenty-five young men was an exceedingly important element in my life. We came to know each other well and to trust each other deeply. We were completely free to engage in any kind of activity and we became involved in many different types of projects. One result was that I acquired a good grasp of parliamentary law and have never been fearful of chairing any type of parliamentary assembly, an ability which has from time to time stood me in good stead. Another experience of that period was that as part of the activity of this Ag-Triangle group, I took on the leadership of a Boys' Club and tried myself out as leader of a group of younger individuals.

During the first summer vacation I began writing personal letters to Helen Elliott, a tall, graceful girl interested in art, whom I had known since grammar school days in Oak Park, where we had ridden our bicycles together. I had dated her a few times during my freshman year at Wisconsin since she had come there to study art, and I found her very attractive.

It was during the Christmas vacation of my sophomore year, I believe, that I went to a conference of Student Volunteers at Des Moines. The Student Volunteer movement had at that time the slogan "Evangelize the world in our generation," and this was a meaningful purpose to me with my religious interests. The speakers were inspiring and there was a great deal of mass emotion engendered. I find it embarrassing to read the highly emotional and idealistic diary I kept during that period. I decided at this conference that I should change my life goal and go into Christian work. Though the Student Volunteer movement was specifically oriented toward the foreign field, I do not recall that I had any particular intention of going into foreign work. I did, however, feel that religious leadership was now my goal. In many ways the movement was the Peace Corps of that day and appealed to some of the same sentiments.

Having made this decision, agriculture no longer seemed to be a very suitable field. I felt that I should shift to some subject which would prepare me for the ministry and decided that history, which had always been one of my interests, was a good background for that type of work. Consequently, I shifted from agriculture to history.

In the midst of my junior year there occurred a sequence of events which had a great deal of impact on me. I was selected as one of ten students from this country to go to a World Student Christian Federation Conference in Peking, China. When I was informed of this I wept with joy and surprise. I couldn't understand how or why they would have chosen *me*. Realistically, I have realized since that my very active work in the YMCA, my good grades, and the fact that my parents would be able to pay most of the expenses of the trip probably accounted for the choice. At the time, however, it seemed like an utterly incredible and exciting thing to be selected from all of the students in the United States for a most unusual experience of this sort.

A delegation of students and professional workers, mostly from the YMCA, went over together by ship. John R. Mott, who at that time was a world leader, Professor Kenneth Latourette from Yale, David Porter of the YMCA, and a number of others constituted the professional group. The students too were naturally a selected group. Here was a very congenial intellectual group and our shipboard discussions and reading constituted a most enriching experience.

I was most privileged to have this whole trip. We met highly cultured and well-informed individuals throughout all our sojourn. The foreign representatives of the YMCA were a statesmanlike group in their approach to intercultural relations. A number of them, such as Jack Childs, became very well known as philosophers, diplomats, and the like. They were not at all evangelical missionary types and I learned a great deal from them.

I was gone more than six months, since in addition to the slow

voyage and the conference in Peking, I was part of one of the delega-
tions which made speaking tours to student centers—in my case to
West China. Following this I accompanied Professor Latourette, who
was gathering data for a book, on a tour of South China and the
Philippines.

This voyage bears curious testimony to the fact that speed of
communication is not always desirable. During the trip I kept a long
typed journal of the various events I was living through and my reactions to them. I was rapidly becoming much more liberal in religion
and politics because of my exposure to a wide spectrum of opinion, to
a wide range of cultures, and to such specifically challenging experiences as trying to understand the interchange between French and
German students and faculty members who were still filled with hatred
and suspicion from the days of World War I. My intellectual horizon
was being incredibly stretched all through this period, and this growth
was recorded in my journal. I sent a copy of this journal to Helen,
who was now definitely my sweetheart, and another copy to my family.
Since we did not have the benefit of airmail it took two months for a
reply to arrive. Thus I kept pouring out on paper all my new feelings
and ideas and thoughts with no notion of the consternation that this
was causing in my family. By the time their reactions caught up to me,
the rift in outlook was fully established. Thus, with a minimum of pain,
I broke the intellectual and religious ties with my home.

This independence was furthered on the return trip, when
shipboard conversations with Dr. Henry Sharman, a student of the
sayings of Jesus, were very thought provoking. It struck me one night
in my cabin that perhaps Jesus was a man like other men—not divine!
As this idea formed and took root, it became obvious to me that I
could never in any emotional sense return home. This proved to be
true.

After this six-month trip I was able freely, and with no great
sense of defiance or guilt, to think my own thoughts, come to my own
conclusions, and to take the stands I believed in. This process had
achieved a real direction and assurance—which never after wavered—
before I had any inkling that it constituted rebellion from home. From
the date of this trip, my goals, values, aims, and philosophy have been
my own and very divergent from the views which my parents held and

which I had held up to this point. Psychologically, it was a most important period of declaring my independence from my family.

Shortly after I returned from the Orient, I was increasingly troubled by abdominal pains which I had had intermittently since the age of fifteen. They were now properly diagnosed as being due to a duodenal ulcer, and I was in the hospital for some weeks and on an intensive treatment regime for six months. Something of the gently suppressive family atmosphere is perhaps indicated by the fact that three of six children developed ulcers at some period in their lives. I had the dubious distinction of acquiring mine at the earliest age.

During this period of medical treatment it was of course expected, by me as much as my parents, that I would work. It seems so typical, both of my own attitudes and those of my family, that the only considered alternative to college, even though I was not too well, was hard physical work. I think that to a considerable extent I shared my parents' views that work would cure anything, including my ulcer. So I obtained a job in a local lumberyard, while living at home. I remember that one time my Model-T Ford—my first car—was hemmed into a tight parking spot at the lumberyard. I simply lifted the rear end of the car and moved it a few inches. I strained my back in doing so. It seemed never to occur to me that I could ask someone to help me. This attitude, too, has been typical of me.

While working in the lumberyard I made no effort to keep up my college work, except that I took a correspondence course from the University of Wisconsin in introductory psychology, my first acquaintance with the subject. I was not particularly impressed. I used William James as a text, but thought our assignments were a bit dull. The only portion of the course I remember is that I got into an argument by mail with my instructor as to whether dogs could reason. It was his claim that only human beings could reason. I was quite able to prove to my own satisfaction that my dog, Shep, was definitely able to solve difficult problems by reasoning.

One advantage of being out of school was that it kept me close to Helen, who had given up university work to take professional art training in Chicago. Consequently, there was much courting during this period, although each visit involved a thirty-mile drive in my Model-T, over roads quite different from modern highways, after a hard day's work at the lumberyard. I returned to the university in the autumn, but during a visit home Helen and I became engaged on October 9, 1922, an event which made me ecstatically happy. I had felt very uncertain that I could win her and floated on clouds for some time after this day.

I graduated in June 1924 with a bachelor's degree in history, having had my one correspondence course in psychology. I had been delayed one year in my graduation by my trip to China and by the half year of illness and work. Because I had shifted from the class of '23 to the class of '24 and because I had shifted from agriculture to history, the close contacts I had built up in my freshman year were greatly weakened. I had few friends with whom I was close during all four years of college.

New York Years

Helen and I were married on August 28, 1924, and set out in a secondhand Model-T coupe of which I was inordinately proud and for which I had paid $450. We headed for New York and Union Theological Seminary. My parents had opposed the marriage, not because they were opposed to Helen, but because it was at that time considered absurd for a man to marry while he was still going to school. Her parents shared this feeling. Helen was at first reluctant to give up her good job as a commercial artist, but I convinced her that we should be together in facing all the new learnings and challenges of graduate work. We both realized later that we had been wiser than we knew in making this decision.

I had chosen Union Theological Seminary because it was the most liberal in the country and an intellectual leader in religious work. Knowing my plan for going to Union, my father had made one offer which was very close to a bribe. I suspect he was not proud of himself afterward for this. Certainly I rejected it indignantly. He told me that he would pay all the expenses for both of us if I would go to Princeton Seminary, which was at that point a center of fundamentalist thinking. Instead, I took some competitive examinations and won a good scholarship at Union Seminary and we made our plans for going there. My parents were then generous in gifts to help us get underway, though it was still necessary for me to earn a considerable amount of money for our expenses.

Helen and I were both very naive at the time we married (though I had loaned her a book on sex life and marriage, a mark of how avant garde I was in my thinking!) Whether in spite of or because of our lack of sophistication we had a delightful honeymoon and it was a great and independent venture to drive all the way to New York City in our own car.

We started our life together in a tiny apartment. At that time there were no dormitories for married students, and hence we were somewhat separated from my classmates as I began to attend Union Seminary. I found it to be a stimulating and exciting place. I made friends, found new ideas, and fell thoroughly in love with the whole experience. Harry Emerson Fosdick was in his heyday, and his course was one which Helen and I took together, gaining a feeling for a modern and liberal religion.

Goodwin Watson and Joseph Chassell, both young fellows at that time, were in charge of a course on Working with Individuals. In addition to their own teaching they brought in psychologists and psychiatrists from the New York area. This course introduced me to the whole field of clinical work and I found it most exciting. Harrison Elliott and his wife (on the faculty of the seminary) were also much involved in both individual work and the group discussion approach. For the first time I realized that working with individual persons in a helping relationship could be a professional enterprise.

I had great respect for Arthur Cushman McGiffert, who at that time was head of the Seminary. He was a remarkable teacher and a profound scholar. He created an exciting philosophical climate at Union. His course on Protestant Thought before Kant and other similar courses introduced me to a new level of teaching excellence. As we heard him present the thinking of one philosopher or theologian we in the class would become convinced that "Aha! This is the person with whom he really agrees." The next week he would present someone else with equal conviction and persuasiveness. In the long run we found that we had to do our own thinking. (Miss Graham in high school and Professor McGiffert at Union were both grave, scholarly, almost scholastic teachers, not at all the sort I would tend to select as faculty members today. Yet they were both highly independent in their thinking and had a deep respect for the independence of their students.)

While at Union Seminary, either during the first or second year, I was involved in an amusing but highly significant venture. Knowing universities and graduate schools as I do now—knowing their rules and their rigidities—I am truly astonished at the freedom which was granted to us at Union. A group of students, of which I was one, felt that ideas were being fed to us and that we were not having an opportunity to discuss the religious and philosophical issues which most deeply concerned us. We wanted to explore our own questions and doubts and find out where they led. We petitioned the administration that we be allowed to set up a seminar (for credit!) in which there would be no instructor and in which the curriculum would be composed of our own questions. The Seminary was understandably perplexed by this request but they granted our petition. The only restriction was that in the interests of the Seminary a young instructor was to sit in on the course but to take no part in it unless we wished him to be active. This seminar was deeply satisfying and clarifying. It moved me a long way toward a philosophy of life which was my own. The majority of that group, in thinking their way through the questions they had raised, thought their way right out of religious work. I was one; Theodore Newcomb was another. Various other members have also gone on in sociology and psychology. The whole seminar was very freewheeling. It took up profound philosophical, religious, and social problems. My own reason for deciding to leave the field of religious work was that although questions about the meaning of life and the possibility of the constructive improvement of life for individuals were of deep interest to me, I could not work in a field where I would be required to believe in some specified religious doctrine. I realized that my own views had changed tremendously already and would very likely continue to change. It seemed to me that it would be a horrible thing to have to profess a set of beliefs in order to remain in one's profession. I wanted to find a field in which I could be sure my freedom of thought would not be limited.

During my second year at Union Seminary I was taking courses both at the Seminary and at Teachers' College, Columbia University, which was located just across Broadway. At "TC," I found my course in philosophy of education with William H. Kilpatrick very stimulating indeed—not only the lectures and question and answer periods, but the small group discussions which were part of the course. This course provided my first acquaintance with the thinking of John Dewey (who has since then been so generally misunderstood) and introduced me to a philosophy of education which has been influential in my thought ever since. A course with Leta Hollingworth, in clinical psychology, also stands out. She was a warm human being, concerned about individuals, as well as a competent research worker. Under her supervision I first came in actual *clinical* contact with children—testing them, talking with them, dealing with them as fascinating objects of study, helping to make plans for their welfare.

By the end of my second graduate year I decided to shift entirely out of Union Seminary and over to Teachers' College, working in clinical and educational psychology. Again this was a relatively painless transition since, as I have indicated, I had already been taking courses there.

Something of my attitudes during my graduate work may be indicated in my reactions to examinations. I look back on these with some surprise myself. Preparation for examinations was a well-organized affair for me. It never gave me any trouble because it never entered my head that I would not be successful. When it came to the matriculation exam for the doctoral degree, I remember my surprise at discovering that some people were frightened of this. I took the examination and passed as I had expected to do. Months later I was amazed to find, quite by chance, that I had the highest score of that particular group on a Thorndike test of intellectual power and also that I had received the highest grades on the content examinations.

Perhaps it would be appropriate to try to describe at this point my very limited experience with educational failure. I remember once in the fifth grade I failed an examination when I had simply loafed and paid no attention to a history class. As a consequence, I had to take a second examination on the same material and I well remember the panic I felt. I even cheated a little by checking one answer with a girl who was taking the same examination. The next failure I can recall was a statistics course at Teachers' College. I had never had a first course in statistics but I was perfectly confident that I could pass the second course which came at a more convenient hour. The instructor was very abstruse in his explanations and I simply could not catch on. It was a totally new experience for me to be in a situation where I could not *grasp* the material. When it came to the final examination I answered it as best I could but I was sure that I had failed the course. Consequently, I took the opportunity of telling him, in the examination blue book, what I thought of the course and his methods of teaching, which were far from the best. Whether because of this personal outburst or in spite of it—I have never known—he passed me.

Our first child, David, was born in 1926 and we experienced all the excitements, apprehensions, and satisfactions of caring for our first born. We endeavored to raise him "by the book" of Watsonian behaviorism, strict scheduling, and the like. Fortunately, Helen had enough common sense to make a good mother in spite of all this damaging psychological "knowledge."

During these two years in New York, I was working as director of religious education at a Mt. Vernon church, spending all my weekends there in order to support myself, my wife, and child. As my interests changed away from religion, I became increasingly uncomfortable in this work. I was pleased to give it up when Goodwin Watson, my brilliant young sponsor, offered me a job. He always had many irons in the fire, and he turned over to me almost complete responsibility for an extensive survey he had initiated. I employed a sizable group of research assistants, conducted the analysis of some very complex material, and organized and wrote the presentation, all under pressure of an unyielding and imminent deadline.

I presume it was in the latter part of 1926 that I applied for a Fellowship or internship at the new Institute of Child Guidance which was about to be formed. Child guidance work was just coming into its own, and an elaborate Institute of Child Guidance was established by the Commonwealth Fund in New York City in order to provide training for such clinical workers. The $2,500 Fellowship would keep us afloat financially and I would be working in a field to which I had become increasingly attached. I was awarded the Fellowship. Then shortly before the year was to begin I received an embarrassed letter from Dr. Frankwood Williams, the psychiatrist who headed the selection committee. He had just discovered that psychiatrists were to get $2,500. The Fellowships for psychologists were to be only $1,200. It was the financial rather than the professional insult which roused my dander. I wrote him a very strong letter, saying essentially that the Fellowship had been awarded, I had been informed of it, I had made all my personal plans on this basis, I needed the money to support my family. On the strength of my letter he made an exception and I received a $2,500 Fellowship. It is interesting and symbolic that I started my professional training—through a fluke—on the same level with psychiatric residents.

The year 1927–1928 at the Institute was extremely stimulating. I was still working toward my doctor's degree at Teachers College where such things as emotions and personality dynamics were completely scorned by Percival Symonds and other members of the Teachers College faculty, and Freud was a dirty word. The whole approach was through measurement and statistics. The Institute emphasis on eclectic Freudianism contrasted so sharply with the Teachers College approach that there seemed to be no common meeting ground. I experienced very sharply the tension between the two views.

I did well at the Institute for Child Guidance. For my doctoral research I developed a test for measuring the personality adjustment of children, building on the attitudes present at the Institute, but also utilizing some of the technical procedures more congenial to Teachers College. It amazes me that this test is still used some forty years later. I also began to realize that I had real clinical skill both in dealing with individuals and with colleagues. I remember one case conference with an uncooperative caseworker from outside, discussing a boy with whom I had been working. I was late because of a sleet storm that morning. When I arrived the conference was obviously stalemated because the outside worker was totally unsympathetic and uncooperative. I won her over by my explanation of the situation, though I was the youngest and least experienced member of the conference group. This boy was the first individual with whom I carried on regular therapy (though when psychologists did it, it was called remedial work or some such name). I made real progress in helping him, though I was full of the psychoanalytic theories which I was trying out at that time.

The eclecticism of the Institute was very helpful to me in the long run. There were different shades of psychoanalytic thinking and other psychiatric and psychological views. Alfred Adler lectured to us, for example, and shocked the whole staff by thinking that an elaborate case history was not necessary. I remember how misinformed I thought he must be, since we routinely took case histories fifty to seventy pages in length. David Levy was chief of staff and a stimulating leader who introduced us to the then new Rorschach. E. K. Wickman, the chief psychologist, was thoughtful, balanced, a good research worker, genuinely interested in discovering the truth.

As this year drew toward an end, the question of what I would do next was a very important one. For the first time in my life I was really seeking a job. By the spring of 1928, David was two years old and our second child was on the way. Jobs for psychologists were not plentiful. I remember I was interviewed for a position at Culver Military Academy and felt I might have to take this. Then I was interviewed for a position at the Rochester Society for the Prevention of Cruelty to Children which had a Child Study Department composed of psychologists. I would be studying children and making recommendations in regard to them. It might even be possible to see some of them for treatment interviews. This sounded like what I wanted to do. There were three psychologists in this department and the salary offered was $2,900 per year.

I look back at the acceptance of that position with amusement and some amazement. The reason I was so pleased was that it was a chance to do the work I wanted to do. That it was, by any reasonable criterion, a dead-end street professionally, that I would be isolated from professional contacts and universities, that the salary was not good even by the standards of that day seem not to have occurred to me, as nearly as I can recall. I think I have always had a feeling that if I were given some opportunity to do the thing I was most interested in doing, everything else would somehow take care of itself.

Rochester Years

The next twelve years in Rochester were exceedingly valuable. For at least the first eight of these years, I was completely immersed in carrying on practical psychological service, diagnosing and planning for the delinquent and underprivileged children who were sent to us by the courts and agencies, and in many instances carrying on "treatment interviews." It was a period of relative professional isolation, where my only concern was in trying to be more effective with our clients. We had to live with our failures as well as our successes, so that we were forced to learn. There was only one criterion in regard to any method of dealing with these children and their parents, and that was "Does it work? Is it effective?" I found I began increasingly to formulate my own views out of my everyday working experience.

Three significant illustrations come to mind, all small, but important to me at the time. It strikes me that they are all instances of disillusionment—with an authority, with materials, with myself. In my training I had been fascinated by Dr. William Healy's wriitngs indicating that delinquency was often based upon sexual conflict, and that if this conflict were uncovered, the delinquency ceased. (This at least was my understanding.) In my first or second year at Rochester I worked very hard with a youthful pyromaniac who had an unaccountable impulse to set fires. Interviewing him day after day in the detention home, I gradually traced back his desire to his sexual impulses regarding masturbation. Eureka! The case was solved. However, when placed on probation, he again got into the same difficulty.

I remember the jolt I felt. Healy might be wrong. Perhaps I was learning something Healy did not know. Somehow this incident impressed me with the possibility that there were mistakes in authoritative teachings, and that there was still new knowledge to discover.

The second naive discovery was of a different sort. Soon after coming to Rochester, I led a discussion group on interviewing. I discovered a published account of an interview with a parent, approximately verbatim, in which the caseworker was shrewd, insightful, clever, and led the interviewee quite quickly to the heart of the difficulty. I was happy to use it as an illustration of good interviewing technique.

Several years later, I had a similar assignment and remembered this excellent material. I hunted it up again and reread it. I was appalled. Now it seemed to me to be a clever legalistic type of questioning by the interviewer which convicted this parent of her unconscious motives and wrung from her an admission of her guilt. I now knew from my more extensive experience that such an interview would not be of any lasting help to the parent or the child. It made me realize that I was moving away from any approach which was coercive or

strongly interpretive in clinical relationships, not for philosophical reasons, but because such approaches were never more than superficially
effective.

The third incident occurred several years later. I had learned
to be more subtle and patient in interpreting a client's behavior to him,
attempting to time my interpretations in a gentle fashion which would
gain acceptance. I had been working with a highly intelligent mother
whose boy was something of a hellion. The problem was clearly her
early rejection of the boy, but over many interviews I could not help
her to this insight. I drew her out, I gently pulled together the evidence she had given, trying to help her see the pattern. But we got
nowhere. Finally I gave up. I told her that it seemed we had both
tried, but we had failed, and that we might as well give up our contacts. She agreed. So we concluded the interview, shook hands, and
she walked to the door of the office. Then she turned and asked, "Do
you ever take adults for counseling here?" When I replied in the
affirmative, she said, "Well then, I would like some help." She came
back to the chair she had just left and began to pour out her despair
about her marriage, her troubled relationship with her husband, her
sense of failure and confusion, all very different from the sterile "case
history" she had given before. Real therapy began then and ultimately
it was highly successful—for her and for her son.

This incident was one of a number which helped me to experience the fact—only fully realized later—that it is the *client* who knows
what hurts, what directions to go, what problems are crucial, what
experiences have been deeply buried. It began to occur to me that
unless I had a need to demonstrate my own cleverness and learning, I
would do better to rely upon the client for the direction of movement
in the process.

While I was in Rochester I had a reasonably comfortable relationship with the psychiatric profession. We had a consultant psychiatrist in the Child Study Department. He was a rather weak person
and for the most part we told him what we thought he should say and
he said it, thus giving our recommendations more force and authority.
Later when I became director of the Child Study Department, I employed Samuel Hartwell as consultant psychiatrist and I had a real
respect for him. He was actually able to accomplish things with chil-

dren which I could not. Later on I employed a full-time psychiatrist on the staff. I also had many colleague relations with psychiatrists at the University of Rochester, which were friendly until the dispute arose which I will mention later.

Because of the interest of another psychologist in the work of Otto Rank, we decided to bring him to Rochester for a weekend. This visit was very profitable. I was not too impressed with Rank's theories but I was very much impressed with his description of his therapy. By this time some of my own staff workers were also interested in Rank's work and some of them had taken courses at the Pennsylvania School of Social Work, which was decidedly Rankian in its orientation. All of this had an important impact on my thinking.

During the summer of 1935 I was invited to teach at Teachers' College. I found this highly rewarding and ego strengthening. I was much surprised that the classes, even though enormous (150 to 300), seemed to respond to me very favorably and had good learning experiences. My approach at that time was to give a lecture but with ample opportunity for questions and discussion from the group. I particularly remember one course which was broken into thirds. I taught the first part, a much more experienced psychologist taught the second portion, and I was to teach the third portion of the course. When I returned for this last portion the class applauded loud and long when I came in. I was bowled over by the message that this contained, namely, that they were glad to see me back and really liked me better than the more experienced faculty member who had been teaching them. I began to realize not only that I loved to get people excited about new ideas and new approaches, but that they loved this too.

During 1937 and 1938, the social agencies of Rochester, in which I took a very active part, decided that a community guidance center was a needed organization and that the Child Study Department, of which I was director, should be its core. The decision was to form a new Rochester Guidance Center. At this point my psychiatric friends made a strong case to the Community Chest, to my board of directors, and to all who would listen that such a clinic should be headed by a psychiatrist. So far as I know there was little criticism of the job I had done. The argument was simply that a psychiatrist was in charge of almost all similar clinics in other cities and must be in charge here. This led to a prolonged battle, with many facets, which I finally won, becoming the first director of the Rochester Guidance Center.

During this period I began to doubt that I was a psychologist. The University of Rochester made it clear that the work I was doing was not psychology, and they had no interest in my teaching in the psychology department. I went to APA meetings and found them full of papers on the learning processes of rats and laboratory experiments which seemed to me to have no relation to what I was doing. The psychiatric social workers, however, seemed to be talking my language, so I became active in the social work profession, moving up to local and even national offices.

I began to teach courses at the university under the department of sociology on how to understand and deal with problem children. Soon education wanted to classify these as education courses, also. Before I left Rochester, psychology, too, finally requested permission to list these courses, thus at last accepting me as a psychologist. Simply writing these paragraphs makes me realize how stubbornly I have followed my own course, being relatively unconcerned with the question of whether I was going with my group or not.

In 1940 I accepted a position at Ohio State University as a full professor. I deeply regretted leaving my newly won position as director of the Rochester Guidance Center and might have turned down the offer had it not been for Helen's gentle insistence in pointing out that I had for a long time wished to have a university position and that these did not grow on trees. So I showed an interest in the offer and finally accepted it. I am sure the only reason I was considered was my book on the *Clinical Treatment of the Problem Child,* which I had squeezed out of vacations and brief leaves of absence. I heartily recommend starting in the academic world at the top level. I have often been grateful that I have never had to live through the frequently degrading competitive process of step by step promotion in university faculties, where individuals so frequently learn only one lesson—not to stick their necks out.

In trying to teach what I had learned about treatment and counseling to graduate students at Ohio State I first began to realize that I had perhaps developed a distinctive point of view of my own, out of my experience. When I tried to crystallize some of these ideas and presented them in a paper at the University of Minnesota in December 1940, I found the reactions were very strong. It was my first experience of the fact that a new idea of mine, which to me can seem all shiny and glowing with potentiality, can to another person be a great threat. To find myself the center of criticism, of arguments pro and con, was disconcerting and made me doubt and question. Nevertheless I felt I had something to contribute and wrote the manuscript of *Counseling and Psychotherapy,* setting forth what I felt to be a somewhat more effective orientation to therapy. I also included the first complete verbatim case, electronically recorded and laboriously transcribed.

Here again I realize with some amusement how little I have cared about being "realistic." When I submitted the manuscript, the publisher thought it was interesting and new but wondered what classes would use it. I replied that I knew of only two—a course I was teaching and one in another university. The publisher felt I had made a grave mistake in not writing a text which would fit courses already being given. He was very dubious that he could sell the 2,000 copies necessary to break even. Only when I said I would take it to another publisher did he decide to make the gamble. I don't know which of us has been more surprised at its sales—85,000 now and still continuing.

I had arrived at Ohio State at an opportune time. Many graduate students had been thoroughly trained in a largely laboratory approach, which they found unexciting. When I came upon the scene— a psychologist interested in working with real human beings—they flocked to my seminars and courses and many asked me to sponsor their doctoral researches. I was too naive to realize that by accepting them for sponsorship I was stirring up jealousies in the other faculty members. On the other hand, many of my lifelong friendships were formed in my dealings with this choice group of doctoral students.

I have been told that the practicum in counseling and psychotherapy which I established in 1940 was the first instance in which supervised therapy was carried on in a university setting—that neither Freud nor any other therapist had ever managed to make supervised experience in the therapeutic relationship a part of academic training. I am not certain that this statement is true. I do know, however, that I had no such brash thought in mind when I inaugurated this prac-

ticum. It simply seemed essential that if students were to study therapy
they must also carry it on and should have the opportunity to analyze
and discuss what they were doing. Nearly all the discussion was based
on recorded interviews, and this was an exciting venture for the whole
group. I realize now that too much of our discussion dealt with individual responses, and with techniques, but nonetheless it was a growing experience for all of us.

I was much involved in professional activities during my Ohio
State years. I plunged into the newly formed American Association for
Applied Psychology, became chairman of its clinical division, and
president in 1944–1945. Meanwhile Robert Yerkes was arguing that
if the parent organization, the APA, could be reorganized so as to be
democratic in its structure, all of psychology might again be brought
together. I was responsive to this and there were many meetings involving Yerkes, Hilgard, Boring, and various others, which laid the
basis for a constitutional convention and the eventual reunification of
psychology. It was a privilege to be involved in this statesmanlike
enterprise.

Though Columbus was our home for only five years, it seems
longer because it was a period of intense growth for the whole family.
We built and enjoyed our own home, and it was a period rich in
friendships. David and Natalie, our children, went through their adolescence here. David pointed toward medicine and has gone on to an
outstanding career as chairman of the Department of Medicine at
Vanderbilt University. Currently he is Dean of The Johns Hopkins
School of Medicine. Natalie became sensitively involved in art, the
teaching of art, and psychology, with a special interest in interpersonal
relationships. She has continued all these interests, adding to them the
responsibilities of a wife and mother. She has been building a career
as an encounter group leader, a therapist with children, parents, and
students. We have had enormous satisfaction in the integrity and
sensitivity of our children. But this gets ahead of my story.

Move to Chicago

I was flattered to be invited to teach at the University of Chicago during the summer of 1944. Toward the end of the summer,
Ralph Tyler, who held several important posts at the university, sur-

prised me by extending an invitation to come to Chicago permanently and establish a counseling center there. This was a very appealing offer. I could not accept it for the coming year because I was already committed to aid the war effort by teaching simple counseling methods to the staff members of the USO, whose staff was being besieged by servicemen with personal problems. I did, however, accept a professorship in psychology and the responsibility of estabishing a counseling center, my duties to begin in the autumn of 1945.

In August 1944, before I left Chicago, Dr. Tyler and Lawrence Kimpton, then Dean of Students, asked me to draw up a memorandum setting forth my views regarding a possible university organization for the counseling of students. This memo was written for university administrators—nonpsychologists all—but I am quoting from it here because it served as the basis for the development of the Center a year later.

The primary purpose of the student counseling organization is to assist the student to help himself, to aid him in becoming more intelligently self-directing. In order to achieve this goal, the purpose of the counselor is to create a situation of deep understanding and acceptance which will enable the student to think through his problems and perplexities more clearly, and to direct himself more intelligently and rationally, as a result of this counseling experience.

It is the purpose of the student counseling organization to deal with the student as a total individual. There is no attempt to treat the individual as a bundle of separate parts—educational problems, vocational problems, social problems, etc. There is a clear recognition that difficulties in adjustment are difficulties in adjustment of the whole individual.

It is not the purpose of the counselor to assume responsibility for the life of the student, nor to control him in the ways which the counselor or others regard as satisfactory. Neither is it the purpose of the counselor to control the student's environment by manipulating the curriculum, rules, or other factors so as to make it possible for the student to adjust.

In short, the counselor controls neither the student nor the college environment. Rather the counselor provides a situation in which the student may work out clearly and independently the adjustment to his college experiences and to later life which is realistic for him and which satisfies his own desire for increasing maturity.

It is the purpose of the student counseling organization to be freely available to the student. The counselor should be physically and psychologically accessible. How many counselors there should be in order to be satisfactorily accessible remains to be seen.

The criterion of success of the counseling organization will not lie in elaborateness or completeness of records, nor in the complexity of organizational machinery, but in the feeling of the student that he has achieved a satisfying plan of action for himself.

Establishment of the Counseling Center

The development of the Counseling Center—its staff, its therapeutic principles, its research, its administrative procedures—was a most exciting process. I believe I learned more and contributed more during the twelve years at the Center (1945–1957) than in any other period. I learned to set the staff free, to make all of us jointly responsible for the work, the welfare, and the future of the Counseling Center. It was a period in which our basic views about the helping relationship came to fruition. These views developed out of a heavy service function. The Center had 2,800 counseling interviews with 605 individuals during its first ten months of work and the number steadily increased after that. It was a time of innovation in our educational methods and in our freewheeling administrative process. It was a germinal period for research hypotheses and theoretical formulations. Although our efforts were essentially task oriented, we were also experimenting with much freedom of expression of interpersonal feelings (negative and positive) in our staff meetings and staff relationships. Hence, without consciously planning it, the staff became a very close and personally nourishing group. Graduate students, clerical staff, and faculty members worked as equals in our undertakings. There was enormous freedom for creativity. I think it is safe to say that anyone who worked for as much as a year in that climate regards his time there as one of the most significant experiences of his life.

Some of the closeness of the group grew out of the fact that though Deans Tyler and Strozier gave us complete freedom and solid backing, we lived in a general university context of skepticism, criticism, and strong antagonism. The antagonism was mostly from the department of psychiatry, in which successive chairmen strongly rejected each of our bids for better relationships and cooperation. Our relationship with the department of psychology was friendly and gradually became close under the chairmanship of James Miller.

For myself, this was the period when I wrote *Client-centered Therapy,* many papers, and formulated a precise statement of my whole theoretical position which was first widely distributed in duplicated form for criticism and was finally published as a long chapter in Sigmund Koch's mammoth series, *Psychology: A Study of a Science.*

It was also a period in which my dreams of research in psychotherapy came true. Up to this point I had been unable to get more than piddling amounts for research, but with Dr. Miller's assistance we obtained a large grant from the Rockefeller Foundation, and this was followed by other grants. These funds enabled us to carry out the dozen or more coordinated investigations which we reported in *Psychotherapy and Personality Change.* Other studies followed.

During these years I sponsored many fine graduate students who have gone on to make significant records for themselves. The staff and students contributed greatly to my personal growth, to the greater depth I was achieving in therapeutic relationships, to my development as a facilitative administrator, and to the enrichment of my theories about therapy and interpersonal relationships.

I would like to mention a few of those who have contributed most significantly to my own thinking and development, listing them roughly in the order in which I came to know them: Victor Raimy, Thomas Gordon, Donald Grummon, John Butler, Oliver Brown, Nathaniel Raskin, Douglas Blocksma, John Shlien, Eugene Gendlin, Desmond and Rosalind Cartwright, Richard Farson, Godfrey Barrett-Lennard, Jerome Berlin, Gerard Haigh.

Professional Activities at Chicago

My manner of conducting courses had never been orthodox, but at Chicago I became more and more radical. The hypothesis which came to be central to me is the first one presented in the chapter on "Student-centered teaching" in *Client-Centered Therapy.* It is that "We cannot teach another person directly; we can only facilitate his learning." This hypothesis had grown largely out of my therapeutic experience, and I endeavored increasingly to find new methods of implementing it. Even in large courses, where some presentation of issues at least seemed essential, I found ways to set students free to pursue their own goals and provide the resources from which they

could learn. My classes became exciting clusters of small groups, in-
forming themselves in depth on topics of real interest. To find
themselves set free was often a shocking experience. One outstanding
student, who later became a leader in the Counseling Center, withdrew from his initial course with me, saying in disgust to his companion, "That son-of-a-bitch calls himself a teacher!" Yet the ferment
he had felt continued to work in him until he returned more than a
year later. This same phenomenon occurred in a Harvard conference
on teaching in 1952. I presented a ten-minute paper ("Some personal
thoughts on teaching and learning") in order to initiate a discussion.
It is hardly correct to say that it initiated a discussion—it set off an
explosion! Yet, constructive reverberations from that paper (included
in *On Becoming a Person*) continue to this day.

      Though I shall not further discuss this aspect of my interests,
my concern with what I believe is a much needed revolution in education at all levels has continued. This is evident in *Freedom to Learn,*
published in 1969. I have tried increasingly to point out, and to
demonstrate, that we do not need *teaching,* as that term is ordinarily
used or defined in the dictionary. What is needed, from nursery school
to the Ph.D., is an intelligent and resourceful facilitation of *learning.*

      Especially during the early portion of my Chicago years, I was
extremely active in professional affairs. I was president-elect of the
APA in 1945–1946, and president in 1946–1947. These were years of
great change and expansion in psychology following the war, and I
was deeply involved in formulations regarding clinical training, the
formation of the American Board of Examiners in Professional Psychology, and the continuing attempt to resolve the tensions between
psychiatry and psychology.

      For my presidential address in 1947, I determined to try to
work out and present my emerging views regarding the importance
of the phenomenological world of the individual as a source of data,
and the centrality of the self-concept as the determiner of behavior.
Because I was in the midst of struggling with these new ideas, the
paper ("Some observations on the organization of personality") is not
a masterpiece of clarity. It did, however, push forward into areas
which have since received much more recognition. I felt it was neither
understood nor well received by psychologists. In fact, I have one
vivid memory of this presentation. Following the address in a beauti-

ful auditorium in Detroit, Chairman John Anderson and I went to the men's room which was crowded with psychologists, buzzing loudly with talk. When I entered, all conversation stopped. The silence was deafening. I felt I had interrupted many highly critical comments. I received very few congratulations, and it is only the increasing number of times that this paper has been selected for books of readings in psychology which has given me the feeling that though it was perhaps a somewhat groping first attempt, it has come to be recognized as at least a significant groping.

Period of Personal Distress

While I was at Chicago there were two years of intense personal distress which I can now look back upon coolly, but which were very difficult to live through. A deeply disturbed client (she would be regarded as schizophrenic) whom I had worked with at Ohio State later moved to the Chicago area and renewed her therapeutic contacts with me. I see now that I handled her badly, vacillating between being warm and real with her and then being more "professional" and aloof when the depth of her psychotic disturbance threatened me. This brought about the most intense hostility on her part (along with a dependence and love) which completely pierced my defenses. I stubbornly felt that I *should* be able to help her and permitted the contacts to continue, even though they had ceased to be therapeutic and involved only suffering for me. I recognized that many of her insights were sounder than mine, and this destroyed my confidence in myself; I somehow gave up *my* self in the relationship. The situation is best summarized by one of her dreams in which a cat was clawing my guts out, but really did not wish to do so. Yet I continued this relationship, destructive to me, because I recognized her desperately precarious situation, on the brink of a psychosis, and felt I *had* to help.

Gradually I realized I was on the edge of a complete breakdown myself, and then suddenly this feeling became very urgent. I *must* escape. I am everlastingly grateful to Dr. Louis Cholden, the promising young psychiatrist, who was working in the Counseling Center at that time, for his being willing to take over the client on an hour's notice. She, within moments, burst into a full-blown psychosis, with many delusions and hallucinations. As for me, I went home and told Helen that I must get away, at *once*. We were on the road within an hour and stayed away two or three months, on what we can now calmly refer to as our "runaway trip." Helen's quiet assurance that I would come out of this distress in time, and her willingness to listen when I was able to talk of it, were a great help. However, when we returned I was still rather deeply certain of my complete inadequacy as a therapist, my worthlessness as a person, and my lack of any future in the field of psychology or psychotherapy.

For a time before I left, I was in therapy with one member of my staff. When I returned I felt my problems were so serious it would only be threatening to ask a staff member to help me with them. I am deeply thankful that one member of our group simply told me that it was obvious I was in deep distress, that he was not afraid of me or my problems, and that he was offering me a therapeutic relationship. I accepted in desperation and gradually worked through to a point where I could value myself, even like myself, and was much less fearful of receiving or giving love. My own therapy with my clients has become consistently and increasingly free and spontaneous ever since that time.

I have often been grateful that by the time I was in dire need of personal help, I had trained therapists who were persons in their own right, not dependent upon me, yet able to offer me the kind of help I needed. I have since become rather keenly aware that the point of view I developed in therapy is the sort of help I myself would like, and this help was available when I most needed it.

Broadening Vista

During these Chicago years, I had many choice opportunities for gaining a broader perspective, both personally and professionally. During various summers I taught at UCLA, Harvard, Occidental College, Brandeis University, and spent a visiting semester at the University of California at Berkeley. While there I counseled a client in front of my large seminar group for about ten sessions, an experience which I think none of us has forgotten.

In these years also Helen and I began to take the winter quarters off, getting away from the cold and slush of Chicago to various isolated hideaways in Mexico and the Caribbean where no one knew I was a psychologist. Here snorkeling, painting, color photography appeared to be my major activities. Yet in these spots, where I almost never put in more than four hours a day in professional work, I have produced, I believe, some of my most creative and solid writing. When I was alone, when neither physically nor psychologically was anyone "looking over my shoulder," I have done some of my best work.

Wisconsin

I was invited to spend one semester in the department of education at the University of Wisconsin in the spring of 1957 as the honorary Knapp Professor for that period. The individual who sponsored this idea, and worked hard to bring it about, was Virgil Herrick, a dynamic professor of education whom I had known previously but who was to become one of my very closest personal friends during the ensuing years.

The five-month appointment was a fruitful one. I held a seminar for faculty members in which I was, I fear, rather rigidly "student-centered." I had not yet learned how to place full responsibility with the group and yet give freely of myself. Nevertheless it was an exciting and unusual experience for most of the participants. I also held a large seminar for graduate students in counseling, psychology, and education. This was highly successful and, judging from letters over the years, had a significant impact on the lives of the members. During this time, Helen and I had many warm personal and social contacts with faculty members in education, psychiatry, and with several of the psychologists.

These months gave me a great deal of time for my own work. I listened to dozens of recorded therapeutic interviews seeking for the elements of the process of therapy. I determined to make this the subject of my paper before the APA, the paper demanded of each recipient of the APA Distinguished Scientific Contribution Award, which I had received in 1956. As with my APA presidential address, I was still struggling with emerging ideas as I tried to meet the deadline, but the paper ("A process conception of psychotherapy") has since stimulated many research investigations and a number of instruments for measuring process movement in psychotherapy.

Meanwhile, Virgil Herrick was working devotedly and selflessly behind the scenes to bring me to Wisconsin. I had assured him that nothing could lure me from Chicago, and he had challenged me to write out the description of a position which would entice me. I described an impossible position—appointments in both psychiatry and psychology, opportunity to train psychologists and psychiatrists, time for therapy and research with psychotic and normal individuals (the two extreme groups where I felt my experience was deficient), and other improbable requirements. To my amazement, he was able to bring this about, though the approval of ten separate committees, besides his persuasive talks with many individuals, was necessary.

I was faced with a difficult decision. I felt I could continue at Chicago along the same lines I had been following, but I could go little further. I could continue to have the encouraging environment of the Counseling Center which had permitted my ideas to grow. Or I could launch out into a skeptical psychology department and a somewhat skeptical department of psychiatry and try to establish myself and my ideas in a more pervasive setting. I could also have the opportunity to pursue research with psychotic individuals, which I felt was my next challenge. In addition, we would have a more pleasant and friendly environment for living. We decided to accept.

The staff members of the Counseling Center were incredulous and greatly upset. They found it hard to understand my view that I had contributed what I could at Chicago, that the Counseling Center was a vigorous and viable organization (which it has proven to be), and that for my own personal growth and development it was challenging to move on. Despite their protests, I held to my decision.

So in the late summer of 1957 we moved to Madison, where for seven years we enjoyed gracious living in a beautiful home of contemporary architecture, situated on the shore of Lake Monona, and where we made many very close and dear friends and thoroughly enjoyed our personal experiences.

Professionally there were ups and downs. For the first time in my professional life I tried to be a *member* only, rather than a leader. I did not do too well in several respects. In psychiatry, I tried to play down any leadership role on my part. This submerging of myself was probably not quite genuine and made some members suspicious of me. I was also frankly appalled at the poor caliber of the psychiatric residents, in comparison with graduate students in psychology. However, by the end of the seven years many changes had come to pass, due in large measure to Dr. Robert Roessler, chairman during most of that period. The caliber of residents greatly improved, I was doing a much better job of stimulating their learning in my time with them, and much research, which had been almost nonexistent at the time of my arrival, was being carried on.

In psychology, I had an ample number of students in my seminars, and under my sponsorship, and I enjoyed them. I had had few illusions about the attitudes of the department in general, which was highly laboratory oriented and very distrustful of clinical psychology. But I had felt that it would be healthy for students working with me to have laboratory as well as clinical training and believed that I could carve out an area of interest in which my students and I could work together, engaging both in clinical practice and in research.

What I did not foresee or recognize was that the department had come to place such stress on "rigorous" examinations, on failing large proportions of students, that no one in any field could turn out a significant number of Ph.D.s. In the department as a whole—though it took me a number of years to recognize this—about one out of seven of our carefully selected graduate students ever received the Ph.D. Some were failed, some of the most creative minds and the best clinicians left in disgust, and I was in the peculiar position of training graduate students who had only a minute chance (a chance which did not have too much to do with merit) of obtaining a degree. I made every effort in my power to change what appeared to me as both an incredibly wasteful and a foolishly punitive system, but without avail. A majority of the department would put through some liberalizing change, only to have it negated by some new policy (all, of course, in the interest of "high standards"). In April 1963, I finally resigned from the department, retaining only my appointment in psychiatry. I felt I would be lacking in integrity to do otherwise. As persons, the members of the department constituted an interesting and often likable lot. Collectively, they were destroying everything I valued in the development of scientists and practitioners.

Meanwhile, I was deeply involved in research. After a considerable period of planning and fund raising, I began assembling a small and devoted staff for the most complicated and difficult research of my life—a study of the impact of the therapeutic relationship upon relatively chronic hospitalized schizophrenic patients. The difficulties of implementing such a study were fantastic but it was at last launched. I am tempted to mention the names of those who contributed the most, but since more than two hundred individuals were eventually involved it is impossible to know where to stop.

But there were flaws in the way I organized the research staff, flaws which were to be nearly fatal. Because I was spread too thinly over many activities, I did not take the time to develop a staff which was unified in philosophy and outlook, as at the Counseling Center. The task was so large, it seemed there was hardly time for this. Although I wished the group to be responsible for itself, I did not devote time enough or energy enough to implement this, so that the staff never felt completely responsible for itself and its activities.

Consequently, when an important member of the group engaged in behavior which most of us regarded as unethical, there was no solid basis for handling the situation. The fact that most of the turmoil which then occurred happened while I was away for a year at Palo Alto multiplied the problems. My difficulty in believing that a person whom I had known and trusted and often admired might be unethical made me vacillate in my own attitudes. Because of the emergency I tried to pull back some of the authority, which I had freely given to the group, into my own hands. This was a grave mistake also. The ensuing uproar, recriminations, disappearance of data, misunderstandings, involvement of many outsiders, constitute without doubt the most painful and anguished episode in my whole professional life. The major portion of the research analysis had to be completely redone, at the insistence of the staff. I agreed to its necessity but was skeptical that we had the time and strength to do it. It was, however, achieved and a fearfully complex investigation, developed and reported by many members of the staff, is at long last published. I hope it has proven to be worth the suffering it has caused so many people.

There were, fortunately for my personal balance, many positive events during this period. In the summer of 1960, I was a leader in a ten-day workshop at the University of Denver for influential young men in the field of college counseling and personnel work. This was successful beyond our hopes.

Following this, Helen and I retreated to a lovely log home near Estes Park, built sixty years earlier, and in a three-week period I drew together the material for *On Becoming a Person,* the book I prefer above all my other writings. This book had been germinating in my mind and my notes for several years but the final selection of the papers, the editing of overlap, the writing of material which would introduce and link the papers was all accomplished in these three intense weeks. Even so I found time to hike in the rocky peaks behind the cabin, enjoying the deer and other wildlife which were plentiful.

The year 1962–1963 I spent as a Fellow at the Center for Advanced Study in the Behavioral Sciences at Stanford. It was in many ways a meaningful and stimulating year, but the greatest single impact on me was my close contact with two Britons, Michael Polanyi, the physicist turned philosopher of science, and Lancelot Whyte, the historian of ideas. I was excited to find that many of my own developing ideas regarding the unfortunate and out-of-date philosophy of science to which American psychology seems committed were not only shared but strongly reinforced by these men, who were much more competent scholars in the field than I. Another important influence was my contact with Erik Erikson, a splendid person whose very appearance is therapeutic, and several other psychoanalysts, foreign as well as American. From them I learned what I had strongly suspected —that psychoanalysis as a school of thought is dead but that, out of loyalty and other motives, none but the very brave analysts mention this fact as they go on to develop theories and ways of working very remote from, or entirely opposed to, the Freudian views.

Before returning to Wisconsin, I had obtained from the president of the university permission to conduct a continuing, interdepartmental, noncredit seminar, open to both faculty and graduate students. After resigning from psychology, I wanted an opportunity to facilitate real learning in a way which would cut across all boundaries and which would be free of the horribly constricting influence of evaluation, grades, and degrees. I decided upon the topic "The philosophy of the behavioral sciences" for the first semester. So many applied that the seminar could accommodate less than half, and still was too large.

It was, partly because of its size, not entirely successful, but it was a stimulating experience for almost all and a beginning experiment in breaking the lock-step of American graduate education.

Western Behavioral Sciences Institute

Quite unwittingly I had had a part in the formation of an adventurous new organization on the cutting edge of the behavioral sciences. Richard Farson, Thomas Gordon, and I had conducted a workshop in human relations in California in the summer of 1958. Dr. Paul Lloyd, a California Institute of Technology physicist who had become increasingly interested in the field of interpersonal relationships, was one of the participants. As a result of many discussions following that workshop, Farson and Lloyd founded the Western Behavioral Sciences Institute, a nonprofit organization devoted to humanistically oriented research in interpersonal relationships, with a particular focus on the manner in which constructive change in interpersonal relationships comes about. At the time of its establishment in 1959, I accepted their invitation to serve on its board of directors. My motive was to encourage what seemed to me to be a pioneering venture in an area in which pioneering is often unwelcomed by established institutions.

From the first Farson, whom I had known for many years, urged me to come out as a Visiting Fellow, or to join the staff, or in any other way I chose to affiliate more closely than as a remote board member. I had never accepted any of these invitations, partly because of other obligations, partly because I felt that my contribution could certainly best be made through a university. While I was at the Center in Stanford in 1963, he repeated over the phone this invitation to join their staff. I gave my stock response but later began to mull over the question. What was a university, at this stage of my career, offering me? I realized that in my research it offered no particular help; in anything educational, I was forced to fit my beliefs into a totally alien mold; in stimulation, there was little from my colleagues because we were so far apart in thinking and in goals. On the other hand, WBSI offered complete freedom with no bureaucratic entanglements; the stimulation of a thoroughly congenial interdisciplinary group; the opportunity to facilitate learning without becoming entrapped in the anti-educational jungle of credits, requirements, examinations, more examinations, and grudgingly granted degrees. As Helen and I talked it over, we were very reluctant to leave our Madison friends and our lovely home, but I recognized that professionally I could now leave university life without too much regret and that from a realistic point of view I would have a much deeper membership in a "community of scholars" at WBSI than at any university I knew. So we decided to, make the move, beginning our new life in January 1964.

Our wildest hopes were exceeded. I could not have believed, in advance, how much relief I would feel on being freed from the constrictions of university life. I have always done pretty much what I wanted to do, but I have had to discover that doing what you want to do, against skepticism and opposition, is a very different thing from doing what you want to do in an atmosphere of encouragement and congenial interdisciplinary stimulation. I became more creative and productive than I had been for years. Curiously enough I had deeper and much more significant contact with faculty members, and more significant contact with eager learners, than I had ever experienced before. This demands a word of explanation.

Having completed our work with schizophrenics, I have been eager to turn to working with "normal" individuals—the other end of the spectrum. A potent way of doing this, as I learned as early as 1950, is through the intensive group experience (often called a workshop, or a T-group, or a basic encounter group). So I have held intensive workshops of from two and one half to ten days in length, with graduate students, faculty members, business executives, groups of blacks and whites, therapists (psychologists and pychiatrists), government officials, executive leaders with their spouses, and others, in this country as well as in Australia, Japan, and France. The impact has been striking for them and rewarding to me. In a very real sense I have been able to adapt my therapeutic approach to the facilitation of learning and the self-enhancement of the well-functioning person. This approach involves feelings as well as cognition, experiencing as well as ideas, learning by the whole person as contrasted to learning "from the neck up." It involves intensive experience in a group rather than the spaced contacts of individual therapy. I have drawn together my thinking about the theory and process of the intensive group, its facilitation, and its results in my recent book, *Carl Rogers on Encounter Groups.*[1]

I have also had the opportunity freely to pursue my second major current interest in the assumptions and philosophy of the behavioral sciences. A seminar with behavioral scientists, psychological practitioners, physicists, philosophers, and others was a beginning. With the assistance of Dr. William Coulson, a small deliberative conference composed of outstanding individuals in the field was held, with much of the focus on a more humanistic approach. This eventuated in the small book *Man and the Science of Man* (1968), which Coulson and I edited.

Center for Studies of the Person

When Farson left the directorship of WBSI, the administrative policy changed sharply to a much more controlling and structured point of view. As a consequence the more humanistically oriented members split off to form The Center for Studies of the Person in 1968. At first out of financial desperation and later as a desire of the group, we have adopted some most unusual policies. What we have become, in essence, is a warmly personal psychological community, from which each of us goes out to organize a project, carry on writing, make films, teach or counsel in a university, conduct a large training program for group facilitators—to name a few current activities. There are approximately forty members, of which more than half are Ph.D.s, representing psychology (and psychotherapy), sociology, education, anthropology, religion, public relations, family therapy, group dynamics, and other fields. There are presently four visiting fellows also.

"Studies of the Person" may convey the notion of conventional empirical research as carried on in psychology departments. This has not been the picture. Two of our members prepared a careful empirical proposal for research regarding young drug users, a proposal which would have had a high probability of acceptance. They finished it just before the deadline. All that remained was mailing it. Then they

[1] New York: Harper and Row, 1970.

discussed it. Did they really wish to spend their next three years doing empirical research of the sort they had already found rather sterile, or would they prefer to work with young drug users, earning their living in some other way? They chose the second alternative and never mailed the proposal. This action is somewhat typical of the Center. We are deeply interested in persons but are rather "turned off" by the older methods of studying them as "objects" for research.

One of our members has become a department chairman, and I recently asked him why he continued his membership in CSP when he had acquired power, prestige, and colleagues elsewhere. His reply was something like this: "Because you provide the courage for me to *be*. When I think of breaking the traditional academic routine, or teaching in an innovative fashion, you're in the psychological horizons of my mind saying, 'Dammitall, you got to be *you*.' And so I do things I wouldn't dare attempt otherwise." I feel the same way, and this is why I prize the Center.

So, as Helen and I turn from looking at our flower-filled patio to the view of surf and coastline and mountains to the north, we feel very pleased that we had the courage to embark on this Western venture which has given us both a new zest for living.

The Meanings in My Career

What meanings, what significant threads, do I see in the events of my professional life and thought? The drafting of this autobiography has made me think seriously about this question for almost the first time, since I have not ordinarily been one to look backward. Let me describe a number of the meanings which I can distill out of my experience.

I have never really *belonged* to *any* professional group. I have been educated by, or had close working relationships with, psychologists, psychoanalysts, psychiatrists, theologians, psychiatric social workers, social caseworkers, educators, religious workers, yet I have never felt that I really belonged, in any total or committed sense, to any one of these groups. When psychology was taking directions I did not like, I joined the social work profession. When psychology became more interested in the human being, I returned to psychology. At the present time, most of psychology seems to me so sterile that I have no feeling of attachment to it. If some new profession were formed which more closely fit my interests, I would join it without so much as a backward glance at psychology.

Because of this attitude, I was deeply touched, to the point of tears, when I was awarded one of the first three Scientific Contribution Awards by the APA. I was astonished that psychologists deeply and significantly regarded me as "one of them." In spite of all the work I had done in professional organizations of psychologists, in spite of working in departments of psychology, I had never regarded myself in quite that way. It should be obvious that whatever its disadvantages, this lack of belonging has left me free to deviate, to think independently, without any sense of disloyalty to my group.

Lest one think I have been a complete nomad professionally, I should add that the only groups to which I have ever really belonged have been close-knit, congenial task forces which I have organized or helped organize, or which have used my ideas as a part of their central core. Thus, for example, I fully belonged to the Counseling Center of the University of Chicago, and I belong deeply now to the Center for Studies of the Person. One may look upon this as evidence of egotism or whatever. I simply mention it as a fact.

I was fortunate in never having a mentor, and thus never had any professional father-figure on whom I was dependent, or against whom I had to rebel. Many individuals, organizations, and writings were important to me in my education, but no one source was paramount. There was no great intellectual or emotional indebtedness to one person or one institution. This too made it easy to think for myself, without any sense of guilt or betrayal.

I was similarly fortunate in having broken from my family and my early religious beliefs, clearly and cleanly, with very little bitterness and only a moderate amount of rebellion. Because the break came at the right time, the differences could be open and aboveboard, not furtive and festering. This too helped me to feel comfortably self-reliant.

The types of isolation or "unrootedness" which I have been describing have made for what I think of as a very positive kind of aloneness. A proverb which has for many years meant a great deal to me is "He travels fastest who travels alone." I feel this has been a central theme for me. I have no great desire to bring colleagues along with me. I am too impatient. I tend to "go it alone," confident that if I am in error my efforts will be disregarded, and equally confident that if I am doing something worthwhile, others will at some point discover this.

I have never felt particularly insecure in regard to exams, degrees, positions, titles, promotions, tenure, and the like. I cannot account for this, for I have often felt *very* insecure as to my abilities, my knowledge, the value of my work or my writings. But I have never worried to any significant degree about whether I could pass an exam, fill a position, or win a promotion. This in spite of the fact that my first positions, held during the great depression, *were* insecure. I have cared so little for permanent tenure that I have on three separate occasions forfeited tenure in order to take a position I wanted.

I have always been inwardly quite certain that I could pass examinations and that I could do whatever was required to hold a job. I have also felt that in any position I could build the job into exactly what I thought it ought to be—and have been naively astonished on the few occasions when superiors have thought otherwise. I have never felt that pleasing my superiors was a major goal. Sometimes they have understood what I was doing, sometimes not. It has never been a matter of great importance to me.

If all of this sounds extraordinarily secure and self-sufficient, it is not. I regard myself rather as having been exceedingly fortunate. I feel very strongly that if I had been continually evaluated as our graduate students are today, frequently failed in such examinations, scrutinized and supervised closely during my early professional years, put through the academic ladder, I would probably have been destroyed as an original worker. I am sensitive to any judgment which I think is a competent judgment, can readily be made to feel that I and my thoughts are worthless and inadequate, and could very easily have been crushed by even the ordinary experiences of academic and professional life in my earlier years. By the time I was forty, I was beginning to have a confidence in myself which would not have been easily beaten down, but before that, negative judgments from competent people would almost certainly have destroyed me.

As a corollary of not belonging firmly to any group, I have never felt myself a part of the mainstream of psychology. Probably the major concern of psychology during my lifetime has been learning theory. I used to be embarrassed by the fact that I found this field totally uninteresting. I felt it was additional proof that I was not really a psychologist, when such highly regarded work seemed to me to be mostly a pompous investigation of the trivial. Now that some others also share this view, I dare to voice it.

I have had some sort of a penchant or gift for being just in the forefront of developments which were on the verge of occurring. I certainly take no credit for this. It is nothing I have tried to do. It seems purely intuitive. Let me explain what I mean with a number of examples.

I became interested in clinical psychology when it was a piddling and insignificant appendage on the fringe of the respectable portions of psychology. I could never have dreamed that in twenty-five years it would constitute much the largest portion of the psychological profession.

I became interested in psychotherapy (the "treatment interview") when it scarcely was a field of endeavor for anyone and when the one certain thing about it was that it was solely the province of the physician. If someone had told me that in thirty-five years psychotherapy would be a major interest of more than one-third of American psychologists, I would have regarded the statement as utterly absurd.

I thought that valuable raw data could be obtained by the electronic recording of therapeutic interviews and made such recordings beginning in 1938 or 1939. At the time, every reputable therapist in the country was certain that it was impossible to carry on any real therapy if either the therapist or the client knew it was being recorded. I sometimes chuckle at the fact that even the psychoanalysts—who were the most adamant—are now involved in and advocating recording and opening the sacrosanct analytic hour to professional scrutiny and study. I became interested in research in psychotherapy a couple of decades before it became fashionable and respectable for psychologists and psychiatrists to invest themselves in this field.

When I first began to realize that a theory of the self and the self-concept might fit the emerging facts of my experience, I felt both lonely and apologetic for emphasizing a line of thought which had died out with introspectionism. I certainly did not foresee today's burgeoning of self-theory.

I was surprised to find, about 1951, that the directions of my

thinking and the central aspects of my therapeutic work could justi-
fiably be labeled existential and phenomenological. It seemed odd for
an American psychologist to be in such strange company. Today these
are significant influences on our profession.

Perhaps these examples will make clear that in many instances
the directions in which I have felt impelled to move are directions
which many psychologists and psychiatrists have later followed. This
has, to me, seemed a strange thing.

On the basis of experiences such as these it is not surprising
that I believe my current concern with the basic assumptions and
philosophy of the behavioral sciences, with the implications of the
prediction and control of human behavior, with the potency of the
intensive group experience, with the development of a humanistically
oriented psychology will also, within the next decade or two, become
central concerns of the whole field of psychology.

I enjoy discovering the order in large bodies of complex experience. This has been a very persistent theme. It seems inevitable that I
seek for the meaning, the underlying order, the lawfulness in every
major area of my interest. I tried to discover the underlying framework
in the conglomeration of things clinicians did for children, and out of
this came *The Clinical Treatment of the Problem Child* in 1939. I
have tried to discover the orderly principles in the work of the therapist and in the process of change in his client. I found it very satisfying
to write the paper on "The process equation of psychotherapy" in
which I tried to describe the interaction in hard, parsimonious, and
general terms. "A tentative formulation of a general law of interpersonal relationships" (Chapter 18 in *On Becoming a Person*) is a
still bolder attempt to sense the lawful pattern which exists in a fantastically complex area of life. I have more recently tried to discern
whatever order exists in the richly varied process of the intensive group
experience.

I have come to realize that both empirical research and the
process of theory construction are aimed, essentially, at the inward
ordering of significant experience. These activities are justified because
it is subjectively satisfying to perceive the world as having order, and
because rewarding results often ensue when one understands the lawful
relationships which appear in nature.

Another theme which stands out is the tension and division

within me between the sensitively subjective therapist or group facilitator and the hardheaded scientist. I suspect I am not as sensitively
attuned to human experience as some therapists. I am sure that I am
not as purely motivated by curiosity as the best of the scientists. Yet,
both this subjective understanding and this detached, objective curiosity are very real aspects of my life. It is the working out in me of the
tensions between them which has been the basis for whatever contributions I have made to psychology. I have expressed this tension most
clearly perhaps in my paper on "Persons or science?" I thoroughly
enjoy the complete immersion in a highly subjective relationship which
is the heart of psychotherapy. I thoroughly enjoy the hardheaded precision of the scientist and the elegance of any truly great research. If I
try to give up either one of these aspects of me, I am not complete.
So some people, knowing me only as a "soft" therapist, are surprised
to learn that I am also "tough." A few, knowing me primarily from
my research, are surprised that I can be at times a delicate artist in
interpersonal relationships. I feel myself fortunate in having these two
sharply different selves. I like both of them, and they are both a real
part of me.

I have often been a so-called controversial person. This has
meant that I have been involved in a variety of professional struggles
and battles. I realize that my strategy has almost invariably been one
of "island hopping." In World War II, General MacArthur—a great
strategist but not otherwise one of my heroes—never attacked the next
island in the South Pacific, which was always heavily fortified and
defended. Instead he slipped a task force through to some island far
beyond and captured and held that. Then the island heavily defended
by the Japanese simply died on the vine, without ever having been
attacked, simply because it could no longer be supplied or supported.
This very well describes my own intuitive strategy in professional
struggles. When psychiatrists have argued that psychotherapy is a
medical function and psychologists should not be allowed to practice
it, I have spent very little time arguing this directly but have simply
gone far beyond it, trying to improve psychotherapy and to strengthen
research in psychotherapy. I was convinced the argument would lose
all its force if psychologists were *doing* good therapy and expanding
the area of knowledge in that field through research. I feel this view
has been borne out. When the psychology department at Chicago had

unreasonably constrictive rules for obtaining the Ph.D., I simply encouraged my students to take their degrees through the Committee on Human Development. As psychology lost students, it modified its rules in a more liberal direction. (In the psychology department at the University of Wisconsin, I was unsuccessful in finding the island to which I might "hop," hence had to engage in a more and more frontal attack on their—to me—antiquated and punitive structure of graduate education, and hence was thoroughly defeated.) In instance after instance in my professional life, I have felt it wasteful and foolish to battle directly to achieve my goals. I much prefer to establish a beachhead far in the future, a beachhead which will make the current controversy meaningless. Thus, for example, it has never been of any importance to me to convince my professional colleagues that what I am doing is significant. This seems to me a most futile endeavor. But to interest *students,* who will be the next generation of faculty members and practitioners, in what I am doing—this has been of the greatest importance to me. I prefer, in other words, to hop the present generation and concentrate on the coming one.

This relates very directly to the next theme of my life. I want to have *impact.* I am not a person who is ambitious in the ordinary sense. It has never made much difference to me whether I have prestige, position, or power. In fact when power has been bestowed on me, I have usually given it away to the group. But it *is* important to me to have influence. I want what I do to *count,* to make a difference somewhere. I am not one of those persons who can do his thinking and research in an isolated corner, with never a care as to whether someone else finds it meaningful. I definitely want my work to have an influence. You can regard this as good or bad—I suspect it is both —but it is most certainly a fact in me.

Very closely related is what I think of as my enjoyment of facilitation. I get great pleasure out of facilitating the development of a person in therapy, the development of growth-promoting interaction in a group, or serving as a facilitative "change agent" in an institution. I realize that my sense of "power" comes from the confidence I have that I can serve as a catalyst and produce the unpredictable! This is truly exciting.

I think this is a rather rare trait. Most individuals who have attained some status tend to dominate a situation—they are brilliant in conversation, tend to be the center of attention in any group, simply cannot be ignored. I, on the contrary, am absolutely at my worst if I am expected to be a "leading figure" or an "exciting person." As my wife can testify, I simply clam up and seem to be the dullest person around. If, however, I am received as a person (by a group or an individual) and can sense an opportunity to facilitate change and growth (in myself as well as the other) I can be a sparkling person whose expressiveness focuses attention not particularly on me but on each person's sensing of change within himself. I feel most deeply rewarded when the group or the individual leaves me, not with the reaction "what a brilliant leader (or speaker, or thinker)" but with "I feel myself changing—within myself and in my relationship to my wife (or my children or my boss, or my thinking and professional interests)." This ability to facilitate change, to free people for change, is something I greatly prize in myself.

Another important aspect of my development is my liking for writing. As a shy boy, I found I could express myself much more freely in writing than face to face. My love letters to Helen, my wife-to-be, are far more eloquent than anything I could express to her verbally. I enjoyed writing stories and essays and poetry, and even my attempts at scholarly papers in college. My work on the college debating team was helpful. The course in homiletics I took at Union Seminary helped me to develop clarity. But the experience which perhaps contributed most to my psychological writing was the twelve years of preparing comprehensive reports on each child we studied or dealt with at the Child Study Department and later the Guidance Center in Rochester. Frequently these reports had to meet a deadline of a court hearing or an agency decision. If they were to have any influence they had to be accurate, penetrating, comprehensive, persuasive in presenting the reasons for our recommendations, clear and interesting enough to be read, and able to stand the test of time, since we would continue to be in contact with both the agency and the child, often for long periods. This was excellent training in writing and strengthened both my desire and ability to write with clarity. I have realized, as the years have gone by, that some writers desire to mystify. They want (consciously or unconsciously) the reader's reaction to be "What is this complex thing you're trying to say? I'll have to read it again." My desire, on the other hand, has been, even from childhood, to be understood. I would like to communicate so clearly that you cannot mistake my meaning. This long-standing attitude has made a difference, and a frequent comment on my writing, even from critics, is that it is lucid.

In more recent years, I have assimilated another learning which has, I believe, improved my writing, my speaking, and hence my impact. This learning is that "what is most personal is most general." I have come to realize that if I can drop some of my defenses, can let myself come forth as a vulnerable person, can express some of the attitudes which feel most personal, most private, most tentative and uncertain in me, then the response from others is deep and receptive and warming. If I can be deeply myself in my expression this sets up a resonance in the other—whether an individual or an audience of two thousand—which is very rewarding both for the other and for me. I have gradually become much more bold in revealing myself.

An important theme of my life is that I have had a personal existence and security quite apart from my professional life. If by some strange circumstance I were completely barred from all psychological practice, research, speaking, and writing, I would still have a full and rich life. I have a security in my relationship with my wife which has been a rich resource to me, and even at times a desperately needed one. Because of early difficulties in sexual adjustment we were fortunate in learning that open communication in problem areas, though difficult, is the only avenue to a better relationship. So we have enjoyed each other and supplement each other in many, many ways. She is naturally social where I tend to be a loner; she dreams up trips and enterprises which I reluctantly accept and then thoroughly enjoy; she has kept our life from being narrow. She has been a true helpmate (a term which is unfortunately growing old-fashioned), in every sense of the word.

In addition, I have many fields of interest. I enjoy color photography, especially close-ups; we both have enjoyed (through snorkeling) the undersea life of the Caribbean; I like to garden and nurse each plant and bud; I like to make mobiles; I have an interest in art and have tried my hand at painting; I enjoy carpentry; I have an interest in foreign cultures, especially primitive ones. All this has meant that my professional work is not the be-all and end-all of my existence.

Somehow I have an inwardly light touch in regard to my work. It is not all there is to life. Sometimes I am struck with the absurdity of my earnest effort to help a person, complete research, write a paper. Placed in the perspective of billions of years of time, of millions of light years of interstellar space, of the trillions of one-celled organisms in the sea, of the life struggle by billions of people to achieve their goals, I cannot help but wonder what possible significance can be attached to the efforts of one person at one moment of time. I can only do my part as one infinitely small living unit in this vast ongoing universe. But such a perspective helps to keep me from feeling too self-important.

There is one final thread in my career which has surely been woven in and out through the years, and that is a great deal of plain luck. Chance and good fortune are elements which should be clearly recognized in the shaping of my career. I do not wish to be unduly modest or to say that the recognition I have received is all luck. But chance *has* entered in, as two illustrations may indicate.

By chance, my book on *The Clinical Treatment of the Problem Child* came out just when Ohio State University was making every effort to establish a major position in clinical psychology. As a consequence, I entered university life as a full professor. I became visible nationally, instead of being involved in a local service agency, and a part of that was pure luck.

When I wrote *Counseling and Psychotherapy,* in 1942, neither my publisher nor I could have foreseen that the minuscule field of counseling would suddenly expand at the end of the war into an enormous field of great public interest. To have written one of the very few books on the subject was to boost me again into national visibility, and again the timing was simply lucky.

As I have been writing this section in which I have attempted to discover the major themes of my professional life, I have been surprised at a certain smugness or assurance which has crept in. At first I thought this was quite unlike me and should be edited. As I have thought it over further, I believe this is a real part of me and should be permitted to remain in the manuscript. It was most certainly not present in my earlier years, when I often felt a great lack of assurance, but it does describe a part of me now. I do believe in what I am doing; I do trust my own experience more deeply than any authority;

I am inwardly sure that the directions in which I am moving are, and will prove to be, significant directions. I do, in some very basic sense, believe in myself. Intellectually, I know with equal assurance that I and my thinking may be shown to be completely erroneous, that the directions in which I am moving may prove to be blind alleys; but in spite of this openness of *mind*, I believe, at the *feeling* level, in myself and in what I am doing.

Selected Writings

The Clinical Treatment of the Problem Child. Boston: Houghton Mifflin, 1939.

Counseling and Psychotherapy. Boston: Houghton Mifflin, 1942.

"Significant Aspects of Client-Centered Therapy." *American Psychologist*, 1946, *1*, 415–422.

Client-Centered Therapy: Its Current Practice, Implications, and Theory. Boston: Houghton Mifflin, 1951.

With ROSALIND F. DYMOND (eds.) *Psychotherapy and Personality Change*. Chicago: University of Chicago Press, 1954.

On Becoming a Person. Boston: Houghton Mifflin, 1961.

Freedom to Learn. Columbus, Ohio: Merrill, 1969.

Carl Rogers on Encounter Groups. New York: Harper and Row, 1970.

How I Found My Way
to Psychiatry

O. Spurgeon English

This assignment is begun with feelings of both trepidation and pleasure. The former is due to the well-known fact that excessive self-
revelation in print exposes one to the varied ambivalent feelings of the
world at large. The pleasure, however, is derived from my belief that
a book such as this is long overdue. Its existence has been much needed
for the stimulation of thought and self-evaluation of the many people
involved in the field of psychotherapy. Consequently there is a sort of
pleasure in joining the ranks of the distinguished colleagues represented in this volume.

Growing Up

I was born September 27, 1901, in one of the northernmost
small towns of the United States, Presque Isle, a town of about 4,500

people. It lies in the rich farming land of Aroostook County in northern Maine. Climatewise, it had a long cold winter, with low temperatures and abundant snow, while the summers were about four months long with a mixture of warmth and rain to make it the valuable agricultural area it has always been. I have been told that I was born in the farmhouse where I grew up and the house still stands in good repair. I was attended by a family physician and a practical nurse, both of whom I for some reason heartily disliked as long as they lived. Part of the reason for this, I think, is that they were like my mother: humorless, overserious people who would periodically put their heads together about my health and activities and generally came up with some bad-tasting medicine or some curtailment of activity, which served to make my life more miserable than healthy, or so I thought.

My mother was one of nine children of Scots ancestry, the daughter of a pioneer farmer in the province of New Brunswick, Canada. In addition to being humorless and overserious she was also overreligious, pessimistic, tended to fear the outside world, never enjoyed being the wife of a farmer, and was distrustful of the morality and good intentions of everyone in the surrounding town and country. My father, on the other hand, came of Irish ancestry. He was unusually endowed with confidence, optimism, overt humor, and courage, did not tend to be distrustful of his fellowman, and was forward looking and successful. In addition to these qualities he played a large role in the activities of the town and gave himself generously to its institutions and welfare.

I was the second child of five children, having an older brother who took first place with my father. However, I had the privilege of working side by side with my father and brother for all the years of my school and college life and even few summers at home during my medical school training. My contacts with these two men, and any other farmhands or contemporaries in the work area, contributed greatly to enabling me to understand and get along with men in all walks of life. Being the second son and four years younger, I was thrown more into the company of my neurotic mother than my older brother. However, through his example, and through the behavior of my father, I was able to avoid a too heavy involvement with her personality, and since I was fortunate enough to obtain a college education and went into medicine and psychiatry, I think I succeeded in keeping myself sufficiently uninvolved with her constricting points of view to possess a few emotionally healthy attributes by the time I reached the age of twenty-one.

I have nothing to say about my infancy and there is little to report about my childhood that seems significant to me now. I have been told that around the age of two or three years I was prone to severe nightmares from which it was impossible for my mother to wake me. However, I was told that my father would hold my hands and talk to me until I would finally awaken and come back to reality. During these nightmares I seemed to be falling off the world into outer space. This sensation was accompanied by terrifying emotions, and at the same time I had the unpleasant taste in my mouth of eating the pasteboard used in the manufacture of shoeboxes. This particular type of nightmare remains very vivid to me to this day, more than sixty-five years later. A nightmare of such insecurity will tell the reader considerable about the effects of my mother's personality, as I have described it, and my early emotional anchoring to security.

There was little about my grade school life that stands out as being significant either in terms of trauma or in peak experiences of the type described by Maslow. The farm on which I grew up was located four-and-a-half miles from town. I attended a one-room country schoolhouse in which all nine grades were taught very effectively by doughty young teachers from southern Maine. We had a different one each year, and on at least one occasion she was invited into the homes of the children she taught. This was custom, along with inviting the minister of the Methodist Church to a family meal which we called supper rather than dinner.

Following my grade school career, I spent a summer being ill with cough and fever which at that time was not diagnosed as pulmonary tuberculosis. However, I recovered sufficiently to be able to go through four years of high school uneventfully. As a so-called country boy, I was required to drive a horse and buggy or a horse and sleigh four and a half miles to the high school. Moreover, I was required to come home after school and help with care of the animals and other duties and hence did not participate in sports or other activities of the high school. I deplored this but could do nothing about it, for it was the accepted custom for children of all farm families to do the same.

Medical School

Even after finishing high school I was uncertain I would be allowed or financially supported to go on to college. However, a few days before college was due to open, my father asked me if I really wanted to go. I responded with alacrity, and after a hurried dispatch of my credentials I was accepted at the University of Maine where I did two years of premedical work. I was taken into a fraternity and my life there was not uncongenial. However, like the rest of my life to date, it was relatively uneventful. I did not catch the attention of any of my teachers and went to classes unobtrusively. Neither did I distinguish myself in campus activities except to try out for assistant track manager and to play in the band. The only noteworthy event in my two years at Maine occurred at the end of my freshman year when I had a second attack of cough and fever and those uncanny chills at four in the afternoon which accompany tubercular infection. I felt I knew what was going on, but again no doctor diagnosed the condition. After returning home for a little rest and another summer working on the farm I was able to complete my second year at the university.

I then applied to three different medical schools and was accepted at Jefferson Medical College in Philadelphia. I felt that my life at the University of Maine socially and academically was not particularly profitable, and I was in a state of mind to pursue medical studies and get my medical training behind me. So I came to Philadelphia in the fall of 1920 and with minor vicissitudes obtained my degree in 1924.

In those four years of plodding away at medical studies I made the usual number of friends, both male and female. One special event in my freshman year was my meeting a student who understood music and offered to teach me to play a musical instrument. I succeeded well enough to become a member of a dance orchestra and played in it for several years. From my beginnings with him I was able to extrapolate upon his training to utilize music as a hobby the rest of my life. This knowledge of music has added greatly to my enjoyment of life and enabled me to make many friends I otherwise would not have made and given me considerable internal enjoyment I could have found no other way.

The first real tragedy struck just on the day of my graduation from Jefferson. I suffered a pulmonary hemorrhage which revealed unmistakably that I was the victim of a third attack of pulmonary tuberculosis. In spite of my understanding of the seriousness of the disease, I was foolhardy enough to enter Jefferson Medical College Hospital as an intern and attempt to overcome this attack, as I had done twice before, in spite of the additional evidence of a tuberculous infection with tissue destruction in my lungs. Naturally, I could not succeed, and in thirty days I was shipped off to Whitehaven Sanatarium in the Pocono Mountains where I remained for fifteen months. During this time I encountered my first depression and my first over-preoccupation with my self, my health, and my future. It all looked pretty dismal from that mountaintop. The evidence of tuberculosis did not resolve very rapidly, and finally my physician said, "Well, English, we don't know which way it's going to go, but apparently you're not making any progress here. It looks as if you'd better go back to your internship and see what you can do. Possibly time and activity and the return to normal life will have a beneficial effect on you and you will emerge healthy."

And this is what I did, although he had not given me high encouragement for a healthy future. All the same, I finished my internship at Jefferson Medical College Hospital in two years, albeit with many misgivings at times about whether I was keeping the tuberculosis infection under control. I also wondered what course my career would take. I had thought of going into general practice in my home territory and also of a career in surgery. However, with my illness I felt I should enter some specialty in which I could control my working hours. Out of the possibilities of dermatology, radiology, and psychiatry, I chose psychiatry and went immediately to the Boston Psychopathic Hospital in July 1927.

Introduction to Psychiatry

There I began to take histories on patients about whose illness I knew nothing, having had during the years 1920 to 1924 only minimal instruction in the field of mental illness. This first year of taking histories and writing them up and listening to discussions of cases left me uncertain about continuing a career in psychiatry. There were some discussions of the psychopathology of mental illness as understood at the time, but more emphasis was put on the disposal of patients than on helping them gain a better and more effective adjustment to their environment. As for types of treatment, we had the malarial treatment of central nervous system syphilis. Carbon dioxide therapy was being applied to neurosis and to psychosis. Soma sodium amatol injection was being tried with catatonic schizophrenia. It was dramatic to see the mute patient liven up and begin to talk, but he soon lapsed back again after the effect of the drug wore off, and nothing over the years has seemed to come from this particular treatment modality. There was to follow insulin shock therapy and metrazol-induced convulsions for depressed patients. These were followed by electro-convulsive therapy, and insulin as well as electro-convulsive therapy ran a vogue for fifteen or more years only to be discontinued except for an occasional case of depression or involutional melancholia.

While I could not see a great value in the application of the dynamic psychologies of Freud, Jung, Adler, or others with their more systematized approach in understanding mental disorders, I was even less impressed with drug and shock therapy. After spending a year in neurology at Montefiore Hospital in New York City, where I studied the extrapyramidal system in the laboratory and gained some expertise in the diagnosis of clinical neurological conditions, I returned to Boston Psychopathic Hospital to continue my preparation for a career in psychiatry exclusively.

In 1928 several Commonwealth Foundation Fellowships were made available by the Harkness family foundation, and I applied for and was given one of these by Dr. C. MacFie Campbell, who was then professor of psychiatry at Harvard and director of the Boston Psychopathic Hospital. This hospital belonged to the state system of Massachusetts and was the admitting hospital for the Boston metropolitan area and the teaching hospital in psychiatry for Harvard University Medical School. Ward rounds were held each day from tenthirty to twelve, and Dr. Campbell and Dr. Karl Bowman alternated in holding these staff conferences on the male and female service. Then, from twelve until one o'clock there was a general staff conference. Here we obtained such knowledge as we could of the dynamics of the cases admitted as well as any suggestions for their treatment. Direct continuous supervision of psychotherapy was to come a few years later after having undergone psychoanalysis and following the program for membership in a society of Freudian psychoanalysts.

I have always regarded my years of training in psychiatry as most congenial, both at Boston Psychopathic and Montefiore. Dr. Campbell was an able teacher, interested in the welfare of his students and residents. His approach was eclectic; he was always willing to apply any system of thought which would help understand a sick or troubled person. Several Commonwealth Fellows were under his guidance at the time and Dr. Campbell allowed each one to decide his own course and how he wished to spend the time. Dr. Campbell did not push us into any field uncongenial to us because he thought it was better for our development to make our own choices. My long-standing friend and apartment mate, Dr. Jackson M. Thomas, who went to Europe with me on the same boat, stayed in Hamburg to study neurology under Jakob while I went on to Vienna to undertake psychoanalysis. Dr. Campbell's approval of what we wished to take never seemed to show any bias, and he trusted us and watched and waited for results. In spite of the different uses of our time in Europe, Dr. Thomas went on to become professor of psychiatry at Tufts Medical School and I to become professor of psychiatry at Temple University Medical School in Philadelphia.

Dr. Campbell's house was open every Sunday afternoon for any students who wished to visit with him and his family or with any visiting celebrities who might be in the city. I recall being able, while on this Fellowship, to attend a conference at Yale University at which Pavlov lectured through an interpreter. Many luminaries came to the Boston Psychopathic Hospital and Dr. Campbell always invited them to make a long or short presentation as they chose. He sought the residents' opinions on cases in addition to those of the older staff members and encouraged each one of us to take a single case of our own and follow it throughout the year's residency. I still recall the name and the symptomatology of the case I treated as well as when I was working with her. I did little to alter the course of her schizophrenic thinking and behavior, but I learned a lot about the tenacity of the condition from her.

Psychoanalytic Training

The Commonwealth Fellowship ran for three years and provided for a year of study in England or Europe. Even though I was not partial to Freudian psychology, it presented the only systematized approach to the understanding and therapy of cases. So I obtained Dr. Campbell's permission to make psychoanalysis the main focus of my year of study on the Continent. In the early fall of 1929 I went directly to Vienna and began analysis with Dr. Wilhelm Reich. There happened to be a congress on sexual science going on in Vienna at the time I arrived. I looked up Dr. M. Ralph Kaufman, whom I had known at the Boston Psychopathic Hospital, and who had preceded me in his undertaking of an analysis. Dr. Kaufman introduced me to various analysts at this meeting on sexual science. I saw nothing to draw me to one psychoanalyst more than another, and since Dr. Kaufman was finishing his analysis at that very time and returning to America, I arranged to take the hour he left vacant with Dr. Reich. My analysis began with six sessions weekly and later was increased to seven times a week. When Dr. Reich suggested this number, I thought it rather much, but he pointed out logically that one hour was as valuable as another, and since I was in Europe to be analyzed and had little enough money to do it, then the more frequently I worked at it the sooner I would be finished. Moreover, since he was willing to work on Sundays and turn the time over to me, I was the beneficiary of the arrangement. During my time in Europe I spent the mornings in some psychiatric outpatient clinic, then went for my hour with my analyst, and spent the rest of the day reading and visiting points of interest in whatever city I was at the time.

After two months in Vienna, Dr. Reich told me he was moving to Berlin. This change mattered little to me, so I accompanied him and simply went on with my analysis and hospital work there. Berlin was as interesting as Vienna and with a little more steam heat—no small item to one who had found the transfer from a steam-heated apartment in Boston to a fourth-floor walk-up without bath quite a change. The chief value of the hospital work was to improve my facility with the German language, of which I knew nothing upon my arrival in Europe. I have always appreciated these years in Europe—in effect a three-year sabbatical during my residency—especially because I was unmarried and could spend my time freely.

Concerning my analysis with Reich, I will recount three incidents of some emotional and developmental import. The first one, which occurred after I had been in analysis about three or four

months, was my first experience of being able to express myself angrily
at him. It centered around a call he made to me one afternoon to ask
me to change my appointment for the following day. I did not wish
to change the appointment, but for no other reason than that I had a
social invitation. Social occasions were important to me, and so in my
next session I reproached him with high emotion about his asking me
if I thought the social occasion was more important than my analysis
with him. I said with some heat that he had made the appointment
and he was changing it, and I did not think he had the right to alter
my plans in such a capricious manner. I said I thought my plans were
as important as his, whatever they were. I talked on for some minutes,
actually being rather afraid to stop and hear what he had to say.
After I had expressed my tirade fully he merely said three words,
"You're perfectly right." My surprise knew no bounds, as I had never
been allowed to express myself this way at home or in any other
situation with anyone in authority. So I had found a new freedom
which seemed hardly believable at the time.

The second matter was important in developing empathy with
people who suffer considerable emotional stress in psychotherapy. I
can remember walking the streets of Berlin to my analytic hour and
feeling sad and discouraged and wondering why in the world I was
pursuing this daily exercise when, as I recalled it, I had felt perfectly
well before going to Europe and undertaking analysis. The cause, of
course, was the force of unhappy memories of my earlier life which
were being opened up and which were crowding in on my consciousness of self. One evening my condition was so severe that I called some
friends and told them I would not be able to meet with them because
my mood made me unfit company for anyone. They seemed to understand, and I recall only this one occasion when I was sufficiently
emotionally distressed to avoid the company of other people. But having experienced this, I have often reassured faltering patients that they
usually need to feel bad before they can feel better.

The third memory is one of unusual significance regarding the
phenomenon of resistance. I was attending lectures and seminars at
the Institute for Psychoanalysis in Berlin and I used to bring material
from there into my analysis and speak about it facetiously and even
ironically or sarcastically as being the greatest nonsense. After listening
to this for a time, Reich told me he thought I was using the courses

for resistance and advised me to discontinue them. I did so, albeit with some chagrin. I felt like a chastened schoolboy, but having been brought up as an obedient New Englander I did as he suggested. While I had scoffed at the courses and their content, I nevertheless did not want to be pulled out of the ranks of my colleagues at the time.

However, my nonattendance at the courses did not seem to be enough, and I continued to ridicule the theory I was hearing around Berlin until Dr. Reich finally said one day, "Dr. English, I have found these theories and formulations of Freudian psychoanalysis to be of value in helping people. After all this time, if you do not think they are going to be of any value to you, and if you think they do not apply to you personally, then I think you'd better stop psychoanalysis and return to America. After all, you can still practice psychiatry without analysis, and if you don't wish to apply it to yourself you shouldn't waste your time and money any longer." This confrontation shook me and brought me to my senses. I had been brought up never to terminate an undertaking until it was finished. I had been willing to discontinue the courses, but I was not willing to terminate analysis and return to the United States a voluntary dropout. So this confrontation caused me to buckle down immediately and Reich had no more trouble with my resistance to psychoanalysis by way of scoffing and ridicule. I went on with analysis and made a more sincere attempt to see its validity. Eventually I was able to see its value in relation to myself as well as others. This incident says something about Reich as well as about myself. There was certainly an integrity within him which I have always been very grateful to have found.

Marriage

During my sojourn in Berlin I met the girl who was eventually to become my wife. Decisions concerning marriage are usually discouraged during analysis, but I had known my wife-to-be well over a year by the time I made my decision to ask her to marry me. I felt I had found an attractive and intelligent and versatile person with whom I was sure for the first time I could live an interesting and harmonious existence and with whom I was glad eventually to undertake parenthood. Reich made no objections to my decision to become engaged in November 1932, and I married the following February in Berlin. I got off the couch for the last hour of analysis at ten o'clock and was married at noon in the presence of Ellen's parents and four friends of long standing. A positive mutual judgment about each other proved correct for we are still together after thirty-eight years and have had an agreeable and richly rewarding time of it most of the way. It would be fatuous to state (and no reader would believe me) if I said that we never had disagreed or gone through periods of either one-sided or mutual disapproval. But these were of short duration; our differences were always resolved, and we never found each other so impossible we had to spend any time apart in what is termed a separation. We became the parents of three sons and a daughter. We had the tragic experience of losing our second son who was killed instantly one Saturday night while on a bicycle on his way to a movie with a friend. He was thirteen years old, my namesake, and a lively, witty, winning boy with many friends and with a sensitive musical talent. I had already been exposed to death, having lost a sister when quite young as well as a brother when I was an intern at Jefferson Medical College Hospital. I had also lost my parents, but they had reached the middle seventies by the time they died. Our grief over the loss of this boy even though we had three other children left is not possible to describe. Only those who have lost an enjoyable and promising young child can possibly empathize with such an experience. Despite every effort to integrate that loss, after twenty years I still can rarely speak of him for more than a few minutes without tears. I was able to turn the loss to some useful ends in that I have been able to speak sympathetically and realistically with bereaved parents and those who have had to cope with death in any form. And ever since that date I have had a keener sense of the value of every human being, and especially every young person in this world.

Learning from Colleagues

I have learned from a few colleagues some positive things regarding psychotherapy, and from others I merely learned that most of them knew no more or even less than I did. This latter was not entirely negative as it gave me the moral support to push ahead and try out some of my own conceptions, and to take the risk of what the result might be. I will mention a couple of the outstanding colleagues from whom I learned a great deal, but before doing so I would like to say that I seemed to be attracted early to attempt psychotherapy with psychotic patients. I usually knew they were psychotic, but I must admit that sometimes in my zeal to help them, or through overconfidence in my power as a therapist, I moved ahead undeterred by any diagnostic label. Had I applied labels to these cases, I would have been reminded of certain admonitions I had heard over the years about getting in over my head in psychopathology. So for a period of about five years I had at least two patients whose inner needs had me all too frequently on the telephone day and night, who would make unexpected visits to my home, who would insist on seeing me at odd hours, and who would throw things or assault me in the office. They would bring in knives to stab me, matches to burn my drapes, and would sometimes simply kick me for not paying enough attention or start hitting me because they thought I was directly involved in their delusional system. Finally it became too strenuous and harassing to treat these people on an ambulatory basis, and so I stopped taking such sick people without having the necessary support of a hospital environment for their all too frequently ruptured ego control. I stopped treating this impulse-ridden type of patient around 1942, but fortunately was able to take it up again in 1955 when Dr. John Rosen joined my staff at Temple University Medical Sciences Center and together we were able to obtain funds for a ten-year study of the psychotherapeutic treatment of psychosis.

In my first years of attempting therapy of psychosis on an ambulatory basis, I fortunately escaped having a suicide or a tragedy of any kind. However, I did carry a heavier load of concern over their welfare and did more things to keep them stabilized than I would ever undertake again even were I a younger man. I now think I was caught up in the belief (megalomanic, I admit) that a concerned adult, armed with the knowledge of the unconscious, could, if he persevered, eventually obtain therapeutic cooperation from anyone, no matter how ill. I do not hold this belief today. But I don't mind confessing the temerity of my younger years. That's the way I was and I wouldn't have missed it even if some of my readers deem it to have been crazy. I never have been an overadmirer of caution. As a child, I used to fret under my parents' cautions of various sorts. I recall that when I was twelve years old I was driving the family car. At that time there were about six automobiles in the whole area and licensing laws were only beginning to be discussed, much less applied. I said to my father, "Why do I have to be sixteen to drive? I can drive as well as anyone right now." He said, "But don't you think a sixteen-year-old boy might have better judgment than you?" I promptly replied, "No, most certainly not!"

Around 1945, a correspondence started between me and a female psychotherapist on the West Coast over a statement I had made in the preface of a book I coauthored with Dr. Edward Weiss on psychosomatic medicine. She and I eventually met when she visited Philadelphia, and thereafter our correspondence flourished for another year before we met again in her territory. In all that time I never asked her about her training. Her ideas were sufficiently interesting and her technical procedure seemed sound enough, albeit daring, that I felt no need to ask her any questions about her background or training. Finally she invited me to interview some of her cases after making me an auditor to her psychotherapeutic method. I decided to lend myself to interviewing for a period encompassing six weeks in all. I thought, after all, the proof of the pudding is in the eating.

I will save a great deal of words and space in this chapter if I merely refer the reader to a book in which the main features of her therapy are described. The book is entitled *The Primal Scream*,[1] and what Janov outlines I had learned from her twenty years earlier. She had extrapolated her approach from Freud's earliest writings on hysteria. She not only tuned in with the patient to his early memories and fantasies but pushed him further into abreacting them and sometimes into memories of an intrauterine existence or a prenatal experience, real or imagined. The treatment encourages the liveliest abreaction, of which therapists of her type are in no way afraid, and also emphasizes a continuing abreaction in each session so that the emotional charges are fully expressed and understood. The connection with an earlier incident eventually becomes disassociated so that it is no longer carried around by the patient as a troublesome burden or an inimical affect. The effort is to relieve pain, shame, and guilt as completely as possible, leaving the

[1] A. Janov, *The Primal Scream* (New York: Dell, 1970).

patient free to live and experience himself in the present and in the most positive and creative way.

Reich had always been a great advocate of the value of abreaction although he never pushed it beyond the confines of the orthodox analysis of that time. So I was open to the added importance placed upon the heavy push toward abreaction by my West Coast colleague. Each city or each area of the country seems to have its mores about the style of therapy, and since my city had been highly influenced by the detached nonparticipation of the analyst in therapy, I rarely found a patient willing to participate in any therapeutic endeavor which went beyond quiet free association or, at best, the unexciting living-room dialogue of "analytically orientated psychotherapy." Now people are reading Janov by the thousands and everyone wants to get into the act. Once they try it they do not find it as easy as they had anticipated because a human being is reluctant to step back into the heat of his earlier life needs, frustrations, and passions. All the same, Janov's case histories open people's minds once more to the importance of Freud's revelations about the importance of early life experience in determining character and neurosis. It remains to be seen whether the Janov style of therapy, or modifications of it, will prevail in the future. It is emotionally and intellectually more taxing than any other therapy I know of for both patient and therapist. But I always felt that my early knowledge of it provided me with an extra leverage when needed or when the patient showed a predilection for it.

The second colleague with whom I found it interesting to exchange ideas and to work was Dr. John N. Rosen, who joined me at Temple University Medical School in the Department of Psychiatry. We worked actively together over a ten-year period—from 1955 until 1965 when I resigned as department head. John's concepts of the meaning of psychotic thought and behavior were uncannily perceptive. His plan of treating each patient by having three young, lively, intelligent, interested, well-educated people taking care of the patient around the clock always worked well. Such an environment of normality created for the patient's benefit, and working under John's instructions, functioned far better than the traditional nurse or attendant care of the emotionally ill. Furthermore, John was strong and persistent in confronting and discouraging psychotic thinking and behavior. It used to be said by many in our field in the thirties and forties that psychotic people were sensitive and easily traumatized and should be treated with great deference and consideration. But work with them shows precisely the opposite. They develop over the years strongly held defensive patterns to which they adhere with the greatest tenacity. Hence it takes a therapist with great strength to get them to understand that there is a more rational and more successful way to think and live. John seemed never to become discouraged and never ceased to expect the patient to modify his trend of thought and behavior in favor of more conventional living. His awareness of the meaning of symbolic behavior and speech in psychotic patients was both versatile and unlimited, and his skills in therapeutic dialogue were unique, unpredictable in any given session, and exciting to witness. After working with him for ten years, I can still enjoy and learn from him. A more detailed discussion of his theories and methods can be found in *Direct Analysis and Schizophrenia.*[2]

Mature Reflections

I can't bring myself to feel there was anything unique in my family life, early education, college life, or medical school that had much to do with my self-actualization as a psychotherapist. I would say my life until age twenty-two was uneventful, even pedestrian. As an intern, that final bout with pulmonary tuberculosis increased my concern about myself because my adult life was just beginning and I had just begun to think that I had been educated to the point of some usefulness to society; if I did not recover all my preparation would have been wasted. But still my concern was more in the nature of plain worry than any truly valuable reflection or philosophical conclusions. The events which were to shape me as a human instrument for healing began with my personal psychoanalysis in 1929. Although I found Reich by chance, I have always been very glad I did find him, as I am as sure as I can be of anything that I would have had a less dynamic and less effective analysis for *me,* my particular personality, had I been in analysis with anyone else of that period (and I eventually came to know most of the outstanding analysts pretty well). I

[2] O. S. English, W. W. Hampe, Jr., C. L. Bacon, and C. F. Bettlage (New York: Grune and Stratton, 1961).

heard them from the platform, I heard them in private, took courses under many, and had supervision by at least five of them. Of course, this opinion may be the unresolved or misconceived transference reaction we are all said to be victims of. Or the reader may ask, "How do you know, since you didn't have a firsthand analytic experience with others?" Of course I don't know. I hold this opinion probably because some of the bold, daring, tenacious, and far out conceptions which eventually branded Reich as insane must have been felt by me, had their influence upon me, prior to February 1933, which was the last time I saw him.

The second most important developmental event would be my congenial married life with Ellen, and the four children we enjoyed living with and rearing to a useful and enjoyable place in the world. The third would be the opportunity given me to develop and lead a department of psychiatry at Temple University Medical School under an unusual man and good friend, Dean William N. Parkinson, as well as my associates there in other fields. Noteworthy among these was Dr. Edward Weiss, with whom I collaborated in psychosomatic medicine. Fourth would be the patients I treated in large numbers from 1933 until the present. As department head I never drew a regular salary because I began under the old custom of clinical professors earning their own income and this was still the case when I left in 1965. I have carried on a private practice of from six to ten patients daily for more than thirty-eight years, not to mention those seen in ward rounds or teaching exercises.

In speaking of positive developmental forces I feel constrained to comment on one or two phenomena which I have always felt did not prove of value. For instance, I cannot recall that I learned anything whatever from psychoanalytic supervision. I went to my mentors and covered the material as well as I could. But no one of them ever said anything or commented on the work reported in a way that has remained with me or served to make me any more useful or wise as a therapist. This may be doing them an injustice, but I have often wondered why such great names in the field seem to mean so little in my training when I can still recall the helpful impact of many an unpretentious clinic patient.

Neither do I recall that meetings on a national or local scale have contributed much to any knowledge or wisdom required by a therapist, although I have enjoyed and profited from their social value and from knowing a competent or genial colleague in some other city to whom I could refer a case if necessary. One notable exception was the Group for the Advancement of Psychiatry. This group of outstanding colleagues was made up of an amalgamation of committees who met twice yearly to give serious consideration to various separate areas in which information or correlation of data was inadequate. The organization is still very much alive and functioning, but the membership slowly rotates. I was one of their number for about twenty years, and a member of various committees in turn, and profited by my work and associations with each committee and every meeting. The liveliest and most profitable meeting on clinical problems exclusively has been for me the American Academy of Psychotherapy.

Growth Through Patient Therapy

While this subject appears late in the chapter, it is by no means least important. Patients have been and still are all-important, for without them I would go unchallenged and stale. And without them I would not, of course, be a psychotherapist at all except in name. I wouldn't know what a retired psychotherapist did with his time or himself. If I meet one, I'll ask him.

I have naturally had all kinds of feeling toward patients, just as toward other people. The difference was that the patient asked for a certain kind of help and, being a professional, I assumed more responsibility for them than for others.

Before proceeding further with this aspect of my self-actualization, I must report some subjective feelings. The first came when I was beginning to recount the experiences of the first half of my life up to and including my personal analysis, up to age thirty-two. Doing so resulted in a couple of days' depression. This occurrence is so unusual for me that I could only conclude that going back over the material had reactivated my emotions in a way similar to analysis. The second thing is that to reveal my feelings about patients over the years has aroused considerable conflict and ambivalence. I have not found that self-revelation is looked upon favorably or treated kindly by either colleagues or patients. The former believe I am naive and showing poor judgment and also regard me as a traitor to the profession, the main body of whom seem to like to maintain an image of human perfection and imperturbability. The patients have actually been kinder than colleagues in this matter. Whenever I was revealing of self to them, they seemed to be disappointed momentarily, then expressed a kind of relieved "You, too," and finally seemed to forget it and work better as a result, in the end appreciating my honesty and admission of human frailty.

So I will be as truthful and factual and honest in my responses as I am capable of being. How much I can fill this requirement will have been aided by the fact that I have followed this design for living for well over thirty years and have never been treated too badly by people. I have been reproached and criticized for stands I have taken but never to a degree which made me consider defection. I have *never* had any impulse to defect from the field of psychotherapy. My only occasional distaste for the work centers around the question, "How does one counter the routinization and arrogant feedback of successful healing?" My answer would be "Diagnose carefully and don't burden yourself with too many narcissistic, arrogant, domineering, controlling patients at the same time. Stagger them with a few nice people, because there are some nice people seeking help with neurotic conflicts who will reward one richly with their friendship and appreciation if we do, as well as paying us. And there are some upon whom you can knock yourself out for ten years and who will still tell you that you have failed them, exploited them, given them little or nothing for their time and money, or they may even say they are worse than before they began therapy.

There have been patients I liked to see and treat and some I dreaded to see, some who amused me, some who bored me to distraction. Some could put me to sleep, and I use the word *put* rather than say I went to sleep on them. Because I would find myself thinking, "How sleepy I am. When this patient leaves I'll take a nap for sure." But when he departed the office I couldn't go to sleep for the life of me. Just how their presence worked on me as a soporific I haven't yet figured out. In my earlier years of therapy I would occasionally get a patient whose hurts of early life took the form of a blistering sarcasm that put to test my ability to keep his assaults upon my pride from making me retaliate in some way. Some of the women were so attractive, charming, and seductive they put to a test my capacity for keeping

admiration at an impersonal or uninvolved level. How much I was
in love with these women patients is hard to say. I can say that I never
encountered one I would rather have for a wife than the woman I
married. I have treated several I fantasied as appearing highly desirable sexually, but the same has been true of many I have met in social
life.

In spite of all my various responses to the variety of personalities who came to me for treatment I do not recall having one I found
it necessary to transfer to a colleague because I found my response to
him inimical to his therapy. No matter how hostile, how angry, how
boring, or how seductive he or she was I felt obliged to think out my
response and bring it under workable control rather than openly or
covertly dismiss or refer the patient. I am fairly sure a certain number
of patients drifted away from me because they found my personality
uncongenial to them. But I have had a few stay for what they said was
that very reason. One woman years ago told me forthrightly she was
going to remain until she made a decent human being out of me if it
took five years. She accomplished it, I am glad to report, in three and
a half years and we continued to be friends until she died recently.
I used to thank her occasionally for her good work on me. All these
differences in temperament help to make psychotherapy interesting, if
for no other reason than the stimulating experience of being involved
with a diversity of human personalities daily. But in order to find it
interesting I must say that a sense of humor is one of the most important qualities for a psychotherapist to possess; a sense of humor, optimism, persistence, and the ability to identify with the patient as well
as to identify the nature of the patient's protest against what life is
requiring of him.

How I See Myself

I see myself as a person who functions as a therapist and a
citizen on the same plane of endeavor and expression. I have said that
I can't tell where English the person leaves off and the psychotherapist
begins, or vice versa. I don't see where English the psychotherapist
leaves off and English the neighbor or family man begins. I live on an
acre of ground with an active stream running through it, big trees, and
a changing panorama of colors in the flowering shrubbery and flower

scheme, as well as a tennis court. All my neighbors know they are welcome to visit, walk around, play tennis, take such pictures as they wish. The little boys play in the stream and on the lawn. The bigger ones use the tennis court and basketball ring. And the patients soon come to know they have the same privilege. Many use it, coming from distances of more than ten miles to do so. If I'm free to participate, I do, and if I'm not they know they are not imposing. I don't find this creates any problem in their therapeutic sessions, and I would gladly invite in any observer to disprove this or submit any random tape session for his comments.

I never counseled a patient about loyalty to parents or spouse any differently from the way I would offer comments to my children, if asked. I have one code of ethics for everyone. I lived and reared my family by the one I used in the office—or it could be said I did therapy with the values I used in living my own life. This approach is not only a much more comfortable way of doing things, it is also simpler, easier on the ego ideal or superego, and requires no special explanations at any time. It also seems to me to be more scientific (whatever that means) in psychotherapy and keeps me in more realistic touch with social action and social change. No one sector of society can be in complete tune with all others at the same time, but to try to have one's value system closely in tune with others' is a step toward the mutual empathy and social accord that every sensitive and knowledgeable person seeks.

My publications have had no remarkable original or inventive quality. They have all tried to simplify complex psychological phenomena, and to put the ideas of more original and complex thinkers than I into a more easily grasped format. How did I know this was needed? By recalling my own previous ignorance and confusion, I think. Because I felt I had emerged from a state of ignorance or confusion I merely tried to describe what pathways of thought I used to achieve this emergence. I really never had an urge to be an innovator, much less a genius, because the field of interpretation offered so many opportunities. Someone once asked me why I never wrote a book solely my own. I thought that one over and replied that my basic interests always lay in the kind of help which required more than one mind. The book on psychosomatic medicine with Dr. Edward Weiss is the outstanding example. That kind of book required a top-notch internist, which Dr. Weiss was, trained in pathology and dynamic psychology, and another physician with psychotherapeutic skills in order to impart both the theory and technique of treating psychosomatic problems. And so it was with all the others, including the assay of John Rosen's work with psychotic patients on which a child analyst, a competent analyst of many years' experience, and another analyst of more recent training collaborated in an effort to define the schizophrenic process as well as analyze Rosen's approach to its psychotherapeutic treatment.

I'm fairly well satisfied with what I am. I would like to have more "life" and more versatility in treatment styles to offer my patients and my family and friends as well. But I feel that I do as well as most, and what is more important, I am always trying to bring these two phenomena to a higher level.

My dedication to psychotherapy undergoes minimum fluctuation, according to my own estimation, as well as judged by the comments of others. When any so-called core conflict is touched, I go to work immediately to identify it and marshal all possible ego forces to overcome its presence. I sometimes become harassed by the routinization of the therapeutic educational process and the arrogant feedback (based on patient narcissism) in the daily healing process. But I remind myself that boring or frustrating as it may be, I still would not want to go back to farming, or take up plumbing, barbering, or trash-collecting—or even law or business—as all those enterprises have their frustrating aspects also.

When I feel in any way dispirited, I play one of my musical instruments, take a walk around my estate, go to a movie, meet with a respected colleague, schedule a meeting in the near future I would like to attend, or share my momentary lack of enthusiasm with my wife. While she was not trained in any ancillary field of psychiatry, she has attended meetings with me over the years, while rearing four children, and has read some of the most dynamic writers in the field; now that our children are no longer in the home she must perforce confine much of her listening and attention to me and my activities and I find her most helpful and supportive. I believe I have considerable basic trust and I thank heartily those who have helped me attain such as I possess. I don't have complete basic trust. I doubt whether this quality can exist in the world today, and furthermore the person who attempted to adopt it in his everyday activities would in due course find himself unnecessarily disillusioned and might, if he pursued it long enough, be pushed into depression or more serious psychosis. Complete basic trust is to my way of thinking a luxury only the man of the future can hope to acquire. Acquired prematurely in our civilization it could, if attainable, wreck him. An absence of basic trust in many areas is tragic, but an excess leaves the individual undefended against the most ruthless exploitation. Let's say I believe I have enough of it for my time and my life style.

If I have a personal demon, it is my need (perhaps even lust) for acknowledgement of *me*. It has and does get me into trouble of a minor nature from time to time. But I would say it is manageable. If I become too demanding, people will usually set me back in case I do not see it well enough myself. Besides, it is not too hard for me to apologize, back up, and start over again on another tack. I would say that demon has more often operated to my advantage than against me.

Challenging Most Patients

Earlier in my career psychotic patients challenged me most. Not any more. I have not repudiated them as too difficult or trying, but I have swung more to adolescent struggles and family dissension. With these cases I feel I can do more to prevent later life stress and possible psychotic or dropout behavior. At any rate, I no longer must tackle the most serious end result of family error. Having seen and struggled with the worst that parental stupidity and arrogance can produce, I'm willing to take papa and mama on before they have done their worst, rather than afterward.

Suffering

Suffering does not attract me more than it should. My problem with it is the reverse. I find myself having to brace myself to cope with it a certain number of hours daily. And the older I get the more suffering I'd like to be spared if I could have it that way and still fulfill my professional obligations.

I have not found that people discover their identity rapidly enough to regard it as a crisis or rebirth. And I don't regard myself as a saver of psyches or persons. Some have told me I had been in their case, but while it was going on I didn't know it.

Healing Encounter

The healing encounter first requires better communication with the patient *self* than ever took place previously in the patient's life. As a result of better person-to-person communication the patient becomes more courageous (less anxious) to be himself. As he becomes more *self* he sees the world in a more real sense (more truly as it is) and can combine his expanding self with the world in a more creative way. As he expands and derives more life from interaction with his fellowman he becomes more effective because he enjoys the life experience more and he feels himself a more important entity meriting more recognition. With these forces started in motion his increased growth continues indefinitely. My part is to bring these phenomena to consciousness and encourage and support their realization.

I do not regard the phenomenology of schizophrenia to be anything unique or apart from the psychology of *every man*. It is the psychology of everyman gone out of bounds and showing itself in its extreme forms. If a beautiful, well-kept home or estate is neglected for as little as a year and is uncared for in any way, it can come to look grotesque and almost unrecognizable. It appears unattractive and possibly uninhabitable. To be useful and enjoyable again it needs much repair work. Abandon it five years and possibly no one cares to restore it any more. This is not an accurate analogy to all that goes on in schizophrenia, but it does point up the sad results of human abandonment of any organism. So I am not influenced by the label of schizophrenia whether it is applied by myself or others. I examine the foundations and consider whether the available price of reconstruction is going to bring results.

Sensitivity Groups

I do not use sensitivity groups, but I allow and support sensitivity group activity as an adjunct to my psychotherapy. I do not rely upon the Freudian model alone and have not done so ever since I first learned it. Psychotherapy is sometimes boring but need never be dangerous. As therapists we are still necessary and will be for several decades yet. No one else in our society fills our function. As society gains more self-knowledge everyone can more and more become his own psychiatrist, aided and abetted by more insightful, altruistic, and creative parents and community leaders.

Since I've reached the age of seventy and have given my philosophy on various aspects of psychotherapy and the living of life itself, I feel that a word or two of my attitude toward death might be a suitable conclusion to this chapter. Whenever I think of my life coming to an end, I am mildly saddened although not disconcerted. I realize that man is mortal and I have had my three-score years and ten; I've had my share of the joys and rewards of life. Consequently, I look upon death as a suitable termination of a life I'm satisfied with, not only with my own productions within it, but also with the way I have been treated by life itself and everyone in it. In fact any reluctance to have my life come to an end is because I have, in the main, enjoyed it so much and not because I have any apprehension about what will come thereafter. I have no strong belief in any life after this one, certainly not in the form of what I know now as myself. I believe in the ongoingness of man in general, but I have never been able to see myself living another life either in Heaven or Hell or Nirvana or any other plane of existence. Should it occur, I have no dread of my ability to cope with it, having coped with this one satisfactorily enough. And if nothing but a quiet stillness surrounds what I've been forever, that will be all right too. I have always found a good night's sleep very restful and pleasant and I could take the same oblivion for an eternity without complaint.

Selected Writings

With E. WEISS. *Psychosomatic Medicine.* Philadelphia: Saunders, 1943.
With G. H. J. PEARSON. *Emotional Problems of Living.* New York: Norton, 1945. (3rd. ed. 1963)
With C. J. FOSTER. *Fathers Are Parents, Too.* New York: Belmont Prod., 1951.

With s. m. FINCH. *Introduction to Psychiatry.* New York: Norton, 1954.
   (3rd. ed. 1964)
With w. w. HAMPE, JR., C. L. BACON, AND C. F. BETTLAGE. *Direct Analysis
   and Schizophrenia.* New York: Grune and Stratton, 1961.

IV

Psychotherapy Without Tears

Albert Ellis

I do not believe that the events of my early childhood greatly influenced my becoming a psychotherapist, nor oriented me to becoming the kind of individual and the type of therapist that I now am. That notion is the psychoanalytic bag, and fortunately I am no longer suffocating in that particular bag. Having nicely survived my own psychoanalysis, and having achieved a reasonable degree of self-realization in spite of my early devotion to the psychoanalytic *mishigas* (with which I not only afflicted myself but also, alas, helped inflict on a good many poor innocent analysands whom I treated when I first became a therapist), I now believe that children bring to their early environments (and to their benighted and entrapped parents) their own powerful innate predispositions to act in highly individualized ways. Consequently, I hypothesize, I was almost as instrumental in raising my mother (and, even to a greater degree, my younger brother and sister) as she was in rearing me. But since the editor of this volume has asked for some material on my early life, and since many readers are likely to be plain damned curious about what happened to me before I began sprinting along psychotherapeutic pathways, let me begin with some of my beginnings.

Poor Beginnings

In many ways, my early life was replete with poor circumstances. For one thing, I was always a semi-orphan. My father, a traveling salesman and a promoter at that time, was frequently away from home for weeks or months on end. When he was living with us, he was so busy with his daytime business activities and his nighttime pinochle games (or running around with attractive women, or whatever the hell else he did) that my younger brother and sister and I literally spent about five minutes a day with him (kissing him goodby in the morning, just before we scooted off to school). Saturday and Sunday were again (as far as I could tell) mainly card-playing days for him, and only occasionally did he take an hour or two drive with us, in our chauffeur-driven electric Cadillac. When he finally was divorced from my mother when I was twelve (my brother was ten, and my sister eight), he was so devoted to our welfare that he came around to visit us literally less than once a year—even though most of the time he lived only a few miles away in Manhattan, while we were being raised on the streets of the Bronx.

As for my nice Jewish mother, a hell of a lot of help she was! Born at least twenty years before her time, thrown out of school in the sixth grade for compulsive talking, and quite unequipped to deal adequately with either marriage or child-rearing, she was much more immersed in her own pleasures and her own ego-aggrandizing activities than she was in understanding and taking care of her children. Her typical day: she arose about eight forty-five (after her eight-year-old son, Albert, had already awakened himself with the alarm clock, dressed, made his own breakfast, and proceeded to walk to school after crossing three of the busiest and most dangerous streets in the Bronx). She sloppily and desultorily did a minimum of cleaning, shopping, and child-tending. She spent most afternoons at her Temple Sisterhood functions or playing bridge or Mah-Jongg with some of her woman friends. She returned home around five or six (long after her son Albert had come home from school, made himself a snack, and helped take care of his younger brother and sister). She cooked or brought from the delicatessen very simple, ill-prepared meals that required a minimum of effort to get together. And she spent most nights with her friends (most of them fifteen or more years younger than she and from a lower socioeconomic strata), quite unrelated to her children (and often out of the house, leaving them unattended, in the charge of brother Albert).

As if all this parental neglect were not enough, I had a few other problems as a child. When I was five, I almost died of tonsillitis and suffered, as a sequel, acute nephritis or nephroses (the doctors are still arguing differential diagnosis about this). During the next few years, I went back and forth to Presbyterian Hospital about eight times, once for a period of ten months. As a result of this hospitalization and my convalescence from it, I was forbidden to take active part in any of the usual childhood games for months on end. Sportswise, I developed into something of a sissy, whereas my brother was easily able to surpass me in every conceivable athletic respect. He also was a courageous, happy-go-lucky extrovert, while I was unusually shy and introverted, and particularly afraid of any kind of public presentation during my childhood and adolescence. Finally, to augment these hassles (and many more like them), my solidly middle-class family was soundly whacked by the Great Depression of 1929 (when I was seventeen), and when my mother's savings were completely wiped out and my father (who was still livingly fairly comfortably) refused to pay her a cent of the tens of thousands of dollars of back alimony he owed her, our family came within a hair of going on relief.

Saving Graces

Despite all this, I somehow refused to be miserable. I took my father's absence and my mother's neglect in stride—and even felt good about being allowed so much autonomy and independence. I ignored my physical disabilities and determined to take care of my health in a rigorous manner so that I would no longer have the frequent headaches and other pains I then had. I decided not to hate my mother for her ineptness and used it, instead, to turn her around my little finger, and even in some ways to exploit her. I allowed—in fact, almost encouraged—my brother to get into one scrape after another (while I played the nice-boy role) and my sister to whine about her sorry lot (while I a little chivalrously protected her from my brother, who could not stand her whinyness and often tried to beat her to a pulp).

I beautifully protected my shyness by refusing to participate in any public performances (even minor classroom plays) and by refraining from risking any overtures to any of the female classmates with whom I kept serially falling madly in love from the age of seven onward. Not that I did not suffer at all: I sometimes had to recite a poem in class or ascend the auditorium podium to accept an award, and at those times I sweated and sizzled with anxiety and desperately looked for (and sometimes managed to cleverly find) some way out. And I never did make it, sexually or otherwise, with any of those girls with whom I was enamored up until my early twenties, because I wouldn't even risk dating, much less pulling up the skirts of any of them.

So I suffered more by omission than commission, and for all my neurotic tendencies, I cannot say that I led anything but a pretty happy childhood. Which, come to think of it, is pretty interesting. For I am reminded that my mother, too, for all her blabber-mouthness, her feelings of inadequacy, and her inability to achieve anything significant in life and work at a level anywhere near her potential (she was always a talented actress-singer-comedienne, as well as a real beauty, and might have got somewhere high in the theatrical world had she ever really tried), was rarely really unhappy for the first eighty years of her life, in spite of troubles and traumas that would have knocked the average woman of her day into severe states of depression. My father and brother, too—each of whom has had his share of worldly troubles, and perhaps a bit more—have seldom been depressed. Only my sister, the most pampered and perhaps least put-upon of my immediate family, has suffered fairly continuously from anxiety, self-hatred, and depression. Which leads me to wonder, once again, about the genetic rather than the psychologically overemphasized environmental sources of emotional disturbance.

Anyway, my difficult childhood helped me do one important thing: become a stubborn and pronounced problem solver. If life, I said to myself, is going to be so damned rough and hassle-filled, what the devil can I do to live successfully and happily nevertheless? I soon found the answer: use my head! So I figured out how to become my nutty mother's favorite child, how to get along with both my brother and sister in spite of their continual warring with each other, and how to live fairly happily without giving up my shyness.

Does this mean that the difficulties I encountered *caused* me to become unusually rational during my childhood? Not that I can see. For my sister had her own share of problems. She was the only female child; she had almost every existent manifestation of allergy (and a host of other physical afflictions); she had closer contact with and was treated more inconsistently by my mother; she was somewhat persecuted by my brother; she was the youngest child and, although always bright, was not able to compete with her two unusually clever brothers; and she had various other handicaps. Why, then, didn't she, like me, develop more problem-solving skills?

My answer—following the longitudinal studies of Stella Chess, Alexander Thomas, and Herbert G. Birch[1]—is that she was largely born with a whiny, demanding, injustice-collecting temperament and that consequently she *chose* to make the worst of her childhood conditions. Later on, as she entered the second fifty years of her life, she worked very hard against her temperamental handicaps, chose a saner (though, significantly enough, still religiously oriented) way of living, and began to be much happier. I, fortunately, was never quite *that* crazy; and in spite of my natural predisposition toward anxiety, shyness, and inhibitedness, I also had a biological tendency toward objectively perceiving, scientifically assessing, and often energetically correcting some of my irrational behavior.

I was also innately inclined to build some consummately clever defenses. My mother busied herself so much with avocational and entertainment pursuits that she left herself little time for overt self-hatred. My brother acted out so many of his frustrations and hostilities —by refusing to do his homework, for example, and sassing most of his teachers when they got after him about it—that he became a noto-

[1] *Your Child Is a Person* (New York: Viking, 1965).

rious rebel and achieved a villainous kind of acclaim. My sister whined so much about my mother's favoring "the boys" (a favoring that was almost completely a figment of her imagination since, by her whimpering, she actually managed to get most of the favors) that some people actually took pity on her. But I did even better: I did so well in my schoolwork, in being tractable and kind with practically everyone, in mastering the art of understanding others, in developing interesting hobbies (especially voracious reading), and in various other constructive pursuits that I could genuinely like myself for my accomplishments, and I did.

In other words, I built a whale of a lot of false self-esteem. So what if I was fairly lousy at sports, in manly aggressiveness, and in asserting myself with any of the girls with whom I was madly (and completely silently!) in love? So what if my brother and most of my close friends were better than I was in these respects? Who was better at English, math, history, and ten other subjects than I? Who would all my friends and classmates come to for practical advice? Who was more favored by practically every adult around? Who better figured out (until, at the age of twelve, he became an unregenerate atheist) what God really wanted people to do to get in His good graces, and who best (albeit with a little backsliding) stuck to this kind of heavenly promulgated conduct?

In sum: the conditions of my childhood were in many ways worse than those of most of my contemporaries. But I basically liked myself for the wrong reasons: because I took these conditions as problems to be surmounted and I rather cleverly, and with a deliberately arranged-for social approval, surmounted them. I based my worth as a human being—which I now realize is quite an error—on my achievements and my popularity; but I did such a good job of using this wrong method that I had a pretty happy, productive childhord.

Back-Door Entry into Healing

When I matriculated for my M.A. (and later my Ph.D.) in clinical psychology at Teachers College, Columbia, I was quite surprised. Just about all my fellow graduate students had entered the field because of their own emotional disturbances. They had suffered from anxiety and depression for many years (not a few were practically psychotic), had gone for some kind of psychoanalysis, had decided while being analyzed that they might enjoy doing this type of work themselves, and had picked clinical psychology as the easiest of the respectable ways to get into the field. Most of them were so batty that they faltered along the road of academic discipline and never got their degrees at all. Those who did get through were hardly eligible for any prizes in the realm of emotional maturity and stability. Perhaps that fact alone should have warned me of the tragic ineffectiveness of psychoanalysis. But unfortunately it didn't.

My case was radically differnt. I had determined, when still in junior high school, to become a renowned writer—particularly, the Great American Novelist. But I was practical enough to realize that writers, at least for the first decade or two of their careers, made little money. So I decided to study accounting in high school and college, to try to make a fortune in the business world in fairly short order, and to retire in my thirties with enough money so that I could devote myself to writing anything I wanted to write without having to rely on selling any of my stuff.

That may or may not have been a great plan; but anyway, it bombed with the onset of the 1929 depression. Because of my family's financial difficulties, I was lucky to get through high school and college at all. When I finally got my bachelor of business administration degree from the City College of New York, good jobs were about as scarce as publisher's acceptances. But that didn't exactly stop me. For the next several years I worked at various unimportant occupations and continued to do what I had already diligently started in college: spending several hours almost every day at writing stories, novels, plays, poems (mostly comic), essays, and nonfiction books. A couple of my book-length manuscripts came within a hair of being published; but at the last minute negotiations broke down and none actually went to press. Nothing daunted, I continued along my writing ways. By the time I reached the age of twenty-eight, I had about twenty unpublished full-length manuscripts (three of which came to about a half-million words apiece) in my bulging files.

By this time, I decided several things. One: I was not going to be the Great American Novelist. Fiction just didn't seem to be my forte. Two: I was going to stick to nonfiction and mainly use it as a vehicle to propound some of my revolutionary views. Three: Since my socioeconomic beliefs were partly shared by a great many writers who were effectively propounding them in print (I was then a liberal-democratic radical, opposed to the Communist Party but still basically a revolutionist), I was determined to devote a good part of my life to promulgating the sex-family revolution, which most of my fellow radicals were sadly neglecting.

I kept working smoothly along these lines, especially gathering material for a massive tome entitled *The Case for Sexual Liberty* (part of which was published almost twenty years later), when something that I would have never predicted happened. Because I was doing so much research in the field of sex, love, and marriage, and spent literally hours every day devouring and writing voluminous notes on hundreds of books and articles in this large area, my friends kept coming to me for all kinds of information and advice. Now this was particularly odd, since I had been so shy and busy up to this time that I had much less actual sex experience than most of these friends. Nonetheless, they were exceptionally worried about such things as masturbation, impotence, frigidity, premarital sex relations, adultery, and a host of other sexual problems. Much to my surprise, I knew practically all the answers and could be extremely helpful to them in a short talk or two.

That discovery set me to thinking that I could do something more in the world than be a sex writer and revolutionist; I could also be a sex-love-marriage counselor. So I immediately set about investigating possibilities of training in this field, found that at that time practically none really existed, and wound up in the nearest thing to it: a program leading to a doctorate in clinical psychology.

A little later on my goals changed. Recognizing that marriage and family counseling was really a subheading of psychotherapy, and wrongly believing at that time that psychoanalysis was the deepest and most effective form of therapy, I determined to become a clinical psychologist, undertake a regular and a training analysis, and become an outstanding psychoanalyst. Which is exactly what, during the next few years, I did. There were no legitimate training institutes which accepted psychologists at that time. But I completed a full analysis with a training analyst of the Karen Horney group (who himself had been analyzed by Herman Rorschach, and whose technique was still largely the classical Freudian procedure). He volunteered to be my control analyst (though the Horney group was then and still is opposed to formally taking in any nonphysicians). Under his direction I began to do, first, classical psychoanalysis and later psychoanalytically oriented psychotherapy with my own clients.

Personally, I never would have chosen to enter analysis at this time since I was swinging along at a fine professional pace, was handling my sex-love life quite well (after one previous marriage and divorce), and thought that I was unusually happy and undisturbed. I did, however, try to take full advantage of my personal analysis and used it to help me decide whether or not to marry my utterly charming and brilliant but abysmally *meshugenah* girlfriend. My analyst and I agreed: "No"; and I worked through this four-year-old intensely passionate relationship very nicely. Some day I shall write up the annals of those years, and boy will the pages emotionally sizzle! By the time I finished with my training analysis, I was well into another intense involvement. And this was even more melodramatic than the previous one—what with my girlfriend's telling me she had left her husband when she was really still living with him; carrying on simultaneous affairs with me, another lover, a lesbian or two, and heaven knows how many one-night drunken stands with strangers; lying to me continuously about various important things; and having alternating fits of mania and depression practically every other week. But I managed to weather that set of storms, too, in fine shape. And that period as well will one day be a steaming autobiographical volume!

During my analysis, moreover, I finally overcame my time neurosis. I had been something of a compulsive worker, who believed strongly that I *had* to get innumerable things done or I was wasting my time on earth. My ego, or self-evaluation, depended on my outstanding accomplishment; and to feed it I had to compulsively accomplish. This, as noted above, worked out to some degree; but, naturally, I was perpetually rushing, looking at the clock, and feeling overtly or covertly anxious about the great mass of things which were not yet done. While I was being analyzed, I finally realized that life indeed was short; that I was not going to accomplish many of the things I wanted to do before I died; and that that was too damned bad—but that's all it was, too damned bad. I began to accept my own limitations and that of humans in general; and although I still wanted very much to accomplish many things before I died, I essentially stopped needing to do so. What my analysis had to do with this drastic change in my outlook I am not sure. Perhaps much; perhaps nothing. But it did occur in the course of my personal analysis, and it may have resulted partly from my talks with my analyst, who was a wise and experienced man and who interspersed his Freudian-Horneyian interpretations with a good deal of existential philosophy and some hard-headed common sense.

How I Became and Unbecame a Psychoanalyst

As for my early psychoanalytic practice, which I started as the 1940s came to an end, I found that a real ball. I always enjoyed what I call "detectiving" and had for years practiced it with my women friends and my other intimate acquaintances. Psychological testing I found something of a bore (though interpreting Rorschachs and other projective techniques was pretty interesting). But uncovering a great mass of information about an analysand, putting this beautifully together and fitting it into analytic theory, and then making clever inductions and deductions about it—that was really the life! I enjoyed it so much, at first, that I considered myself very lucky to be paid for this kind of mental jigsaw-puzzling, and I was utterly delighted to have chosen this kind of a profession.

I must also say that I was damned good at psychoanalysis. My clients acquired all kinds of positive transferences toward me; they usually were able to see and agree with the interpretations I made about the connections between early experiences and contemporary complaints; and they seemed to improve as well as, or perhaps somewhat better than, the usual 60 per cent of continuing analysands who are significantly helped by treatment. Unfortunately, however, they tended to feel rather than to get much better, and their original symptoms or their tendency to create new symptoms largely remained. Moreover, when I was forced, largely because of their monetary difficulties, to see them only once a week or once every other week (instead of from two to five times a week as classical analysis requires), and when I consequently resorted more and more to psychoanalytically oriented psychotherapy instead of to orthodox analysis itself, I was shocked to find that most of my clients did as well or better with this "superficial" procedure than they did with "deep" analysis. This discovery was one of the first things that made me skeptical of the hypothesis that psychoanalysis is the deepest and best form of therapy extant and that other techniques are relatively shallow and palliative.

Even worse jolts followed. Because I had been doing marriage and family counseling for several years before I started doing analysis, and because the direct methods I employed in this counseling at times seemed appropriate with my analysands, I from time to time began interspersing these methods with my more passive analytic procedures —even though the classical texts in the field insisted that this was definitely not the thing to do and that it was only sidetracking the client away from his deep unconscious feelings and attitudes. But I had to honestly admit to myself, after awhile, that the more active, the more quickly and directly interpretive, and the more advice-giving I was as an analyst, the quicker and more completely my clients tended to get better. That discovery really made me stop and think!

Another important thing gradually happened, especially with my more disturbed and recalcitrant clients: I began to use myself, my own experiences and ideas, as part of the therapeutic process. For I saw that many of the things that bothered my clients were also part of my own repertoire of nuttiness. Since I had personally conquered some of them myself, I thought I could help considerably by explaining how I had used these processes and what they could do in this respect.

Take, especially, the matter of my early shyness. By the time I went into analysis, I had worked through this problem almost completely and hardly even discussed it during the years I was on my analyst's sofa. How had I worked it through? Mainly by reading and practicing philosophy—notably that of Epictetus, Marcus Aurelius, Spinoza, and Bertrand Russell. Thus, being terribly afraid of making contact with new girls until I was in my early twenties, and maneuvering my male friends into making the initial contacts (and then, once the overtures were made, often taking over and talking like a blue streak), I realized that I was maintaining and even exacerbating my anxieties by that kind of evasive behavior.

I therefore laboriously taught myself, first, to challenge my anxiety-creating philosophies—namely, my beliefs that it would be awful if I got rejected, that I absolutely must not fail in making sexual-social overtures, and that if I did fail I was indubitably a lousy person who was therefore doomed to fail forever in this kind of somewhat risky pursuit. I kept fighting these internalized and long-held beliefs until I truly started to believe that no matter how many times I might fail or how foolish I might look to others while failing, I was still only a person who failed rather than a Failure with a capital F.

That was, theoretcially, all well and good. But what really cured me of my shyness in this respect was thinking plus action. For before I could get rid of my fear of being rejected in making overtures to girls, I had to force myself, scores of times, to approach strange females, to make friendly overtures to them, to get rejected on many occasions, and to convince myself that the world did not come to an end, that I was not a shit, and that it merely was too damned bad that I wasn't getting accepted as I would like to be. After enough of this deliberate practice at risk-taking, I got to be one of the most accomplished woman-chasers and overture-makers in the Bronx Botanical Gardens (one of my main hangouts during my younger days) and (later) the world at large.

So the more I saw that psychoanalysis was *not* working very well, and the more I shared with my clients some of my own risk-taking practices that had worked to get me over my fears of failures and my self-downing hangups, the more I found that this kind of teaching did far more therapeutic good than did the analytic interpretations. Thus was the core of what later became rational-emotive (or active-directive, cognitive-behavior) therapy born. I gradually gave up almost entirely on psychoanalysis (and, in fact, became highly anti-analytic). I have always loathed inefficiency—whether it be personal, political, economic, or social. And my being devoted to revolution, in the first place, and to psychotherapy, in the second, stems largely from my strong desire to help myself and others achieve individual and social effective living.

Becoming a More Mature Healer

I have been a professional healer for almost thirty years. How do I now feel about that and about me? Exceptionally well, I must say. For my therapy has helped me as well as many others, and one of the best empirical proofs of its workability has been the changes that it has wrought, over the years, in my own thinking and behaving. Moreover, these changes have occurred as much or more in the course of my working with others as they have during my deliberate attempts to use therapeutic procedures on myself—which is an interesting phenomenon that I accidentally found, during the first few years of rational-emotive therapy, and that I have used to good account, especially in my group therapy activities.

Let me give a specific example. As noted above, I began life with distinct problems of shyness, inhibition, and constriction in emotional expression. I deliberately worked on these years before I was a therapist, and actually a decade before I was psychoanalyzed, and I became much less withdrawn. But vestiges of the old coarctation remained, and, if anything, some sentiment crawled back under my skin as I practiced, passively and controlledly, along psychoanalytic pathways.

Things got a little better when I began being more actively psychoanalytically oriented rather than classically analytic. For I was then more alive and outgoing in my procedures. But when I became rational-emotive, my own personality processes really began to vibrate. For one thing, I became far more honestly confronting and risked telling my clients things like, "You say that you really don't give a shit what your friends think when you act unconventionally. But you also say that whenever you go to a party with them you slug down a half pint of whiskey within the first half hour you are there. What kind of a nonshit do you think you are when you are doing that?" And I learned, while I was doing this increasing confrontation, that it wasn't horrible for my clients to fight me, to hate me, and even to quit seeing me when I was telling it like it was (or at least as it seemed to me to be, for of course I was not always correct about these confrontational interpretations and sometimes made the most asinine errors).

I also gradually began to lose most of my natural irritability. My father, as I noted at the beginning, was rarely around when I was a child and had about as much to do with rearing me as my other relatives (most of whom lived in Philadelphia and whom we saw, maybe, once every year or two for a few hours at a time). My mother, on the other hand, was almost my sole mentor, until I began to teach myself to read at the age of five. But where my mother was rather compliant and ass-licking (more to her peers than her own children) my father was easily irritated, dogmatic, authoritarian, and angry. I was afflicted, in some ways, with the worst of both their traits—I was ingratiating (most of the time) and underlyingly impatient and irritable (to a lesser degree, but quite often).

When I first developed rational-emotive therapy (RET, for short), I squelched a good many of my negative feelings toward my clients; but inwardly I often felt impatient at their latenesses and other irresponsible behavior toward me, impatient that they did not quickly see and use the marvelous self-accepting philosophies I was vigorously trying to help them acquire, upset about some of the cruel ways in which they continued to treat others, and angry at their reversion to psychoanalytic, Rogerian, and other magical and boy-scout-ish outlooks which I, of course, knew were full of pernicious hogwash.

It was the second of the two most important RET outlooks which soon began to help me mightily in this respect. The first RET theory, which virtually all my clients are actively shown how to accept, is that humans are irretrievably human—fallible, fucked-up, and full of frailty—and that they therefore would better never damn nor devilify themselves no matter what they foolishly do. The second mainstay of RET is that, because of this same human errancy, one would better not condemn, decry, or cast into hell any other person than oneself—no matter what he or she nastily does to oneself or others.

As I kept practicing rational-emotive psychology during the middle and late 1950s, and as I kept showing my clients how crazy they were behaving when they felt angry, resentful, hostile, revengeful, or vindictive, and how they would invariably lose (especially in the long run) by following this kind of Jehovahistic thinking, I couldn't help stopping on many occasions and saying to myself: "Hang it! Don't *I* do the same thing, too? He says he's trying to help his wife, but he's thoroughly impatient with her. Well, aren't I, who am supposedly trying to help him, equally impatient when he comes late, doesn't do his homework, or resists me with this psychodynamic horse manure? Face it! I am often doing the same thing as he does. Now what am *I* going to do to change? Healer, heal thyself!"

The same thing happened at some of my public lectures and workshops. Some hostile questioner, especially a devotee of analysis, would try to put me on the spot and make me look foolish. Whereupon I would first flash to myself: "Idiot! How can he be so dense! Here I worked through that crap a long time ago and he still devoutly and bigotedly subscribes to it. Now let me see how I can quickly fix his wagon and make him the laughingstock of everyone in the audience." And, being witty and bright, I usually did pulverize him—much to the amusement of most of my audience, and much to his own horror. Naturally, that was one of the best possible ways for me to lose friends and uninfluence people, and some of the worst enemies I have to this day I nicely made in this manner.

Immediately after my clever retorts, however, I would tend to revert to my own theory and at least inwardly recant. "Look," I would tell myself, "stop the nonsense! You supposedly teach people that no one is a bastard, not even a benighted psychoanalytic religionist; and then you do your best to blast this poor individual out of his seat and make him a laughingstock even to his best friends in the audience. What kind of tolerance is that? You show people how to deplore people's traits and not their being, but you clearly were attempting to put him down as a person. How rational-emotively sane was your own behavior?"

You can well imagine that my self-criticism—or, more accurately, criticism of my own acts—did not perform instant miracles. For quite a number of years thereafter I still could not—er, did not—resist the temptation to make my public opponents look foolish. To be honest, I still don't resist on more than a few occasions. But, as many people have said to me who have heard me speak on the same topic both a decade ago and more recently, I have significantly improved in this respect. RET works even with its originator! I still have, and think I am strongly disposed biologically to have, much of the irritability which my father displayed for the full eighty years of his life. But as I keep working against it, and keep asking myself, "Why shouldn't benighted people think the way they do about my theories? Why are they screwballs for having a few screwing ideas? What can I learn, for my own benefit and that of my theories, from their valid and invalid objections?" I keep becoming increasingly patient and less irritable, and I gain more from objectionable objections to my views than I previously did from my angry counterblasts.

The more I practice RET with others, the more I automatically tend to use it with myself. This is why I favor group therapy so much. In my regular weekly groups, and in the many marathon weekends of rational encounter that I lead in various parts of the country every year, I train most of the group members not only to use the RET philosophy of tolerance, scientific validation, and openness with themselves but to actively, determinedly employ it with other group members. My theory states that if they thereby keep talking others out of their bullshit, they will automatically and unconsciously tend to talk themselves out of their own. As I write this hypothesis, I can see that it could be empirically tested. I could arrange an experimental group where a participant only tried to use RET methods with other group members and a control group where he (or other clients who had similar disturbances) only brought up his (or their) own problems to RET-oriented group members and never tried to help these other members with their upsets. Then I could see whether, as I hypothesize, the individual who only (or at least mainly) worked on other people's problems with RET made as much emotional progress himself as the individual who only (or mainly) brought up his own problems for discussion. Well, maybe I shall do this experiment someday (for, unfortunately, I have almost innumerable things to do for the dear old cause of RET before I die, and exceptionally little time left in which to do them). Until that day, I still maintain the hypothesis that talking others out of their magical, self-destroying philosophies tends to help one appreciably surrender one's own tommyrot. If anyone is the living proof of that thesis, I think it is I.

Another problem that keeps coming up in my own life and that RET helps me with is therapeutic routine. I enjoyed, as I previously said, psychoanalytic "detecting," because it is a fascinating form of problem solving; and there is virtually nothing in which I delight more than throwing myself into a good and difficult problem. But RET, fortunately and unfortunately, is (in my estimation) a much more efficient theory and practice than analysis, and consequently anyone who practices it well can zero in on a client's problem in record time—often within a few minutes of meeting the client—and discover his or her most important hangups and what could be done to alleviate them. This means, as you might expect, that RET can get relatively boring as far as understanding the client is concerned, for humans really are not as complicated, at least in their disturbances, as the analysts (and many other kinds of therapists) wrongly perceive them as being, and a great deal of detecting does not have to be done to comprehend and help them.

Well, suppose it does get somewhat boring at times? What can I do about it? And the answer, in RET terms, is, first, accept the routines, in so far as they are part of the whole system of doing therapy; and, second, try to arrange to minimize them. This I have done pretty well for the past several years. I have seen myself at times doing the same thing over and over with clients and have recognized that this is a pain in the ass, this is something that I don't greatly like. But I have also looked at what I am doing in perspective, for I do like therapy as a whole, and I immensely enjoy those challenging cases that frequently come along. While I don't enjoy half so much the routine, nonchallenging cases, why do I have to enjoy every minute of doing therapy? I don't!

Taking this attitude, I am then able to go on to make what I do far more interesting and challenging than it would otherwise be. I deliberately take on, for example, some of the most difficult clients— such as outright psychotic or psychopathic individuals—because they are exceptionally hard to work with and therefore present more intriguing problems. And now that I know—or think I know—pretty much what is bothering most people soon after they open their mouths, I focus more on how I am going to induce the individual to change his basic disturbance-creating philosophy than on what that philosophy is. No matter how similar people are—and I often frankly tell my clients that, individual though they be, they are nauseatingly similar to other easily upsettable people in their core philosophies—I can try for some unique, and preferably quick, way of attacking and uprooting their self-repeated drivel. That process I still find interesting and at times fascinating.

Besides, whoever the client is and whatever his difficulties may be, I creatively make him a part of my own theorizing and experimenting. If I can enjoy myself with solving his particular problems and significantly helping him, great! But if he is a little too rigid, too run of the mill, or even too easy for my particular tastes, I can still do my best to help (and perhaps get him out of my office in as few sessions as possible) and also use his behavior to help my own theoretical bents. For I like psychologizing—which to me means inventing theories and then testing them. And I am not only a practical therapist (who perhaps sees more clients than virtually any other therapist in the world, since I regularly have as many as a hundred individual and nine group therapy sessions a week), but also a theorist of therapy. I am passionately devoted to devising new methodologies of treatment and new explanations of why people behave the way they do and what can be done to help them improve their behavior (that is, become less anxious, guilty, depressed, and hostile). I can consequently use even "boring" sessions as grist to my theorizing mill and thereby make myself much less bored.

I also use in psychotherapy some of the discoveries I began making some time ago in my sex life. I realized that no matter how much I loved a female and how attracted to her I might be in general, I often felt wholly unturned on about making love to her when we presumably had plenty of time and energy to fuck each other to a fare-thee-well. But at some of those very times, when I was about as excited as a three-toed sloth, she was bursting at the panties and ready to take on almost any penis-wielder in town. What to do? Well, after giving the matter some thought, and reminding myself of my sexual-social responsibilities (for we were in bed together, partly at my behest, and it would have been damned inconvenient for her to go out at three A.M. and look for a homeless sailor), I usually decided, at these times, to throw myself into active lovemaking whether I wanted it or not and experimentally see what would happen.

Almost always, when I did so with a no-nonsense-about-it, and nothing of a poor-me-look-what-I-have-to-put-up-with approach, decidedly good things happened. Within a few minutes of my catapulting myself into action, my previously limp pecker soared to heights of newfound glory and I really wanted—and, man, I mean wanted—to ream it into any one of her eagerly awaiting orifices, and there we were, wildly whacking away on eight or ten cylinders for some of the best ten or twenty minutes of her and my life.

Making an analogy between how one can make sexual and psychotherapeutic participation maximally exciting may seem a little farfetched, but I insist that the two goals can significantly overlap. For in my group therapy sessions, I frequently find that things are getting somewhat dull—that Joel S. is whining again in his irritatingly high voice; that Marilyn F. is screaming at him, as usual; and the rest of the group members are morosely sitting around and saying practically nothing. Whereupon, I am sorely tempted to withdraw into my own shell, dream about some pleasant pastime that has nothing to do with the group; let the Fellow at our Institute who assists me in the group take over the leader's burden for awhile; and nicely cop out.

But, except for a minute or two, I rarely do. For, just as I have discovered in sex-love play, if I forcefully thrust myself into the group process, insist on opening my big mouth about something (such as actively getting at the philosophic sources of Joel's whining or Marilyn's screaming), I quickly become absorbed and vitalized. Although the group material may still be "boring," *I* am not bored. In fact, as I resort to humor, to logical analysis, to insisting that Marilyn and Joel present empirical evidence to back their awfulizings, to role playing, to encounter exercises, to assigning homework tasks, and to various other cognitive-emotive-behavioral methods of stirring things up, the group itself usually tends to awaken from its lethargic state and to become truly interesting. Then I subsequently, spontaneously turn on still more

Maybe that, in fact, is one of the main reasons why I escaped from the shackles of psychoanalysis and why I was equally repulsed by the early Rogerian nondirective therapy, which I was specifically taught at Columbia University and which I put to the test for awhile in the 1940s. People often tell me, "Oh, I can see that you gave up analysis and developed rational therapy because you naturally have a very logical mind and you just cannot personally tolerate any kind of irrationality." Maybe so, but the irrationalities—even in regard to RET—which I have beautifully tolerated for many years of my life would tend to belie this hypothesis.

What is truer, perhaps, is that I damned well cannot—or at least will not—tolerate hours per day of passivity or inactivity. These are bad enough for the clients—who have their own natural passivity, usually, and would better overcome it—and probably worse for me. I have always been exceptionally active, which, once again, I do not think I was trained or conditioned to be by my early experience with my parents, but which I believe is basically an inherited trait. My father was vocationally and socially on the go until the day of his death. My mother, in her late eighties, literally ran me around on a tour of her new nursing home when I came to visit her shortly after she had moved into it. And she will probably dance herself, say in her late nineties, to death. Their scores of close relatives are similarly vigorous and constantly astir.

So if anything has predisposed me in favor of active-directive, evocative-emotive, forcefully confronting methods of therapy it is probably my high energy level and my allergy to sloth and uninvolvement. This same energy level—freed by the RET-abetted beliefs that I can enjoy, that there always is something I can find and make significant to my existence, and that even the greatest possible disadvantages and inconveniences that can befall me are only that (and are never awful, horrible, terrible, or catastrophic)—helps keep me tirelessly seeking for exciting new ways to work and to live. Most, though hardly all, of the psychological things that Sigmund Freud said were, alas, woefully exaggerated or false. But he did say, with much truth, that if an individual would be happy and mentally healthy he had better be dedicated to love and work.

I concur. Except that I would change his proposition somewhat to read: Being healthy and happy is most often achieved by dedicating oneself to loving (rather than to being loved) and/or to working (rather than to needing to achieve). And since loving is a major form of involved activity and working is (or can be) a form of active involvement, I wonder whether the two endeavors are not different aspects of the same basic life process. I am sure they have been in my own life, since as a therapist (and as a theorist, a writer, and a speaker about therapy) I intensely love my work and work at my love. And as a man I can hardly think of myself, any longer, becoming and remaining too involved with any woman who is not concerned (as my present long-term inamorata is) with the theory and practice of what I consider to be effective (and probably rational-emotive) therapy.

I repeat: I love my work and work at my loving. That is the secret of my present unusually happy state. Let me conclude with a recent application of RET to my own living, an application which may indicate how utterly determined I am to enjoy life and to avoid needless, self-defeating anxiety and hostility. I shall couch this illustration in the now fairly famous ABCs of rational-emotive psychology.

At point A, a dramatic and noxious Activating Event (or Action or Activity) occurred. I am diabetic and take forty-three units of insulin every morning on arising. Two days ago, on a Wednesday morning, I rose an hour earlier than usual and foolishly took my regular dose of insulin immediately. Perhaps because I was sleepier and more bleary-eyed than I generally am in the morning, I probably misread the syringe markings and took five or ten extra units. I called one of our secretaries to my office when he entered the building at eight-fifty, gave him some things to do, and that is all I remember until I woke, an hour and a half later, in nearby Lenox Hill Hospital's emergency ward, after dreaming that I was getting a blood transfusion and that I was in danger of dying because the nurse in charge had left me alone and might not come back in time to save me from an overdose of infused blood. After waking, I discovered that I had gone into an insulin coma while talking to the secretary. He (not knowing what was wrong with me and thinking I had gone pretty crazy because I was acting quite irrationally) had delayed in getting help. By the time other people at our Institute had realized what was going on and got a nearby physician, I was incapable of imbibing any sugary liquids. An ambulance had to be called to take me to the hospital. At the hospital, they gave me dextrose intravenously, and I came out of the coma.

At point C, or what is called the emotional Consequence, I felt (at least momentarily) some inappropriate or disordered responses directly related to the Activating Events at A. They were: (1) feelings of panic at awaking in the hospital, feeling perfectly all right physically, not remembering any of the events leading up to my being in a hospital, and wondering why the hell I was there (in a restraining bed, no less, with firm bars imprisoning me in the bed!); (2) a little later, when I realized I had taken an overdose of insulin and not warned our new office people about my diabetic condition, feelings of shame because I had acted so stupidly; (3) feelings of some anger toward the secretary who had acted so stupidly when he saw I was acting bizarrely and had not immediately realized that there was something physically wrong with me and that medical attention was quickly required.

Now, according to RET theory, the noxious Activating Events that occurred to me, at A, could not have possibly really caused my disturbed feelings or emotional Consequences at C. Instead, my Beliefs, at B, about the Activities, at A, truly caused C. What, therefore, were these Beliefs?

First, I obviously had a set of rational Beliefs (rB's) about A. In regard to my panic at awaking in the hospital, I first believed: "How puzzling! What am I doing here? How annoying to be in a hospital bed, with bars up its side, and not know what happened to get me here! I wish to hell I could understand this! What a pain in the ass to be so confused and in doubt! Maybe there's really something wrong with me. And how unfortunate that would be!" If I had stuck rigorously to these rational Beliefs, I presumably would have felt the highly appropriate emotions of frustration, annoyance, puzzlement, concern, and displeasure, but not panic. What, then, created the panic?

Obviously, according to RET theory, my additional set of irrational Beliefs (iB's). Probably: "How awful! Here I am in a hospital and have no idea why I am here or what is wrong with me. Suppose it is serious? Suppose they don't let me out? Suppose I have gone nutty, or something like that, not to remember at all what happened to me or why I am here? How horrible that would be! I couldn't stand it! My, what a weak and incompetent person I'd prove to be if I kept on being confused and puzzled like this and never got over it!"

In regard to my feelings of shame about acting stupidly about the overdose of insulin and not notifying our office people about my diabetic condition, I again had a set of rational Beliefs: "What a stupid thing to do! How unfortunate! I certainly don't like behaving so idiodically, and I'd better watch these kinds of things next time." These rational Beliefs, had I stayed with them, would have again made me feel frustrated, annoyed, concerned, and displeased, but not panicked.

My shame almost certainly resulted from a set of irrational Beliefs: "What a total idiot I am! I should have acted more intelligently about the insulin and notifying our employees about my diabetic condition. I really deserve to suffer for behaving so asininely! Maybe I'm such a nincompoop that I'll always keep acting like this, and that would be awful!"

My anger at the secretary who found me is the state of insulin shock arose because I originally had a set of rational Beliefs, probably along these lines: "Shit! Isn't it too bad that he didn't act more observantly and intelligently! How unpleasant to have him make a stupid diagnostic error like that! I wish he had behaved more perspicaciously." Again, had I believed only these sane thoughts, I would have felt appropriately frustrated, annoyed, concerned, and displeased, but not angry.

I almost certainly went on, however, to a set of highly insane or irrational Beliefs (iB's): "What a dolt he is! How could he have

Carl R. Rogers
at age nine.

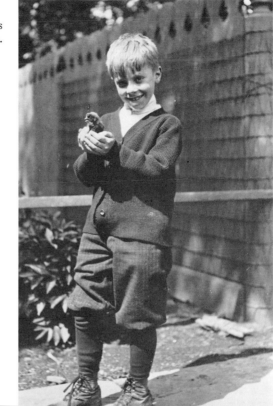

Carl R. Rogers today.

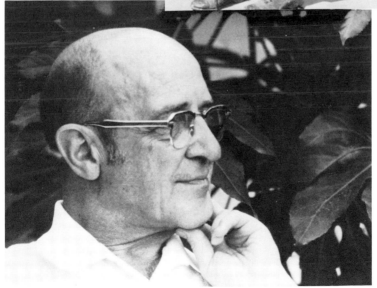

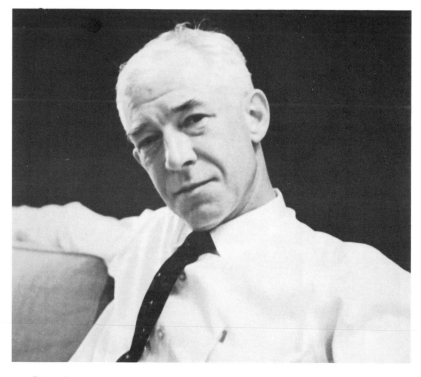

John Warkentin today (above), and, standing in back, at age ten, with family (below).

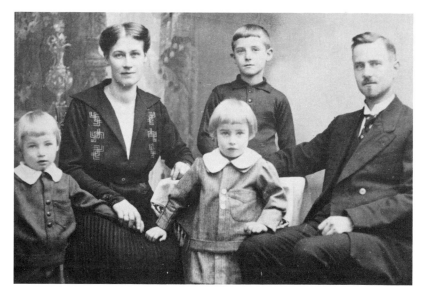

Rudolf Ekstein at age eighteen (below) and today (right).

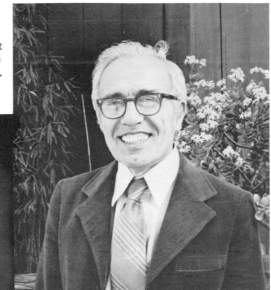

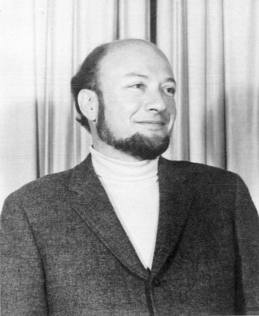

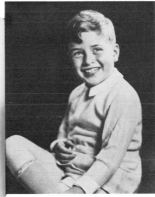

Werner M. Mendel today (left) and as a child (above).

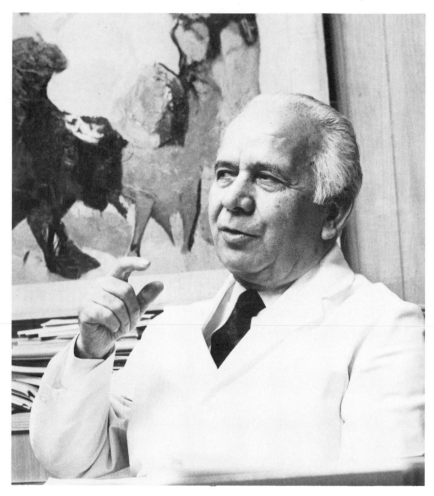

Juan J. Lopez-Ibor today.

behaved so stupidly! He shouldn't have been so careless at jumping at wrong conclusions! How horrible it is for me to be afflicted with stupid people such as he!"

Fortunately, having worked through such irrational Beliefs many many times with my clients and myself, I automatically went to work on my own in this instance and vigorously Disputed them, at point D. Thus, I challenged:

"Why is it awful to be in the hospital and not know what is wrong with me? Even if I have acted bizarrely, to get myself here, and I am off my rocker, where is the evidence that that is horrible?" And I quickly answered myself: "It's clearly not awful, but only inconvenient, to be here. I'll soon find out what's wrong with me. And if it is serious, it is. Tough!" So I almost immediately lost my panic and merely felt puzzled and concerned.

"What makes me a total idiot, just because I screwed up (for the first time in about thirteen years) on my insulin dose? Why should I have acted more intelligently about this and about notifying our employees about my diabetic condition? In what way would it be awful even if I kept making mistakes like this and eventually foolishly killed myself?" And I replied to myself: "Obviously, *I* am not a total idiot just because I did two foolish things. There's no reason why I *should, ought,* or *must* act more intelligently, even though it would be better if I did. It's not awful, but merely quite unpleasant, if I keep making mistakes like this and even finally kill myself by them." Whereupon I lost all my feelings of shame and considered the objective problem of how I would act more intelligently in the future and not repeat these silly errors.

"Why is our secretary a dolt just because he diagnosed my condition wrongly? Why could he not, or for that matter why could not any other human being, behave so stupidly? Where is the evidence that he should not have been so careless? What makes it horrible for me to be afflicted with fallible human beings in our office?" I directly answered these questions: "Of course, he's not a dolt just because he did one mistaken act. He easily could behave wrongly in this instance, and there is no reason why he shouldn't. It's certainly troublesome for me to be afflicted with fallible human employees; but I can still refuse to make myself childishly angry and miserable because of that difficulty." Within literally a few seconds, I lost all my anger at our secretary and, in fact, I felt grateful to him for doing as much as he was able to do for me when I was in insulin shock and for at least calling in others who better knew what to do.

After the entire experience was over, and I had rid myself, by prompt use of RET methods, of my feelings of panic, shame, and hostility, I actually felt fine about the events of the day. For I thought as follows: "It certainly was a damned nuisance to go into shock, to inconvenience and help stir up the negative emotions of so many people. But this sort of thing has never happened to me before, and it was a fascinating and interesting experience. In fact, in some ways I'm happy it occurred, since it adds to my repertoire of intriguing things that have happened to me and that I can remember and learn from. Moreover, now that I've almost killed myself with my careless behavior, I can profit from my mistakes and make pretty sure that something similar will never happen again. You know, I'm rather glad that it, or at least certain aspects of it, happened."

Well, there are many, many more things I could now say about RET and me—about how it helps me, almost daily, to cope enjoyably and unupsettedly with my clients, my public appearances, my writing, and virtually every other aspect of my life. But my space has run out. I now have learned, in writing this piece, that it is highly enjoyable to review some of the major aspects of my own practice and my own being and to see how they tie up with rational-emotive psychology. You know, I think I really will do that lengthy autobiography I have mildly thought about doing for some time. Meanwhile, happy thinking!

Selected Writings

Sex Without Guilt. New York: Lyle Stuart and Lancer Books, 1969.
Growth Through Reason. Palo Alto: Science and Behavior Books, 1971.
Reason and Emotion in Psychotherapy. New York: Lyle Stuart, 1962.
Homosexuality: Its Causes and Cure. New York: Lyle Stuart, 1962.
How to Live with a Neurotic. New York: Crown Publishers and Award Books, 1969.

V

Self-Actualization and Philosophical Awareness

Helm Stierlin

This autobiography, like any other, distorts while it reconstructs. Moreover, it is sketchy and leaves out many data that an analyst would consider crucial, particularly data which refer to my early life and family. But since I had to make a choice about what I should cover in the allotted space, about what would interest the reader, and what I could reveal comfortably, I decided to focus on how my self-realization as a psychotherapist went hand in hand with my quest for philosophical awareness, or *Selbstbesinnung*, a quest that still goes on and reflects my indebtedness to various thinkers and their ideas.

Such *Selbstbesinnung* seemed to come naturally to a child like me who was ill for long stretches of time—I spent approximately one school year in bed after I contracted diphtheria, scarlet fever, and tuberculosis in rapid succession—and who therefore had much time and cause to think about myself and the world. (It seems to me now that my later personal psychoanalysis repeated an earlier condition when I was trapped in bed and could do nothing but think.)

As a German growing up in Hitler's Reich, I was young enough to be spared major complicity in the Nazi crimes but old enough to be drawn into the holocaust. By the time the war was over, I had lost my father, brother, and home (which was located in the eastern part of pre-war Germany). Much of my adolescence had turned into an acted-out wild West story, made "real" by the madness of times. Günter Grass, my agemate, has described in his novels what such an adolescence was like. For me it implied, at the age of fifteen, compulsory service in the air defense of my hometown of Stettin, now in Poland, which at the end of the war was almost totally razed by bombs. It implied also a last short bout in Hitler's army when this army was already crumbling; and it meant that I witnessed a post-war doomsday world wherein long-held values collapsed and ever-new horrors surfaced.

It was in Heidelberg that I could take stock of what had happened, where I stood, and where I wanted to go. The seat of Germany's oldest university, Heidelberg had miraculously remained undamaged. Hence classes could start here soon after the war had ended and I was one of the first students to enroll. (I still remember how the inscription over the portal of the new university—"To the German Spirit"—was changed back to "To the Living Spirit," as it had been originally conceived by Gundolf, the famous literary scholar.) In our times of affluence I find it difficult to recapture the climate of students' lives that then prevailed. Those were the years when food had finally become scarce for many Germans, as it had been earlier for other Europeans. Hence there were long queues in front of grocery shops, and there was a black market that fed on the flow of American cigarettes and other consumer goods. Students ran around in army clothes that were barely shorn of military insignia. But, despite or because of the prevailing austerity, the intellectual life was intense. I remember countless discussions with teachers and fellow students on almost any conceivable subject. As a member of the student government, I contributed to these discussions by arranging seminars on such topics as the origins of nazism, problems of modern art, and the rele-

vance of present-day science to modern life. I discovered Hegel and
Nietzsche and both have remained my favorite philosophers. And it
was in this intellectual climate that I became introduced to the challenges and problems of psychotherapy—presented to me in a charac-
teristically conflictful and polemical fashion. Karl Jaspers, Alfred
Weber, Victor von Weizsaecker, and Alexander Mitscherlich became
the most important figures in my world. Let me briefly comment on
each of them.

Philosophical Influences

Of the four, Jaspers was then the shining star. Like many of
my fellow students, I was held spellbound by him. As a result, I chose
philosophy as my main subject—which allowed me to participate in
Jaspers' advanced seminars—and under Jaspers' preceptorship I began
soon to write my philosophical thesis on "the concept of responsibility,"
in which I evaluated and integrated ideas of Immanuel Kant, Max
Weber, and John Dewey. Jaspers was also the first one to teach me,
albeit polemically, about psychoanalysis. Jaspers saw Freud, along
with Marx, as the evil geniuses of our times, and he imparted this
view freely to his students. Yet it was he who led me to study psychoanalysis more objectively and to eventually become a psychoanalyst.
He did so by recommending my going into medicine. I followed his
advice, because I always had wanted (though ambivalently) to enter
this field and because after three semesters spent as a bookworm I had
become afraid of getting lost in the never-never world of philosophical
speculation. (Jaspers himself had studied medicine before he had
taken up philosophy proper.) I began to study medicine in Heidelberg,
after my third semester at the university, but continued with philosophy at the same time. I became a doctor of philosophy in 1951, at a
time when Jaspers moved to Basel, Switzerland. Kurt Rossman, who
later succeeded to Jaspers' chair at the University of Basel, helped me
to finish my thesis.

Alfred Weber, then in his seventies, the second major figure to
influence me in Heidelberg, was holding private seminars in his home.
I attended several of these. Alfred was the younger brother of Max
Weber, the noted sociologist, and it has been said that he lived in
the shadow of Max, but I found him impressive and courageous in

his own right. Alfred Weber was one of the few Heidelberg professors
who from the outset rejected Nazism by surrendering their academic
positions. Not even Jaspers did this. Yet notwithstanding his stand
against Nazism, he seemed more burdened by the Nazi past than most
others I met. I still remember how he, shortly after the war, broke
down in tears while listening to the conciliatory talk of a French professor who had been a concentration camp victim. He commented to
me, while crying, "Oh, that this must be said to us Germans!" (In
contrast, many of his academic colleagues, who in one way or the
other had held out under, or cooperated with, Nazism, seemed casual
and unmoved.) I found his seminars immensely stimulating. Here I
was introduced to the world of William James and John Dewey whose
ideas I tried to incorporate into my thesis. Alfred Weber also aroused
my interest in psychoanalysis when he referred to it as one of the most
potent intellectual currents of our century.

It was, however, up to Victor von Weizsaecker and Alexander
Mitscherlich to introduce me more expertly to the fields of psychotherapy and psychoanalysis. Von Weizsaecker, then holding a chair in
internal medicine, is little known in the United States although he,
along with L. Binswanger, E. Minkowski, and E. Straus, must be
counted among the major European thinkers who developed an analytically oriented medical phenomenology.

Mitscherlich, after returning to Germany from his Swiss exile,
had reopened in Heidelberg the first German post-war psychoanalytic
training center. While pursuing this objective, Mitscherlich attacked
some of the most revered establishment figures in German medicine,
such as the surgeon Sauerbruch and the physiologist Rein. Mitscherlich had made it known that these two professors had been implicated
in the crimes of Nazi doctors and hence were disqualified as medical
teachers. Subsequently, he published several books on the complicity
of medical doctors in the Nazi atrocities. These publications intensely
antagonized large parts of the German academic community. More
recently, Mitscherlich has published *Die Unfähigkeit zu trauern* (The
Inability to Mourn), a book whose main theme is central to my own
life and personal analysis. That is the weakness and corruption of a
generation of German fathers who failed their sons in helping them to
become fathers to a new generation. I feel now that the unusually

militant and self-destructive features of the present German student unrest derive partly from this failure of the father generation.

Through my contacts with Mitscherlich and his associates at the "psychosomatic department" in Heidelberg, I finally gained firsthand knowledge of Freud's writings and came to publish my first article in the newly founded psychoanalytic journal *Psyche*. In this article I analyzed critically some of Jaspers' epistemological assumptions which had led him to treat psychoanalysis as a nonscience, that is, a concoction of fictions and beliefs. This article then led Jaspers to disavow me.

A short time later—while still studying medicine—I became interested in the research of Konrad Lorenz and other animal psychologists. I wrote then what was, to my knowledge, the first paper that brought together Lorenz's ethological and Freud's psychoanalytic approach to instincts. (Freud was then not yet accepted by many German scientists. I found this out while studying at the University of Freiburg, when I contacted a prominent German professor of zoology for advice on my paper. This man listened to my proposal—to compare critically Freud and Lorenz—and then said disdainfully, "I advise you against your project, as a good scientist would not want to have anything to do with a swine such as Freud." At that time also, approximately seven years after World War II, quite a few German publishers still refused to print anything Freud had written.)

In 1953 I finished my medical studies in Heidelberg and moved to Munich. Here I underwent my first psychoanalysis and began to see patients, first as an intern at the university outpatient clinic and later as a resident at the psychiatric hospital. Around that time I discovered Sullivan's *Conceptions of Modern Psychiatry* while browsing in the library of an America Haus. (I noticed I was the first reader to borrow the book.) Sullivan, at this point in my life, made instant sense to me, much more than Freud had done when I had read him as a medical student. (Only much later could I fully appreciate Freud, whom I now consider the more penetrating and innovative thinker of the two.) Thereafter, if there ever was one person leading me to seek my self-realization as a therapist, it was Sullivan; and it seems no happenstance that I later followed Sullivan's trail when I first moved to Sheppard and Enoch Pratt Hospital in

Towson, Maryland, and later to Chestnut Lodge in Rockville, Maryland—two places with which Sullivan had become associated. Particularly, Sullivan's concept of the participant observer found meaning with me. Subsequently I contrasted this concept with that of the "distant observer," one which I found dominating the German psychiatric scene. Also, the more I read Sullivan, the more I came to see Jaspers, my philosophic mentor, as the reactionary prototype of the "distant observer."

My dim view of post-war German psychiatry and psychotherapy was confirmed when I served my first year of residency at the University Clinic for Nervous and Mental Diseases at the University of Munich. Kurt Kolle, its director, was of a mercurial temperament and his outlook was much influenced by Jaspers. He lorded over a psychiatric operation that to me seemed as disorganized as it appeared anti- or a-psychotherapeutic. Schizophrenic patients were still given shock treatment in large numbers, while "refractory" hysteric patients were given painful electrical treatments. Although I personally liked Kolle, who had suffered much from the Nazis, I found unacceptable the way he ran his hospital, treated his patients, and viewed psychiatric illnesses. Thus I waited for my chance to leave Munich and go to America.

Sheppard-Pratt and Chestnut Lodge

This chance came in the summer of 1955 when, with the help of Edith Weigert, I found a position as a psychiatric resident at the Sheppard and Enoch Pratt Hospital. SEP was then a rather sleepy and idyllic place. It was surrounded by many acres of park and farm land on which one could roam freely. (This no longer holds true, as much of SEP's ground has been sold in the meantime.) It housed approximately 250 patients who were cared for by about twelve residents and four or five senior physicians. Like the rest of the residency staff, I carried approximately ten to twelve patients, most of whom I saw in psychotherapy three times a week. I learned a lot from them, as I have from my subsequent patients, to whom I feel deeply indebted.

It was at SEP that Sullivan had pioneered his treatment of schizophrenia in the late twenties, and his presence could still be sensed. Will Elgin, for example, the hospital's associate medical director, could tell delightful stories of Sullivan's life; but there was also Lewis B. Hill, a powerful person in his own right and who for me embodies the tradition of Sullivan. I cherished my weekly supervisory session with Hill who, I felt then, could teach me more about schizophrenia and human life than I had ever learned before. This, without doubt, had to do with his own bouts with pain and suffering. (When I met him, though, he had weathered his major life crisis.) I was fortunate to meet him at the height of his career and I was often awed by his brilliance and diagnostic acumen. I remember how he once, on the spur of the moment, dictated a full-length paper in which not one sentence had to be changed. Even today I consider Hill's *Psychotherapeutic Intervention in Schizophrenia* one of the seminal books in the psychiatric field, an absolute must for anyone who tries to actualize himself as a psychotherapist. Unfortunately for our profession, he died much too soon. I tried to pay homage to him by translating his book into German.

Around the time of Hill's death, I moved to Washington, D.C., where I had found a position on the staff of Chestnut Lodge. Chestnut Lodge seemed then at the height of its fame. Sullivan, although never on the staff of the Lodge, had lectured there extensively and had powerfully shaped the philosophy of the place. He had deeply influenced Dexter Bullard, the medical director of the Lodge, and had left his imprint on Otto Will, Jr., and Frieda Fromm-Reichmann. (Harold Searles, however, another prominent alumnus of the Lodge, seemed less influenced by Sullivan and formulated many of his ideas within the framework of psychoanalytic theory.) Frieda Fromm-Reichmann, unfortunately, died shortly before my arrival at Chestnut Lodge. I had met her a number of times at lectures and at private parties and, like so many others, had become immensely impressed by her. Beside Lewis Hill's book, it is her *Principles of Intensive Psychotherapy* which most lastingly has influenced my own views and attitudes as a psychotherapist.

While working at Chestnut Lodge, I developed those ideas on human relations and schizophrenia which I have since put forth in my *Conflict and Reconciliation.*[1] Otto Will, Jr., and Clarence Schulz were the two persons who influenced me most at Chestnut Lodge. Both

[1] New York: Science House, 1969.

have now left the Lodge and are active elsewhere in administrative and psychotherapeutic practice. Although I owe them much, I shall not comment on them now. Instead, I would like to reflect briefly on the theme of this presentation—the self-actualization of the psychotherapist—as I came to look at it through my Chestnut Lodge experience.

Self-Actualization as Conflict and Reconciliation

Since Freud, we have come to equate a psychotherapist's self-actualization with his self-examination. This self-examination, according to Freud, has to occur on two interrelated levels: on the level of ongoing analysis wherein the analyst is required to check his patient's activities and projections against what transpires in his (the therapist's) own unconscious; and on the level of his personal life in which he—assisted by his personal analysis—is expected to strive for ever-increasing self-insight and self-accountability. In this way, Freud had given new meaning to the Socratic credo: The "unexamined life is not worth living." Since Freud, the therapist's self-actualization had thus come to imply and require a self-examination that in some respects had to be even deeper and more encompassing than that which Socrates himself had envisioned.

Such self-examination and self-actualization as I found at Chestnut Lodge required the therapist to become aware of various areas of inevitable conflict and needed reconciliation. I have dealt with these areas in my book on this topic. The therapist of schizophrenic patients, I found, is likely to become subject to unusual frustrations and temptations. He may feel challenged to achieve the impossible, that is, to succeed where others have failed, to be a rebel in his profession, to remake a dependent patient in his own image, to penetrate deeper than others before him the uncanny, unexplored world of madness. Like an artist, the therapist seems called upon to achieve the extraordinary in terms of self-perfection and self-abandonment and, in so doing, again like an artist he seems to court unusual frustration and despair. In this situation, the therapist must, I came to believe, achieve two things: He must expand his awareness of his own motivations and conflicts, and he must make use of balancing

and reconciling features in his personal life and in the hospital structure.

Along with making these insights possible, my work at the
Lodge made me aware of the deep and intricate interdependence of
the needs of patient and therapist. We can distinguish here between
repair needs and growth needs. Repair needs come into play when the
therapist realizes he needs his patients in order that he can be confirmed as a therapist. He thus becomes aware that *his* self-esteem depends on his seeing his patient thrive (or actualize himself) just as a
mother feels confirmed by seeing her child thrive. Winnicott has specifically made this point. He emphasized that a doctor usually em-
barks on a lifelong career of doing repair work—work he has to do
because of his own psychological needs. Obviously, he could not do
this repair work without recruiting a patient. Therefore, without his
patients, he could not be a doctor, analogous to a lawyer who could
not exist without his criminals, or a minister who could not minister
without his parishioners.

In addition to becoming confirmed as a parent and doctor, the
therapist needs his patient in order to realize his growth potential.
Here growth needs, rather than repair needs, seem important. Thus, a
deeply anxious schizophrenic patient may bring his therapist into
closer touch with areas of dissociative, disintegrative anxiety which the
therapist can now experience, "own," work through, and allow to contribute to his growth. Yet, when we reflect on our own repair and
growth needs as therapists, we find that we have to steer a narrow
and precarious path from which we can stray in either of two directions. Either we can need our patients too much, unconsciously tending to keep them dependent and needy, or we can need our patients
too little and then lack the needed motivation for investing ourselves
deeply in them. In other words, when we need an "interesting" patient too much for our self-actualization, we will tend to feed too
much on him and become exploitive. The patient will be the worse
for it. But, if we require too little from the patient in terms of our
own growth and repair needs, we are likely to be insensitive and un-
empathic to him. Again the therapeutic process, that is, the interde-
pendent self-actualizations of therapist and patient, will suffer.

Another angle to conflict and reconciliation has to do with

how, and how much, the therapist can or should provide his patient with values and models for identification. The modern-day patient, according to Erikson, is beset by the problem of finding out who he "should or might be or become" and therefore, overtly or covertly, turns to his therapist for answers. The therapist can choose not to face this issue openly. He can say—as did Freud and his early followers— that he only wants to assist his patient's liberation (to assist the resolution of neurotic conflict and suffering) and does not want to serve as a supplier of values and identities. However, as a matter of fact, he cannot *not* serve as such a supplier, just as a parent cannot *not* supply his children with the vital ingredients that make up their identities and values. Again the therapist must attain a difficult reconciliation. The more he is a child of his times and is affected by the breakdown of current value systems and identity support structures, the more likely he will be to flounder around himself and perhaps covertly turn to his patients for identity and value guidance. But if he does so, his patient will be hard-pressed to have *his* identity and *his* value needs fulfilled through the therapist. There is no easy answer to this problem which, on a theoretical and practical level, has preoccupied me much in past years and which has, in slightly different form, intruded into my present work with disturbed adolescents and their families. These parents, overwhelmed by social change and unrest, tend to cling to their established identities and values. Yet, it is precisely these identities and values which their children attack as obsolete and unviable. But while attacking their parents, the children at the same time ask desperately for a firmness and rightness of parental identities and values against (and with) which they can define themselves. The parents therefore must reconcile firmness and flexibility, strength of principle and ability to listen—qualities that seem to exclude each other and yet are required in order that dialogue and mutual growth can occur.

Binswanger and Jung

In the fall of 1962 I left Chestnut Lodge. The time then seemed right for this move. Originally I had intended to take on a position as "Oberarzt," under my friend G. Benedetti in Frankfurt. But this plan fell through when Benedetti became ill and decided to stay in Switzerland in his professorship of mental hygiene in Basel. I then accepted a position as senior supervising analyst at the Sanatorium Bellevue in Kreuzlingen, Switzerland. But before doing so, I made a trip around the world during which I lectured in New Zealand and Australia. I started my work in Kreuzlingen on January 1, 1963.

This was the sanatorium which Ludwig Binswanger had headed for nearly half a century. By the time I arrived, Binswanger, then in his late seventies, had resigned as its medical director and left its administration to his son Wolfgang and his Oberarzt Dr. Fierz. Yet he was still alert and interested in the patients and affairs at the sanatorium.

I do not want to comment on my experience at the Bellevue per se but merely to offer some reflections on Binswanger and Carl Gustav Jung, who both then became important to me. I had run into Binswanger's work while studying philosophy and psychoanalysis in Heidelberg. I believe von Weizsaecker was the first to mention his name to me. He alluded to Binswanger as the founder of "Daseins-analysis," an important philosophical development which attempted to integrate the insights of Martin Heidegger and Sigmund Freud. I heard Binswanger's name often mentioned along with that of three other authors who were all said to represent a new "medical phenomenology": E. Straus, E. V. von Gebsattel, and E. Minkowski. Gebsattel, Binswanger, and Minkowski have since died, and Straus alone is still alive and active, in Lexington, Kentucky.

Binswanger's major work, *Grundformen und Erkenntnis menschlichen Daseins,* has often been compared to Heidegger's *Sein und Zeit.* The book was clearly inspired by Heidegger's seminal work but took off in a somewhat different direction. Among many other things, it made *love* and not *care* (Sorge) its pivotal concept. I believe anyone who reads the book cannot help being impressed by its immense humanistic erudition. So was I when I read it for the first time in my twenties. In subsequent years, after reading more of his writings, and in particular his correspondence with Freud, my personal admiration for Binswanger had grown. My overall assessment of Daseinsanalysis, however, had become critical. I express this criticism in an article, "Existentialism Meets Psychotherapy," published in 1963 in *Philosophy and Phenomenological Research.* Thus, when I finally met Binswanger in person, I did so in a spirit of admiration mixed with critical skepticism. While talking with him, I did not hide my

critical views. My critique reflected my conviction that Binswanger
had either never grasped or lost touch with many of those psychodynamic insights that have, in the last decades, so enriched and perhaps
revolutionized our understanding of human relationships and schizophrenia. Yet never—and this seems striking even to me in retrospect—
did Binswanger seem to resent my critical view of his works. Indeed,
in some way he seemed to cherish my opposition, although I doubt
that it caused him to revise any of his own views. Like any complex
person, Binswanger presented many different sides to different people.
I felt fortunate that he offered me his perhaps most likable side, the
wise humanist who was generous, attentive, curious, engaged. Whether
we talked about Adalbert Stifter (the German novelist Binswanger
esteemed so much in his late years), about life in America, or about
his early encounters with Freud, it was always an enriching and stimulating experience for me. Binswanger clearly shared a quality of great
people—the ability to learn in old age, to be affected by an experience
as if it were made the first time, and to remain constantly alive and
questioning. I remember, for example, how elatedly he once returned
from visiting an exhibition of French impressionists. From his en-
thusiastic description one could have assumed that he had encountered
French impressionism for the first time in his life.

During his final year, Binswanger's physical and mental powers
declined visibly. He stayed frequently in bed, usually with bronchitis,
if I remember correctly. Still, even in this last year he completed a
book on the paranoid's experience of the world. He died approximately half a year after I had left the Bellevue. I was myself sick at
that time so I could not attend his funeral. Since his death I have
reflected on how the same qualities which I found so attractive in him
—a warm, lively humanity that allowed him to engage intensely with
a person who disagreed with many of his views—might also have attracted Freud. For Binswanger's relationship with Freud is perhaps
unique in that it could last for approximately three decades despite
the fact that the interests and theoretical positions of the two thinkers
grew increasingly apart.

My two years at the sanatorium also introduced me anew to
the world of C. G. Jung. Before I came to Bellevue I had read a fair
number of Jung's works. I had also heard and seen Jung on several
occasions, at one time exchanging a few words with him, but at Belle-

vue I worked for the first time with Jungian psychotherapists. The most prominent of these was Dr. Fierz who presently heads a small hospital in Zurich. (This, according to my knowledge, is the only mental hospital in the world whose psychotherapeutic orientation is explicitly Jungian.)

Over the years I had come to feel rather critical about Jung's works. I also felt repelled by his one-time attraction to the Nazi mythology which paralleled Heidegger's sympathizing with the beginnings of the Nazi movement. However, I came to appreciate at least some aspects of his work and thought. For one thing, I could not help noticing how several therapists of the Jungian school did exceptionally well with seriously disturbed schizophrenic patients; for another, I began to understand better some of the historical and cultural forces which shaped Jung's ideas. I began to see common elements in the works of Binswanger and Jung. Both came from that German-speaking corner of Switzerland where the democratic cosmopolitanism of the Helvetian Republic intertwined in a curious way with a sectarian, brooding investment in theology and philosophy as well as with a rather narrow provincialism. (The more I have read Heidegger, the more I have also found in him this provincialism, a background feature which to me explains much of his antitechnological and antidemocratic stance.) Deeply steeped in the cultural heritage of this milieu, Jung found his personal road to salvation by immersing himself in the world of symbols, myths, and dreams. Such salvation clearly had a theological dimension, as it had for Binswanger, who seemed to seek his salvation through contemplating the essence of human *Dasein*. Yet further: Such search for personal salvation appeared a creative and unique way of mastering a possible schizophrenic fate, the potential for which both seem to have possessed and sensed in themselves. Of the two, Jung more than Binswanger has enlarged our psychotherapeutic horizons with regard to the schizophrenic disturbance. He did so mainly, I believe, by focusing on the enriching and healing potentials inherent in the schizophrenic's subjective experience, thus anticipating a view of schizophrenia which later was popularized by Ronald Laing. Through his teaching and personal example Jung has, we can say, advocated the "trip into our psychic interior," a venture that can not only bring us in touch with our individual and cultural heritage but can also lead us to rebirth and growth. Such experience, according to Jung, can become useful or even necessary when we have passed the halfway mark of our lives and are inexorably moving toward death. By advocating such venture into the psychic interior for the middle-aged and elderly, Jung has in effect held out options for growth to large numbers of patients who so far had been unaware of this possibility and had been left stranded on the periphery of psychotherapeutic concerns.

These, however, tended to be patients who were relatively well-to-do and untroubled by their social standing in life as were, for example, those individuals who attended (and still attend) the "Eranos" meetings in Ascona. Not surprisingly, we note that where Jung's ideas continue to attract followers in the United States, social status and affluence seem more or less taken for granted. From this vantage point, it is not surprisnig that Philip Rieff, who has written one of the most insightful books about postFreudian developments in psychotherapy, made Wilhelm Reich into Jung's ideological counterpart. Whereas Jung lived and advocated a largely apolitical life of introspective contemplation devaluing or neglecting the social and political determinants of human behavior, Reich, the one-time Marxist revolutionary, became obsessed with breaking up and transforming society's exploitive structure. In our days, Jung and Reich continue to find their unwitting followers and popularizers. All those who advocate the "greening of America," that is, seek rebirth and growth through heightened subjective experience (be this through contemplation, drugs, engineering of peak experiences, alpha waves, or other means), can be viewed as latter-day followers of Jung. Those who want to radically transform or erase exploitive social institutions, such as David Cooper, can be viewed as followers of Reich.

Contemporary Issues

In 1965, after a period of writing, traveling, and lecturing in Europe and Asia, I returned to the United States where I took a position as research psychiatrist at the Adult Psychiatry Branch, National Institute of Mental Health. Lyman Wynne, then chief of the Adult Psychiatry Branch, whose seminal research in schizophrenia and the family I had long admired, made possible this move. Thus began a new phase in my self-actualization as a psychotherapist. Since this phase is not yet completed, I want to touch on it only briefly. Suffice it to say that in the last six years I have become preoccupied with studying and treating the family. Though I continue to see patients in individual psychoanalysis and psychotherapy, this work has taken on a new perspective. I have become much more aware of family tensions and family issues that enter into any individual's problems.

Studying and treating whole families meant learning a new craft, and it was not always easy. Particularly the shift from dealing with one individual patient to dealing with groups I found difficult to make. Group processes have become immensely important facts of our lives, but, like pollution, are not necessarily welcome facts. Yet they have to be confronted and will remain one of the greatest challenges in the overcrowded decades ahead. Again, we face here a critical task of conflict and reconciliation on the theoretical as well as practical levels, a task that requires us to do justice to the individual as a center of subjective experience, executive control, and responsibility and also to the group and wider human environment wherein this individual is embedded, on which he is dependent, and whose rights and power he must respect.

The One and the Others

In thinking about the individual's relation to others, I have come to appreciate anew that philosophical writer who, over the years, has intrigued me most, G. F. Hegel, a philosophical giant who, quite apart from inspiring Marx and countless others, as an interpersonal psychologist was more than 150 years ahead of his times. My latest book, written in German, has as its title a phrase from Hegel's *Phenomenology of the Spirit: Das Tun des Einen ist das Tun des Anderen.* This statement on the interconnectedness of human lives condenses into one brief sentence much of what I have tried to convey and seems therefore most suited to conclude this autobiographical sketch.

Selected Writings

"Existentialism Meets Psychotherapy. *Philosophy and Phenomenological Research,* 1963, *24,* 215–239.
Short-term versus long-term psychotherapy in the light of a general theory

of human relationships. *British Journal of Medical Psychology,* 1968, *41*, 357–367.

Conflict and Reconciliation. New York: Science House, 1969. (German translation in preparation.)

"The functions of 'inner objects.'" *International Journal of Psycho-Analysis,* 1970, *51*, 321–329.

Das Tun des Einen ist das Tun des Anderen. Frankfurt: Suhrkamp, 1971. (One chapter published separately under the title "Die Familien-beziehung." *Psyche,* 1970, *24*, 678–961.

VI

Stolen by Gypsies

Erving Polster

When I was four my mother, transplanted from Czechoslovakia, used to tell me stories about gypsies who steal children. Standing head-high to her ironing board in unblinking absorption, I heard about children with fairy names, such as Jobbela-Bobbela. They were always transcendentally dear to their parents. The stories I remember best are the ones in which the gypsies stole these children just because they loved them and had no inhibitions about stealing them. They reared them as princes. The children, nevertheless, always longed to find their lost homes where their primal familiarity would be restored.

Mother got me right there, entering my psyche with her own homing surge. Even now, at fifty, I still struggle between my love for what is familiar to me and my search for novel experience. My internal dialogue between familiarity and novelty would go something like this:

Familiarity: I know the old days well. I never have to make it with the people I knew a long time ago, family or friends. They never judged me except momentarily, nor I them. That's how I like life to be. If anything I do doesn't include that, forget it.

Novelty: Bullshit. You could rot that way. Unjudgmental loving is overrated. You have always been too impressed with that. You're just too lazy and scared to do the things necessary for changing your world. People can judge me any way they want. I want new and I'll take care of the consequences.

F: Lazy, my ass! You misjudge serenity for laziness and you have made a god out of ambition. Where do you think you're headed? You must know none of us will get out of this thing alive and the constant struggle for new worlds won't get you any closer to what you want than the basic ways you're familiar with. Ambition!

N: Yes, of course we are all going to the same place but I want to be fresh until I get there and not hang onto staleness and safety just because I am going to die someday. I would like death to represent a change in my life.

F: Well, you have a point there, but you should know that if you don't pay attention to me you can very easily get frenetic and grow, grow, grow without ever tasting your experiences.

N: I know. That's not really how I am, though. I feel fresh only when I taste my experiences and then when that happens they all seem very familiar to me. Familiar at the roots of me.

F: There you are, familiar, that's me, and I am the ticket. Not whether something happened before but whether the feelings are the ones I know from deep inside. OK, if you and I can keep getting those familiar feelings I don't care whether the events and places are the same or not.

N: Now you're talking more like a person I can live with.

Even in the face of mother's unwitting brainwash it is plain that what I am calling primal familiarity can only be recycled through new events, old sensations being repeatedly reincarnated. The basic sensations accompanying such qualities as absorption, awe, shame, or delight may remain the same all through life. Since such universal awareness is polymorphously present, having no predetermined subject matter, it is possible to feel the same agelessness at eighty as one does at eight. I am recurrently mystified by the fact that my age keeps changing and yet I remain the same in my native awareness, not counting the aches and pains. I experience myself differently now but not so much in my primal quality as in the content of what I am doing, like appearing on TV; or in new perspectives, like not wanting to work for a living, or in specific sensations, like the taste of a new Indian dish. I surely would not have been doing this, typing these words, when I was eight. Instead, I would have been throwing a ball up against the point of our front steps trying to catch the rebound and counting how many times I could do it in a row. The inner striving, attentiveness, and even adventure are quite the same, though. The details of what I am doing are important only because I could no longer get that old sensation throwing a ball against the steps, except perhaps as a momentary nostalgic act.

There is an infinite range of experiences that will give me the basic sense of familiarity, and paradoxically the more novel the experience is, the more likely it is that a primal familiarity will be part of it. I may get it with a stranger on an airplane. It may appear in awesome physical settings, such as the place where the Mediterranean and the Alps join. It may happen with someone I fall in love with for an evening at a cocktail party or with breaking into second wind while swimming. I felt it in my parents' bedroom when they were making love, when I was making butter in the kindergarten, on the roller coaster and the ball yard, on a holiday in the synagogue, when I first touched a girl's breast, meeting my brother in Little Rock, seeing my sister married, driving to the hospital knowing my mother had just died, seeing my wife rolled out of the delivery room or even just seeing her as I walk into the house, the birth of our two children and the death at birth of another, coming down from altitude after a bombing mission, a beer after sweating, a surprise meeting with an old friend, an ice cream cone. Then, of course, there is the experience as it may happen every day, like sitting with my feet under me, smiling at a light word, or remembering something that builds on another person's story.

All I need for this sense of primal familiarity is a favorable climate. When I am in a hospitable climate, my whole range of behavior is okay, whether I am hollering, lecturing, joking, listening, or even blanked out. However, when I am alienated from my surroundings or when I am ashamed of something I have done, there is no sense of familiarity in me, only an out-of-it foreignness. Then I have to live through the sense of isolation. Until familiarity returns, I am in purgatory. Frequently, it is a silent purgatory, my very own; sometimes bereft, always alone.

The compulsion for a favorable climate is a root poison I have sucked on a long time; yet, paradoxically, as you will see, it mobilizes my movement in psychological theory and action. Until my adult years, I accepted life pretty much as it came, never creating new climates but operating tolerably well in those which were already hospitable. Under those conditions only half my cylinders were necessary, which was all right with me because I had very little ambition for life to be different from what it was, and in the still waters I lived in, half was plenty. When my own directions began to take root and my need to effect decisions appeared, abrasions came too. I began to care about things that were happening around me and I felt an urgency to be in the center of these happenings. In my first fights, during the early years of our gestalt institute, I lost two friends who left the institute. This was an unsettling experience and through it one aspect of me died and another was born. My exhilaration multiplied but my serenity took some severe lumps. Until I became an in-the-world professional and occasionally got my back up about this or that, I had been playing out an internal bargain to be a nice guy. Even in my early years as a therapist my patients rarely got angry with me and I wondered how that could happen. My colleagues didn't get angry at me either. Alas, I succeeded, at least somewhat, in working out my unavailability to anger. Again exhilaration and anxiety played in-out games. Not a bad bargain, says my presence, but my nostalgia doubts it. Nowadays, I am glad about anger, no matter how painful, when resolution results, but my existential friends can have it when the alienation comes. For many of the people I have admired the most, a conflict here or there adds spice to living and, as for resolution, they can take it or leave it. Apparently for me, utopia still goes a long way.

I did have an early utopia as the first grandchild in a tiny Czechoslovakian village of a man who had twelve children, the oldest of whom was my father. The celebration lasted six months, I have been told. What else was there to do in that village? Then, about time, the novelty wore off. Still, in spite of starting out in a rose garden and having lost my place in it, I never thought one way or another about love as I was growing up. No trouble, except that when it was absent, I simply didn't produce the way I could otherwise. That was safe enough because at home love was about as unconditional as it could be and I didn't have to produce. Such easy acceptance flowed like mother's milk—but what I really needed was a stiff potion that would galvanize me into producing. Not that we didn't have a zillion hassles in our house, but love was never at stake in them so they did not have emergency quality. Mother could be angry, and frequently was, sometimes out of simple irritability and sometimes about charming improvisations like playing basketball in the living room. Her anger was a ripple in the water, though. She never placed any of us in a corner we couldn't get out of. Demands from her and protests from us were standard. Very often her demands would be met as a result of the fights. But hardly always. Nevertheless, there was never an ultimatum or a punishment in our household. I remember that she never even said a word about the pyjamas I wore when I masturbated in bed. When they dried they would look like crackled paper. In my own innocence it never occurred to me that she would know. I would have been mortified. Now I realize that she could not have been *that* innocent and that she was simply remarkably decent to leave me alone in grace with my private discovery and not to spoil my fun, as she could have by intruding her own morality. A friend will do that, of course, giving the loved person the benefit of the doubt. That is something I really like with my friends and I think it is basic to friendship. Among people in the psychological world, generally, I have experienced over and over that kind of openness to another person's way, and whenever I do, I feel a glow, I feel I am in the right place.

A faraway land and a very little boy looking at his mother, she, fresh, ready to hold him when his movement brings him into her fold. As he rides into this seat of all, a message is breathed into the soul of his youngness, indelibly wafted into fresh nostril, and he will know such fragrance always.

Then, one day safety leaves and future comes. A lively gypsy, from an always foreign land, steals the inwards of his life and, though he loves the boy well, the bounds of his gypsy-otherness crease the future and trace a new course. Betraying the boy, in truth, the gypsy also blesses him later with a new primacy, showing him ways into the princely life as gypsy, unfettered by mother-will, beloved anew. The boy fills his well with waters always foreign; rich, but made, not born of self.

Split Between Worlds

My high priority for primal familiarity was not fertilized, of course, only by mother's gypsy stories and her easy love but more pervasively by a split between being a foreigner and an American. I was brought to this country at two and stayed European for a long time thereafter because my home, family, religion, and neighborhood were all European. My sister, one year younger, and I were jokingly referred to as the Europeans and my brother, four years younger than I, was the American, having been born here. This country had charisma, which probably means there was a lot of food, drink, gangsterism, a newspaper in every household, radio, movies, masses of people, excitement and action, informality, and so on. Also, our vast extended family was reunited here. Furthermore, a person had a chance. I used to think about how lucky I was to be here and felt sorry for those who weren't. In my milieu it was always America this and America that, much as an anthropologist might describe a curious primitive island. I only caught glimpses of America, though—in the movies, the department stores, in school, and at the ball park. After I entered school, the split grew and I lived in two worlds, home and out there. Out there all of us spoke English but I understood little of what was going on. At home, my mother always spoke Yiddish to me and I always spoke in English. Nevertheless, we understood each other perfectly.

The differences between my parents and me were just givens, hardly worth notice even though the split was a crucial one. For one thing, my parents knew next to nothing about most of the events of my life. Though this seemed okay, like breathing, it unconsciously accented the novelty of the world out there. Whereas we all grow up spellbound by new *experiences,* for me these were transformed into new *worlds,* accentuating not only the spell, as new experiences naturally would, but also emphasizing my own awkwardness and nonbelonging. When I first saw Santa Claus and later when I first played basketball in a Christian church or hitchhiked or heard stories about marijuana or talked to kids who had been to reform school, I was not only growing up but I was entering new worlds. When I would occasionally over the years relate "American" experiences to my parents or guests at home, they would smile at the incongruity or sometimes laugh hilariously, tickled by the ludicrous unreality, as though the stuff of movies had entered right into the house. Consequently, although I didn't verbalize it, even to myself, I always knew that I was on my own. This circumstance was underlined by the fact that I got my bachelor's degree, spent three years at war, and was already in my second year in graduate school when my father talked to me for the first time about my future. He asked me what this psychology thing was about and was I going to be able to make a living at it. I reassured him that it was going to be all right and he was satisfied, blessed with a strange faith in my own self-regulation. I wish I had had as much faith as he did.

He was a self-possessed man who struggled to support us all and tightened every muscle to keep his body and soul together during the depression. He asked for no help, guidance, or sympathy from anyone and he never gave me any, either. A war story about him, possibly apocryphal but probably literally true, is that he was sent to a Polish regiment in World War I. While living in the trenches he would pull out his Jewish prayer shawl and philacteries daily, binding them liturgically around himself, and pray. The fact that he did this among people, some of whom required only small arousal to slit a Jewish throat, didn't prevent him from doing what was a simple indispensability to him. Life was as simple as that. Fortunately for him, he was never a greedy man. He worked very hard, doing what he could, but never lusted for the world beyond, as I have. Even the most cunning gypsies would never tempt him.

My mother never had to venture into "America" as he did, nor did she ever try to. She was at home in our familial home, in our extended family, and in our neighborhood. In the thirty-four years she lived in this country, she never went outside the neighborhood alone. Not that she felt deprived because all she seemed to want existed within her familiar environment and she was not about to be taught the new possibilities by any of us. At home she could familiarly cook, beautiful; laugh, like music; scream, from a transparent mind, in panic, rage or exasperation; and tell stories, soft. She projected her inner nature reflexively and would sometimes rue the fact that, as she put it, what was on her lung was on her tongue. This also meant, though, that all she had to do was say my name and I could feel her love. But she never was at home in "America" right up until the day she died, when she refused to accept the hospital's oxygen mask.

Somewhere along the borders of my awareness, I frequently felt a gnawing responsibility for my mother, and my sister, too. My father wasn't around because he worked too much. My brother was a simple pleasure, always a luminous person. He would often join in the games of us older boys. I would teach him athletics and just play with him. But I never needed to "do" anything for him. My mother and sister, though, wanted something from me which I could not identify. I was affected by my own feeling that women had a lousy fate in this world and I felt sorry for them. They seemed hemmed in. Nevertheless, I just copped out on them, anyway, going my own way most of the time. Later on, I had some of my warmest conversations ever with my sister. But in our earlier years all I felt was a lingering undertone that I should be more helpful and that I was defecting from my own basic urge to make everything right for her and mother. This urge, maybe more like an obligation then, may have been the psychotherapist budding in a corner of my life, waiting for its instrumentality. But what could I do then? Now I speculate that in my mistaken heart of hearts I was immobilized by the belief that making love was the unavailable instrumentality that would make it all okay.

I knew about the magical possibilities of sexuality in my crib, hearing my parents make love. I didn't know what they were doing but I did know that my mother made sounds altogether outside of my repertoire, strangely deep and from an opening that had to go beyond her throat. I was spellbound and probably fainted dead away but I experienced a pureness of attention in that room which is always present in the most fulfilling experiences in my life, especially, as it happens, in my therapy work. Nevertheless, I forgot about these experiences until I grew up and was left only with a nameless fantasy that one could press the good-life button which in one stroke would bring radiance to people. I still have to say "down, boy," to that one. As for sexuality, it was so far removed from my actuality in childhood that, though I slept in the tiniest of rooms with both my brother and sister until I was fifteen, I never even saw her naked. Such a feat of legerdemain I have seen paralleled only on the beaches of France where, presto, people change in and out of their bathing suits without nudity. Needless to say, my sister and I both missed out on a good thing and I experienced an indispensable distance between me and girls even though I always longed for them.

It is still tempting to think that good sexuality will straighten out one's world and I have no doubt that the Reichian recognitions are magnificent insights into the urgency of orgastic potency. However, where they view the orgasm as the basic requirement of good life, to me it is only a prototypical event. That is, the conditions which accompany orgastic potency are also necessary for all other human potency. Muscular release, engagement of all relevant aspects of one's self, movement through resistance into smooth, exciting function, building then through climax and into release are all essential ingredients in moving to the greatest levels of human potency. This would apply not only to orgasm but also to functions as disparate as vomiting, planning a conference, or even writing a chapter for this book. Though sexual experience is nevertheless a central surge for me, I am also aware that I am at least equally nourished by scintillating conversation, a job really well done, or a time of hilarity. Invariably these register on a par with the most luminous orgasm. Even so, I would always choose the latter.

Moving beyond the home side of me, grade school came as the first of my other-world requirements. During my years in grade school I could not understand the contrast between my school behavior, on the one hand, and my behavior in my neighborhood or at home, on the other. At school I was vastly shy and uncommunicative, daydreamed a lot about saving girls from burning schools and other kindred exploits, and watched the clock interminably. I own a clock like that now and it hangs beautifully in my kitchen. School then was agonizingly boring. But in the neighborhood or at home there was always a lot of action and I was organically involved, more quiet than most but very absorbed and probably strangely serene. I excelled in nothing, yet because of some odd combination of incongruities in me, whenever there was a continuing grouping of people, like a ball team or a social club, I would find I was central, being voted captain or president. The major incongruity to me was between being a spot in the background at school, unnoticed and noncontributing, and being in the clear foreground in my home territory. Only in writing this now do I realize that I was making sure the gypsies couldn't catch me.

Not until graduate school, at Western Reserve University in 1946, did I find a scholastic metier where I experienced the primal familiarity I needed. Not only in school but also for the first time in "America" I finally became a meaningful participant as well as an awed observer. Luck was with me because I went into a beautiful department led by Calvin Hall, who was the most brilliant and inclusive man I knew and who was the person who turned me on to psychology in the first place. My cup ranneth over when I was recognized and included in the workings of that department. I was offered a responsible and exciting assistantship, doing therapy with undergraduates, and later a fellowship. I also became part of a psychoanalytic repartee that blew my mind open to the knowability of persons. Nothing was sacred in that department. I operated there within an altogether new frame of mind, exploring unconscious sensibilities which had ripened long in me and broadening my view of nature almost unassimilably. We, faculty and students alike, presumptuously applied our recognition of each other's deep characteristics, adventurously and incisively confronting each other. We only barely escaped from hideousness by the hilarity of our humor, our abiding affection that transcended specific remarks, and our hardiness. The image of my being affected by castration anxiety or wanting to screw my mother or growing through the psychosexual stages was both ludicrous and compelling. When someone remarked about how deeply hidden my homosexuality was, I was profoundly shocked. I almost swallowed the psychoanalytic message hook, line, and sinker, a risky business but worth it to me. Even though I no longer accept the psychoanalytic perspective, I owe a lot to my willingness to be uncarpingly fascinated with it. Learning happens best for me when, through my intuition, I am willing temporarily to set aside my interferingly critical faculties, absorbing messages as given, as mother's milk or a nursery rhyme. Chewing comes later and is, of course, just as necessary. But my mind expanded by approaching psychoanalysis with the innocence that was native to me and by allowing my sophistication to develop organically. In any case, the new liturgy had timely relevance and was far more exciting to me than the orthodox Jewish liturgy had been even before I gave it up five or ten years earlier.

Once, at a family party, I explained to my uncle that I had

been learning how we all pass through the oral, anal, phallic, and genital stages. He, unschooled and a man of great earthy exuberance, laughed with wide-eyed bawdiness at this ineffable union of the shit-house story and the advanced college education. He beamed in pride that I had been able to pull off such a union. Forever thereafter, even in the face of later missed contacts between us, he marveled at me, as though inexplicably I had become wise in ways he could not under-stand but which nevertheless must reflect indelible marks of my hu-manity. In our experience together at this party we bridged the two-world quality which is a major theme in my life.

The two-world notion is, of course, the natural view of the foreigner, which is to say me. An idyllic view in one sense, because it is simple. Incongruities are not confusing. They are just set apart, each side in its own compartment. But for me, this view was doomed. Once I ventured into the gypsy world I became grandiose. I wanted to go beyond professionalism and exercise my commentary on the world out there. I wanted to experience my power to change it, to have a hand in creating it.

In spite of a new focus on the world out there, I continued to live at home through graduate school. Strangely, though I was already twenty-four when I entered, it never occurred to me to live anyplace else. For one thing, I was dead broke. For another, I had just finished a stint in the Air Force, and after bombing missions, it was a serene pleasure to live at home, where my movements were always my own anyway. In spite of the vastly new experience I was soaking in at school and the new camaraderie with other graduate students, my lifelong friends and my family were still the core of my community. The psychological world was becoming more and more compelling, though, and furthermore, at the end of graduate school I got married. Then I left Cleveland to take a job at the University of Iowa, and though I came back to Cleveland two years later to go into private practice, my two worlds have never meshed well again. One might say I grew up, but I have often felt more like a renegade. Nevertheless, my directions were indispensable. I had married Miriam, who was lovely and added new dimension to my life. She sang beautiful songs, made household lovelies, smiled like sunshine, told stories, and left me trails of funny notes and other endearments. I was spellbound when I was with her. The new home with her was as primally familiar to me as the old, only it was far more exciting. But Miriam did not have the investment in my family or my old friends that I did. Besides, I was up to my ears in new "professional" directions and I didn't have enough energy left to continue also with life as usual.

Gypsies!

The giant step in my new direction came in 1953, two years after starting my practice in Cleveland. Fritz Perls gave a workshop in gestalt therapy and he was a revelation. He was an undulating mushroom of a man, with a large, transcendent head and lithe underpinnings which wrapped themselves into the space he occupied. He was a breathing freedom, like a respirator, and he had a voice that made every word feel like the final accent with which life itself would be endowed. He had a radar sensitivity and a simple faith in the power of staying with people step by step as he worked with them. He could also be trusted in a clutch. I experienced that one day when I raged at him. He had inspired my rage with instructions which finally led to shouting and which left me open to spasms of crying and a return deep inside myself to primitive aloneness. All of a moment, focused on the only light left, inside myself, I felt his warm hand and there he was as I opened my eyes, so tender. I loved him and I embraced him. He said some soft words I can't remember and I felt damp and lubricated all through me.

He was a very tough man, was Fritz, as many people have said, and he is widely known as a person who was cutting and rejecting whenever the spirit happened to move him. It may not be as widely known that he had vast capacity for tenderness, and indeed it was this quality, as well as his unparalleled imagination and sensitivity, that made his work go. One knew that he knew both the authentic agonies and delights of life. Once, during a break in a workshop, he asked me why I was so silent. I told him I was afraid. He said he knew about that, too; that up to a few years earlier, he could not say a word publicly without reading from a paper, so shy did he feel. I was amazed and felt the gift he was giving me. Later, he named me interferer in the group because I had not wanted to say things that might interfere with whatever process was going on. He instructed me to interfere at any point. I wanted to. I did it to a faretheewell, free associating out loud to whatever was going on. Finally he got angry with me. Someone said, "You told him to interfere." Fritz said, "Yes, but I didn't tell him I would like it." I continued to interfere, though, and discovered that what started out as interference wound up as lively leadership, one of the more important lessons I have learned. In spite of his great tenderness, Fritz could turn into a first-class son of a bitch when he felt people trying to capture him or foist a sense of obligation on him. His own unwillingness to inhale environmental poisons communicated the vital message he was always sending: one creates one's own life.

Fritz was an eye-opener in Cleveland as he later was throughout the country. Among us, he found the first place where he had a substantial breakthrough in teaching his method of therapy. He was counterintellectual and, as I now realize, he moved fast into primal familiarity. He described the nature of good contact and exercised it, stripped of amenities and professionalism. He showed how good contact joined with techniques for heightened awareness could provide new leverage into developing profound emotional experiences. The resulting emotionality was a rarity in those days. Even to cry in public, among fifteen people that is, was remarkable then and, in fact, quite suspect for the rest of the community who saw his methods as dangerous and irresponsible. We got a lot of flak in Cleveland in those days about what we were doing, but our new community had too much discovery and excitement in it to leave much room for worry about how well-liked we were by those who spread and heard rumors about our bacchanalian rites. I should have had it so good as the rumors had it.

The basic novelty to me was the accentuated possibility for entering into the *experience* of therapy rather than trying to *understand* the therapy. This simple change in orientation seems old hat now but at the time it presaged a core change in my professional existence. I gave up being merely professional and permitted myself to become as deeply absorbed as is necessary for the sense of primal familiarity. I moved from the periphery of people's lives, which was a tease away from the personal absorption I wanted. I moved out from behind my desk and began to allow myself authentic centrality. Whatever intimacy developed I no longer felt as a professional applique irrelevantly administered by the transferring patient but rather as a just response to my participating artistry, a joined thrill in the creation of fulfilling drama. One of my first patients with whom my gestalt flow became noticeable said to me, "It's not so lonely here anymore." I was teaching another patient how to bark and I succeeded so well my psychiatrist neighbor across the hallway teased me in the elevator the next day about my patients bringing dogs to therapy. When I told him it was no dog, that it was me, he was shocked. Nothing more was said but there is no telling what rumors followed that one. I liked going crazy like that, and my patient learned more from barking than a whole stream of words would have taught him.

Perls was not the only eye-opener. Our gestalt community in Cleveland was, too, as were the other teachers we invited from New York, including Paul Goodman, Paul Weisz, Laura Perls, and Isadore From. When I first saw Isadore From he looked like a scholarly Arabian jockey—tiny, exotic, and elegant in his language and mind flow. He is hardly known outside gestalt circles because careerism is incidental to his life. He only accidentally fell off the psychotherapy tree, ripened by therapy with Fritz and Laura Perls and their wide knowledge of phenomenology. In spite of the great impact of all our teachers from New York, Isadore was the most important to us. They came in for the most fertile workshops four or five times a year, but Isadore stayed with us for six years, coming to Cleveland twice a month at first, then once a month later. His visits were like holidays, not recreational but the kind of holiday which is a harvest of sensation and which addresses itself to life's primary forces. With Isadore, in my private therapy, I talked, cried, screamed, touched, whispered, walked, saw, heard, remembered, fantasied, laughed, and loved. He had a remarkable knack for what was organic between us, never contriving an experiment and never resorting to theoretical fiat. I became a poetic patient, respectful of my inner flow, always moving from initial confusion and verbal constipation into the most heartfelt and eloquent statements I had ever been able to make. He was exquisitely tuned in to my character and his learnedness and wisdom were the fulcrum around which my life grew for ten years after I met him.

Our gestalt community had weekly leaderless meetings for two years, at which time, in 1955, we formed the Gestalt Institute of Cleveland, one of the early growth centers. At first we set up training experiences for ourselves as a learning community, and as we grew, we took on the training of others who wanted to learn gestalt therapy. I was central in this process, leading our first workshops, teaching our first courses, doing private therapy with many who are now our leading people, and being a prime mover in establishing our postgraduate training program. We carved out our own style of function through our joined enterprise, and my part in this has been a major radiance in my work life. This was a place in "America" where what I contributed and what I received were comparable. Being at home among these people was therefore another recycling of my early primal familiarity, joining the old feelings of familiarity and the new associations, restoring the old environment without imitating it. *Le plus que ce change, le plus que c'est le meme chose.*

Present Leaning into Future

What I see as a result of growth centers which have subsequently appeared all over the country is that psychotherapists and their brother workers are now in the midst of developing a populist psychotherapy, by which I mean a psychotherapy which moves beyond patients and offices and addresses the general population.

The traditional psychotherapist's view was the naive one that with good therapeutic experience we would all—those of us who were successful, of course—be enabled to manage the society we live in. Presumably the society had such range within it that anyone in sound psychological form could find a rightful place for himself. Only those who were filled with distortion and obsession could fail to fulfill the requirements of their own directions. It is apparent now that these assumptions were pure pollyanna and that the reality is closer to the graffiti sentiments of our young people who say Horatio Alger eats shit. We wanted only to "cure" people until it became clear that sickness was an obviously inadequate word to describe most of the people we worked with. Then the term *growth* came into phase.

New people came on board, more of them than ever and more who were seeking better forms of living, thinking little of cure and a lot about self-improvement and personal discovery. Excitement became more central than ever as a motivation and the forms of interaction did induce great excitement, leading over and over to experiences of primal familiarity.

A central factor in the induction of this excitement has been what I have called the synaptic experience. This is the experience of personal unity and vibrancy brought on by joining together an individual's awareness with his actions. Since we are all sensory-motor beings through neurological predetermination, we are most complete when our sensory and motor sides are both represented in our existence. There is a variable preference among us for the sensory side over the motor side or vice versa. Under certain conditions, either may cover over the other, thereby causing blockage of our full sense of presence. The restoration of the unity of awareness and action is one of the general directions that growth-oriented groups have taken, calling attention over and over to the specific feelings, wants, values, and assessments which exist for people in groups. The accompanying actions— mostly talking but also including non-verbal acts—come as a result of knowing what is going on inside, such as dancing when one recognizes his wish to dance. Or the other way around, the actions artfully developed may make us newly aware of what is going on inside, like feeling scintillated because one has danced. Whichever way the union happens, a heightening of personal presence develops with an accompanying sense of the primal familiarity involved in being in fresh contact with other people.

Another quality of the growth groups is in the condensation process, which through its power to heighten excitement also reproduces primal familiarity. Condensation is man's way of creating brief but faithful representation of vast stretches of his experiences. Through condensation one expresses poetic as well as literal truth, achieving clarity, parsimony, and meaningfulness. Thus, for example, a person who is large and silent in a group sees himself poetically as an elephant. When he plays out the elephant, he gets into a wrestling match where, in mindless aggression, he nearly injures his partner whom he vanquishes with far greater force than necessary. He is faced with the dismay and fear of people in the group. He thus feels what it is like, perhaps for the first time, to exercise the elephant in himself and he can then fathom the fact that people are frequently frightened of him even though he does not usually do frightening things. The transition from a condensed, surface experience to the underneath behavior results in a whoosh of excitement, releasing the energy subsumed within the symbolic shorthand.

A further quality of the growth group is sanctification, which means setting the group apart from the usual conditions which, in everyday life, are inhibitory. The risks of being fired, divorced, ostracized, misunderstood, punished, and so on, which exist ubiquitously in everyday life, are minimized in these groups. Most of us cannot manage the world of unremitting sequentiality without withdrawing to sanctified opportunities for experiencing that which is usually forbidden. There is no surely desirable proportion between that which is sanctified and that which happens every day, but it is clear that there must be a continuing relationship between the two. Otherwise the sanctified experience would wind up tricky and cultish, splitting the world in two again. Instead, the world out there must be changed by the new experiences of our groups, as will inevitably happen when enough people insert their new discoveries into our everyday world. The more timely and vital the sanctified experiences are, the more revolutionary will be their effect on the population.

Given these conditions for fostering primal familiarity and for developing revolutionary effect, we come to the sociological step which moves not only beyond cure but also beyond growth and into the development of *new climate*. Since none of us can escape the psychological pollution of our surroundings, until we create psychologically necessary changes in our communal climate we in our groups or therapy continue a two-world existence. New ways of communicating; new values; new priorities; changing institutions, such as marriage, schools, and government; new vocational requirements; new reward systems are all parts of a necessary change in the spiritual atmosphere of our society. In a society based on the indispensability of change, as ours is, changes just naturally happen. In this time in history the psychotherapist and his kindred workers are feeding their perspectives and wishes into our sociological stream. They are currently having great impact but are hardly assured at this point of having the most effective voices. The greatest challenge comes as always from the materialistically oriented people who, sometimes through greed, sometimes through habit, and sometimes through the most fundamental need, believe that a chicken in every pot will give us what we need. Materialistic needs, such as eating, for one, are so primordial that in truth they outweigh all other considerations and draw the attention of people and governments. The psychological facts of life, of course, recede into the background, a slight homage being paid through the workings of faded religion. It is therefore from a position of poor leverage that we from the psychotherapy milieu are making our mark. Yet we are doing it and I believe will continue to, without necessarily ignoring basic materialism. Perhaps our move to expand into materialism has already begun through the extensive work of psychologists in industry and the growth of consultations with governments and other social institutions. A further unknown force in the future of our movement may be the effect of pharmaceutical discoveries which, though they could aid the populist cause by fostering the experiences of our new climate needs, may also become a formidable handicap, hindering the populist cause by serving as an easy soporific or as a source of delusion for those who could wind up defused.

In the meantime, through a concern with climate as well as personal growth, we are coming into a more fully holistic view of man, who is not only whole within himself but inseparable from his community. The loosening up of poisonous taboos is happening all around us. Boys are wearing very long hair, young men and women live in the same dormitories, black people appear on TV commercials, communal living foreshadows new forms of family life, peaceniks slow down a war, nude people are seen on stage and screen, men's clothes have become a riotous delight, and so on. Psychotherapy has had an important place in all of these creations, having sent out the message over the years for people to experience their actuality rather than to swallow the stereotypes and distortions which have always made deviations from the norm seem like pathology.

The messages are continuing at an increased rate. One can hardly keep up with new technological prospects that are emerging. Large group innovations have led the way, adding the concept of *design* to the interactive illuminations which were discovered in the open-ended small groups. The designs have supported leaderless interactions, allowing us to work with as many as one thousand people in a room. Large groups have been used in setting up new designs for interaction in conferences, coffee houses, growth centers, housing projects, industry, universities, welfare agencies, town meetings and other normal groupings of people. Our technology now also includes recordings, TV, and self-administered instruments. Furthermore a sociological architecture is developing, as reflected in the new-town movement in particular and in new design philosophies generally. For example, an intimate friend of mine, Philmore Hart, who is a professor of architecture, takes as his fundamental theoretical base the inextricable unity of the psychological side of man and his built environment. He has designed one school without interior walls, wiping out the cellular structure of classrooms. The sense of community is vibrantly apparent to pupils, teachers, and visitors.

Obviously, these brief words about new opportunities for spreading the populist message are only a lick and a promise, hardly doing justice to what requires extensive exploration and critique. They are perhaps enough in this context to suggest why I believe that widespread innovations in humanist technology will inevitably affect the society at large, moving it further into directions which people within the psychotherapy milieu have inspired. For me, during the past twenty years, this entire movement, beginning with my place in the development of gestalt therapy and including my many experiences with people throughout the country, has been a communal home. It is my gypsy home and I have been repeatedly fascinated in it. When I next visit my mother's grave I should tell her about my gypsy experiences. She would have a harder time believing my story than I did hers. After all, what's a mother for, if not to come back to?

Selected Writings

Trends in Gestalt Therapy. Cleveland: Gestalt Institute of Cleveland, 1967.

"A Contemporary Psychotherapy." *Psychotherapy,* 1966. Reprinted in D. Pursglove (ed.), *Recognitions in Gestalt Therapy.* New York: Funk and Wagnalls, 1968.

"Encounter in Community." In A. Burton (ed.), *Encounter: Theory and Practice of Encounter Groups.* San Francisco: Jossey-Bass, 1969.

"Sensory Functioning in Psychotherapy." In J. Fagan and I. L. Shepherd, *Gestalt Therapy Now: Theory, Techniques, Applications.* Palo Alto, Calif.: Science and Behavior, 1970.

The Nature of Gestalt Therapy (in preparation).

VII

Mystery of Self and Other

Bernard Steinzor

I savor the correlation, imagined and real, between the widely acknowledged affirmation of the sixties as the decade when unpredicted libertarian movements arose to deauthorize establishments and the more immediate happenings in my life. These past years, following so suddenly on the so-called apathetic, satisfied fifties, are those when Catholics began to walk out on cardinals, blacks threw the color of whites in their faces, women proceeded to shed their masochistic innocence, and youth became much more than a transitional phase between childhood and the family of procreation.

In 1960, I became forty and life really appeared to begin. Luciana (my present wife) and I met on 1950's Thanksgiving eve, the feast I was taught blessed the native red men and the foreign whites meeting as brothers. Our marriage the following spring appeared to me at that time to justify all the scenes in my own version of Fellini's *8½*, the elapsed time of a four- and five-times-a-week psychoanalysis. The

162

growth of my feverish devotion to Dr. Ellen S. began at the Menninger Clinic in about 1949, where she had come as a training analyst with the impeccable credentials of having been analyzed by Max Eitingon, one of the secret seven ringmates of Freud. She was an outgoing, highly intelligent woman who appeared to have no regard for status. Her qualities must have touched me deeply when she befriended me and even sought me out for advice on group dynamics. Encouraged by her clear interest in me and my family, I became aware of my affection for her and sought her help, outside the formal channels of institute and clinic, to ease my marital discord. The possible advantages of serving a patient apprenticeship I considered secondary, with even the smug thought that I was not sneaking in my neuroses behind the rationale of a training analysis. Perhaps I am still falsely proud, since I continue to think of myself as a maverick who made his way without any of the benefits accruing from membership and certification in any training institute.

I satisfied the first motive for becoming a patient by divorcing Shirley after about the seventh year of the analysis. I should have done this long before. My regret is, I suspect, only because I always feel the poignancy of wasted time whenever I do something which sharply increases both relief and pleasure. (Luciana anticipates that my dying complaint will be "why haven't I done this before!") My only acceptable rationalization left now for sticking in the marriage for twelve and a half years is the fact that the birth of Rena—just now graduated from the University of Wisconsin, where she was editor of the student paper *The Daily Cardinal*—made me a father.

I've accumulated many grievances toward Dr. Ellen S. but few are as sore as my swallowing her dismissing my affection for my young daughter as a crucial variable in debating the wisdom of divorce. Instead, I was told to adhere to the requirements of analysis regarding the elimination of acting out. I had entered treatment, I thought, because Rena's birth precipitated the worst of a difficult marriage, but in the course of treatment she became a figure in my head.

The common sense cliché about the significance of parenthood I can attest to by many memories, including the ambition, formulated clearly when I was sixteen and a well-liked camp counselor, to have six children of my own. Undoubtedly, this ambition had been forseeable, given my mother's appreciation for my help in taking care of my only sibling—a younger brother—and numerous other children she "day cared" during the early depression years when many women sought some work to keep the family from going on relief. During the past ten years, my attachment to Rena has been affirmed through the first book-length manuscript I wrote which in discussing the problems of divorced parents also served as an intense effort to clarify my relationship with her.

Regarding the second motive for entering an analysis, to experience the role of a patient, I have drawn two correlated lessons of dogmatic proportions. Do not trust any system and its proselytizers. Do not give yourself to any person whom you cannot look straight in the eyes and inquire into the condition of his soul. I try to balance my grievance against the years I endured in aggravated anxiety with the depth to which I now feel these dogmas. They have become the rationale for coming into "my own" and helped me feel congruent with the youth identified as the New Left. Compared with the Old Left, their radicalism is antisystem. Power to the oppressed correlates in my book with power to the patients. We are a shifting confluence of systems and we emerge into the mystery of freedom as we become critically aware of all the social (and biological) systems that make us human.

Though there is much evidence that long before the analysis, which I consider the most critical part of my formal education as a therapist, I had developed a strong suspicion of authority, the analysis drove home to me that I must always be embarrassed if I hear myself becoming defensive against challenges to my authority, certified or not.

All the therapeutic denominations have in common the proselytizing of procedures and techniques. In doing so, in the name of a distinctive orientation, the spokesmen certify psychological distance between persons. I try to play only one game in my treatment work: reciprocity of self-revelation. Any feeling and thought I ask the person to share with me I am ready to expose myself.

Perhaps I am especially ready to accept the convenient correlation between events and decades, because I was born right at the beginning of a decade, January 1, 1920. Yet I think it is more than my imagination when I realize how I spent the apathetic fifties in analysis and have emerged in the sixties as a proponent of the equalization of power between patient and therapist. I cannot believe I would have remained prone for so many years had there been in the fifties the noise we now hear so often in the streets. As I have become increasingly guiltless in expressing my selves, I have encouraged persons to carry on wherever they find they can serve the goals of social justice —in the home, in school, at work, and in bed. Encounter groups are wherever we meet people, and it is not necessary to establish them to speak one's mind and heart. Love is increased as clan, caste, sex, and age hierarchies are broken.

Family Romance

I have retained from my studies emphasizing life history an appreciation for the memories of my own. Thus, I think it is evident that I am stirred by the exposure of political values in all our professions because I grew up in a radical home where political questions did move people to make and break long friendships. The contest between my parents for my loyalty, a rather ordinary event in most lives, comes to me vividly in the question my mother would pose to me, "Which flag do you like better, the American or the Red Flag?" Though she was in sympathy with my father's Communist ideology, she continuously felt deprived by his distance from family affairs. I presumed she embraced the American flag more with antagonism against her husband than with devotion to a country where only much later, in the years of Roosevelt, did the government appear to be in league with the common man.

I do not recall the aggregate of my answers to her query about flags, but she continuously bid for my interest and help in ameliorating her loneliness. (It was she who introduced me to better books to read, even though she, like my father, had little formal education.) In her despair, she would often beat me, yet the cat o' nine tails hanging behind the kitchen door (where an occasional salami also appeared) hardly threatened me as did my father's disapproving look. He never raged at me, but a muttered insult—"Animal"—set me wailing. Though I've considered every variant of oedipal interpretation, the facts of my repeated experience with my parents lead me to conclude that though I often became angry wtih my mother, I could appeal to her reason and need for me. With my father I felt hopeless in reaching him and this has been in the depth of my shudders. It is credible to consider that my becoming a therapist who proclaims the virtues of intimacy with fathers as well as mothers was first reinforced by my mother's rewards for being a kind of man who was different from my father.

As the years of the depression accumulated in growing bleakness, my memories began to include my father's energetic devotion to improving the lot of oppressed garment workers and his courage in meeting the vile responses to his apostasy from the Stalinist dogma. Poppa was always at meetings. He has literally devoted his adult life to the labor movement, from the age of fourteen, when he went to work in the pre-World War I sweatshops of New York City, to his recent retirement at seventy-eight, ill and somewhat embittered after serving for long decades as a second-rank administrative officer for the International Ladies Garment Workers Union.

I am certain that much of the passion I manifest for fairness in all relations I absorbed from him. His ideals and his actions in putting his body on the line became a significant part of my idealism, though at a distance, because of his emotional distance and coolness toward all of us. The longing for reconciliation with one's parents, which I think we take to our graves, I've felt sharply with him. Yet despite many frustrations and my recognition of its impossibility, I am surprised at the lift to my spirit when he praises me. No doubt I have overworked my decision to become independent of authority out of my fear that my father and all like him whose approval I search for will finally dishearten me.

Of course, this struggle for love from one's father may mask what I am also supposed to be possessed by: my rivalry with him and need to outdo him. I do not believe that at all despite an awareness of intermittent fury toward him. I wished to be close to him and was puzzled by the disparity between his place in public life and his silent retreats at home. The lively engagement between himself and his friends and colleagues, always in evidence, stood in marked contradiction to the stillness when the four of us were together. So I continue to be preoccupied with the question in all our lives: the distinctions between our public behavior and our private postures, and at times I realize how I become overbearing in my insistence that how I carry on in my vocation should not differ in quality from the mutuality I respect with my family.

I feel heartened by social critics who discern that human relations are developing away from loyalty to designated titles and roles toward the pains and joys of intimacy. Why should a parent and child go on together? Because we should honor our fathers, or because friendship across the time separating a generation is vital to both young and old? If the growth between a parent and a child is not possible, then why shouldn't they divorce, each to seek the possibility of rewarding caring with other children and other adults. I consider it good fortune that most of my close friends are under thirty, and I am affirmed in my aspirations by the fact that Rena and I have become intimate friends after we both chose to break the silence of a few years of complete separation.

Social Categories and the Self

Freud is reported to have once exclaimed to the effect that "They will not be able to call psychoanalysis a Jewish science" when Jung expressed his desire to join the Vienna group. I recalled this story again when reading *The Fifth Profession*,[1] which provides evidence for the common but not openly discussed fact that about half of all those seeking an identity as psychotherapists are from a Jewish background.

Why should we be surprised that the traditions of the groups in which we become ourselves affect our values and actions with those who seek our help? Is it the difficulty in accepting that whatever marks us as different from another, the personal self, is essentially a mystery and that whatever energies we commit to what we call our free choices are often enough derivative? Why do we demean those attitudes and experiences whose essence is held in common by people with similar cultural origins? Repeatedly I have discovered that a precious conclusion I have settled on with considerable cost has been absorbed from others. At such moments, I try to be grateful, and if the experience is painful, I struggle to be tolerant toward my forebears and my colleagues.

[1] W. E. Henry, J. H. Sims, and S. L. Spray (San Francisco: Jossey-Bass, 1971).

Yet what is clearly a logical derivation from our studies in culture and personality, what has come to be called the social psychology of the relationships, whether it be a laboratory experiment, a clinical contact, or the dialogue of friends, was hardly part of my education as a therapist. Of course, my fellow students and I reviewed the differences among the various schools of therapy, even as we became immersed in a particular brand. We were trained to debate and give witness to the system which possessed the truth, yet to be fully revealed, of course. I received the texts first of Rogers and some years later of Freud, always with the stress on their differences. However, both shared the distortion, in seminar or clinic chamber, of simply ignoring the facts of the social origins of the teacher and his disciples.

I studied theory and technique as if these were unrelated to the images I used to evoke the revelations of the "other," who by calling on me took on the social category of client or patient. Even my personal therapy did not seriously address my Jewishness, my being a first-generation American, my working-class consciousness, or my faith in human progress toward a world of brotherhood. I lay at the chair of a refugee from Hitler, a woman whose ambition must have been formed in an aristocratic German-Jewish household. Yet our respective ethnic and class sensibilities were never considered as forces in the transference and its counter.

Sexuality as psychosexuality, of course, but as social sexuality? Was my very limited sexual experience prior to my first marriage only due to mother fixation and father castration? I have come to envy and respect the young and their readiness to exclude the pleasures of sex from the question of marriage and to include them in friendship.

Who can quarrel with Rogers' emphatic moral: Respect the person's capacity for self-development.

I recall the early months of 1942, in the Saturday morning seminar on counseling at Ohio State. We were privileged to read, in manuscript form, Rogers' *Counseling and Psychotherapy* which a few months later announced the emergence of the first genuine American approach to the treatment of troubled people. At one point, in those first exuberant weeks, I exclaimed with some passion, "But this non-directiveness is really rugged individualism!" My remark was met with no more than momentary laughter. Today, my pleasure in its recollection is also increased when I read of Rogers' advocacy of encounter groups. Still, I remain critical of the leaders of the encounter movement because of their nondiscussion of how their groups bear a resemblance to religious revival meetings and to the methods of a variety of action groups determined to erode the power of the state.

There is hardly any analysis of the historical determinants setting many people on this road to personal salvation. Philip Rieff[2] has helped me understand how leaders, bound to their ambitions to create a movement, drift into a demand for commitment and thus fail to realize the intractable paradox between salvation and objectivity. My favorite fairy tale has become "The Emperor's New Clothes." I fancy myself playing the little boy's game and this is one way of explaining why I welcome the politicization of our profession, whether it is expressed in radical criticism of all our dispositions (as medicine men versus wise teachers) or expressed in some outrageous action (nonviolent, I insist). We are all on an ego trip, contained in a struggle for power and for love. It behooves me, when I call on the public to call on me, to be continuously self-critical regarding the manifestations of power granted to me by the groups in which I have developed and by the inherited temperament and energy which give thrust and resonance to my opinions. I must first consider my good fortune in having had the background, and the relatively good health, which brought me into a vocation of being human. Our historical times have been most propitious ones for the growth of the spirit and practice of our work. We have been very well rewarded in finding our ways as healers. Sought after and recently consolidating our position in law, our ways appear as secure as anything can be in the forseeable future.

My Parents' Parents

I never met my mother's parents. She was fourteen when she, her older sister, and older brother left them in Bialystok, never to see them again. My mother has hardly talked about them, an omission I ascribe not only to the pain of her depression over separation but also to a lack of an education which gives value to personal history. Now, I always counsel parents to reveal their own stories to their children.

My father also did not speak about his parents, but I knew

[2] *The Triumph of the Therapeutic* (New York: Harper and Row, 1968).

them well, both having died in their middle nineties in a New York City old-age home. My grandfather came to the United States because the streets were paved with gold, earned enough to send for his oldest son, my father, and after a few years was able to bring over his wife, to whom he was married by arrangement, and four other chlidren. An orthodox rabbi, he worked as a sexton of a large synagogue in the Bronx. Reb Eli was a dominating, intolerant, and self-righteous man. I cannot remember a single incident of compassion from him. My own difficulties with my father were often eased when I remembered what a father mine had.

My Bube, in contrast, was the only person from whom I ever felt unqualified love. She was an extraordinarily kind person, and I may have benefited also from being the first son of her first son. We never talked much to each other but I always felt happy in her presence. As a child, I often was left in her care. My earliest memory is of being at her home in possession of her devoted attention during the days when, I later learned, my mother was in confinement with my brother. His birth is noted in my recollection on the day of his ritual circumcision at my grandparents' home. The sense of displacement was strong. My first awareness of loneliness and terror dates to that June afternoon when I was four and a half.

Though both my parents rewarded independence, my father by noninvolvement and my mother by her hearty approval of my initiatives in helping her with household chores and the care of my brother, it was my grandmother who provided the sense that independence need not be lonely or exploited. The last time I saw her she was in the hospital ward of the Beth Jacob Home for the Aged, almost deaf and blind, complaining why God did not take her. She did not recognize me when I came to her bedside. She caressed my face and after some minutes she spoke, "Boruchel, you who always have been independent."

Jew and Christian

When my father was in his late teens, his father threw him out of the house for nonobservance of orthodox ritual. He had become a Marxist years before I was born and I was brought up to consider God as the needle through which opiates were shot into the people. Yet my brother and I were raised as self-conscious Jews, required to attend nonreligious Jewish language schools after we were dismissed from public school. I did not speak English until I was four or five years old.

My parents have experienced anti-Semitism much more than I have. I felt comfortable in the cultural ghetto, persuaded as I came of age that the worst oppression was from capitalism. Yet the consciousness of Jew and Gentile was always sharp, and only since my early thirties have I become fully at ease with non-Jewish people. An obvious factor in this point is that my second wife was raised a Catholic.

I am accenting my preoccupation with Jewishness, a feature I believe I share with all Jews of my generation, because of a most unexpected turn in my career line which markedly influenced my work as a therapist. In 1958, through a series of quite *ordinary* events (a diagnostic test referral and an invitation to a panel discussion) I came into contact with Dr. Earl Loomis, then the director of the Program of Psychiatry and Religion at Union Theological Seminary. (I stress the word *ordinary* because I am convinced that we never can tell at the time the significance of an event.) Shortly after our meeting, he began to refer seminarians to me, which also helped much in the early period of private practice. Quickly I was drawn into thinking about liberal Christian young men and women. For the first time, I began to read in religion and the Bible. Earl also invited me to teach in the program, and shortly after I began as a lecturer at the Seminary, Dan Williams asked me to join him in presenting a seminar on psychiatry and religion in the spring of 1964.

That spring, with Dan and Union students, I celebrate as the time I fully found my voice, in a paper whose title, "On Faith, Doubt and Suffering," conveys something of the impact of theological categories in my thinking about healing. I had always felt defensive in discussing intellectual questions with my professional colleagues and religious questions with Jews. My father and I, for example, never discussed religion. But Dan and the others received me with grace. I had found a fully encouraging intellectual father figure who even surprised me by suggesting I expand the paper into a book. I then wrote *The Healing Partnership*.

I like the image of an apostate Jew finding his way among

liberal, social gospel Christians. I, to whom a cross had been a sign of
a pogrom, learned much in the presence of the thought of Dan Williams and of Reinhold Niebuhr. (Interestingly, my father had long
before become a coworker with Niebuhr in the Liberal Party.) From
these thoughtful men of nondogmatic faith I came to feel the con-
tingencies of man's judgments and pride. Though a scientific training
did help me to be skeptical about any psychological theory, it was not
until I worked with religious humanists that I deeply felt the sins in
my work with people and understood in detail how the self is itself
always under judgment and always emerging in relative mystery. My
character and my history make it impossible for me to convert to any
institutionalized faith. At times I wish I could speak of God with the
measure of belief with which some of my devout friends speak of Him.
But the pressure of transcending forces in relationships besides those
recognized by the persons has become real for me, often in that sudden
rush of feelings when we break into open ground previously marked
by a no-trespassing sign.

Youth in the Age of Roosevelt

My brother and I were well protected from the severity of the
depression. We never went hungry or ill-clothed. I was aware of the
unpaid rent and my parents' preoccupation with unemployment,
and the increasingly bleak prospects as the months of hard times added
up to years.

My teens began almost exactly with FDR's election to the
presidency. How often I've remembered his sentence, "We have
nothing to fear but fear itself." The leader of the American people
talked to them and acted for them. Radicals, unionists, liberals, and
the common man began to feel integrated with the government of the
people. Adolescent and youthful self-consciousness was tempered in
hope for the future, in the belief in American progress and American
goodness. For the first time I began to feel I was an American. The
Stars and Stripes had won out over the Red Flag, for my father as
well as for me.

My sense of being spoken for by the president and my faith
in the honesty of our government were disturbed only for a short period
just as the war in Europe began. Elements of pacifism, and Marxist

analysis of wars among capitalist states, led me to join in the Oxford pledge never to support my government in war. I think the mobilized fear of death had much more to do with this distortion of the necessity of sacrifice to stop Hitlerism.

I still regret that I did not seek a more active role in the fighting. By the time I was drafted in 1941, I had completed my master's with Carl Rogers at Ohio State. I sought to continue my career as a psychologist in the service and was soon assigned to the Psychological Research Unit of the Air Force, which developed and administered selection tests for pilots, bombardiers, and navigators. It was a frantic yet really easy time for all of us serving in a safe position as the ferocity of the battles in Europe and Asia increased.

We were a large group of psychologists, a large number of whom were already prominent in the field and many of whom were to go on to make significant reputations. The images of Laurence Schaeffer, Neale Miller, Nicholas Hobbes, Urie Bronfenbrenner, John Harding, Harold Proshansky, George Klein, Donald Super, Gerald Blum, Herman Freifel, and Leo Srole come to mind most easily. Also being married, as I was one year after Pearl Harbor, made it possible to live in town and commute to the jobs at the camp. Much of the world was ablaze, but we chattered ungratefully about the light discipline we had to endure and enviously watched the promotion lists.

In 1944, I began to suffer from an ailment in my left eye whose origins were never diagnosed. Treatments and surgeries only led to my being discharged in early 1945 almost blind in one eye. I became a disabled veteran, never having fired a shot at the enemy. A sense of cowardice still comes to me, as well as the apprehension over bodily failure, particularly blindness.

Though less and less, I still find myself arguing with younger friends about the possibilities of this land and people of ours. I call up historical perspectives about the rise and fall of such imperial powers as Sweden and the Italians. But my optimistic convictions come, I'm sure, from the years in which my social and vocational identities were developed in unified feeling with men who had the highest authority over us. It is these memories and my own chagrin at not having taken risks enough in being with my country against Satan's incarnation that serve to temper my rage against the lies which have spewed from our leaders in the past ten years. I have always been very

intolerant of what I sensed was a distortion. I recollect with some
pleasure that in the sixth grade I called my teacher a liar when she
accused me of soiling a book. I am too often overbearing in pushing
people for clarity and self-disclosure. But again, what I think has
helped me much in recovering whatever tolerance I muster toward the
ambiguities and injustices inherent in social life is the fact that I, a
first-generation son of a Marxist Jew, came of age in years of increasing identity with America. My hopes for the American system seem
to me to have been personally amply fulfilled. My capacity to identify
with oppressed people has always been strong and rather quick. I
think I can empathetically understand the rage of prisoners and blacks.
Yet the relative affluence, educationally, materially, and emotionally,
which my loved ones and I have attained stands in marked contradiction to the awareness of social injustice. Feelings of hypocrisy arise
mostly around my applause for those who struggle against injustice and
my relative inaction buttressed by fears of losing my good fortune. I
suspect that I partly compensate for these conflicts by taking large
risks with people I care for. When Rena, whose radical interpretation
of world events sometimes takes me aback, says that I live a revolutionary existence in the ways I relate to people, I feel comforted.

Teen-Age Peers

We were at first the Red Pirates (of course, Red!) and then
as we became accustomed to the wish to go on together as friends, we
called ourselves the Incas, choosing that name to demonstrate that we
knew that others than white men could develop a great and peaceful
civilization. There never has been a question in my mind that what
I believed was our superiority as a group was actually so. Though we
took our share of championships in punch ball and basketball, we
displayed our special powers by raising whatever money we needed by
producing plays written by one of our members. The other clubs
merely sold raffles.

For me, the companionship was also a great relief since the
usual young person's apprehension over being accepted by peers was
aggravated by the vitriol peculiar to the party politics of the Left. In
one of the twists of the Communist line, my father had been expelled
from the Party and became a target of political hatred from the
majority of our neighbors in the cooperative apartments where we

lived through my adolescent years. But the differing political attitudes of our parents did not affect the Incas' loyalty to each other. I recall all these friends with a very special fondness even though I am no longer in touch with any of them.

Vocational Decision

I was never brilliant, though always a good student, and generally dutiful even when bored with the required studies. To begin with, going to school and learning something was a privilege, so the relevance of what I studied was rarely questioned.

Jeb Barmack taught the first course in psychology I took, in 1938, in a style composed of highly organized lectures, assignments, and quizzes. This was just right for me as was his making available the work of Freud, Klineberg on "Race Differences," and Dashiell. I did well, yet a concern to choose a field where I could make a living persuaded me to become a high school teacher, first in math and then, when I lost interest in that, in physical education. The wisdom of my body prevailed through various injuries, and so I went on in psychology where my pleasure in being with children, as a camp counselor, could be disciplined.

Gardner Murphy came to City College in 1939 to head the newly formed department of psychology which until then had been a section of the studies in philosophy. His reputation as well as his presence generated enthusiasm among faculty and students. We were pioneers in the development of a new department whose director was a man with an international reputation and who wrote books with his wife. I met Lois Murphy briefly when they entertained the honor students, and a decade or so later taught and researched with her at Sarah Lawrence.

We took courses amid the clatter of the conversion of the top floor of Townsend Harris into laboratories and special offices for honor students doing independent research. Among these students, I recall Daniel Lehrman (who even then was already at work on the problem of instincts and impressed me as the one most likely to become famous), Mervin Freedman, Morris Stein, Herbert Krugman, Herbert Zucker, and Harold Proshansky. When I graduated, I had completed a research on personal tempo. I recall with amusement that the younger psychology major, quiet and diffident, who assisted me in statistical work was Roy Schaeffer.

For many years I did not appreciate this work on tempo, which I investigated as an example of the questions psychologists then were heavily into: whether traits were generalized or specific. It turned out to be a fine introduction to what is always a dilemma in an interpretive mode of psychotherapy. I'd like to think these first data became a source for the present skepticism I insist must accompany any generalization I offer to a person about his character. I have become convinced that such generalizations, in clinical categories or whatever, are largely loaded with attitudes of superiority and have both the covert intention and effect of controlling the patient. I have thus become concrete problem-feeling oriented. I maintain that abstractions about styles are useful only when they serve to open a new understanding in the reality of a particular relationship. Of course, a later exposure to diagnostic procedures also served to increase my circumspection in the use of categories. Yet my undergraduate training provided a strong intellectual base of scientific skepticism. Even the learning of the Rorschach from Max Hertzman I recall now as occurring in the spirit of something to play around with rather than use as a fabulous instrument. (I asked my girlfriends to come up and see my inkblots.)

One other experience brought the psychology majors together at a time which I realize now was the last period in my life when I felt I was a full participant in a community. Many of us joined to protest the 1940 harbingers of the McCarthy period, the Rapp-Coudert Committee investigating subversives at City Colleges. Bertrand Russell was denied a professorship at City College through a taxpayers' suit accusing him of subverting the morals of youth. And a short time after a number of regular college staff, including some psychology faculty, were fired, accused of belonging to subversive organizations. Our protests were to no avail, but I cannot believe that any of us who tried to combat the philistines of those days could ever lose sympathy with the efforts of students interested enough in their education to wish to join in the formulation of educational policy and the university's relation to the surrounding community.

Three Years at Chicago

After the medical discharge from the Army in January 1945, I chose to study under the G.I. Bill at the University of Chicago because

I had learned that Carl Rogers would be coming there in September. By the time he arrived I had discovered the Committee on Human Development. The feeling of good fortune for my intellectual development I felt at the time has increased with the years. Not only was the psychology department moribund, but here was an interdisciplinary program calling for preparation in all the social sciences and in biological study as well. Robert Havighurst administered the program in the spirit of the university which had for some years encouraged students to work at their own pace. Now, whenever I bewail the parochial developments in psychology in the name of standards and credentials, I am gratified to the Committee which educated students in the non-parochial spirit in which psychotherapy itself should be practiced.

After Rogers arrived, I learned that he had come to establish a Counseling Center. Though he soon asked me to join the staff, I did feel strung out because he hadn't directly invited me to come to Chicago as he had some others of his students. That was the first time I felt hurt in not being among the favored few, and it was a forerunner of repeated struggles to keep my jealousy over the success of others in balance. I now feel that my conflict over being recognized by people I admire has contributed to my departures from institutional affiliations into a work setting essentially solo—private practice.

I cannot attribute to Rogers anything but fairness and encouragement of his students and associates to develop in their own ways. He worked with the Counseling Center staff in a truly democratic way as we developed policy, discussed our clients, or decided how to furnish the waiting room. I realized much later that the very first expression of what became my major hobby, woodworking, grew out of the spirit with which we met together. I designed and built a playhouse for the play therapy room, the one that Virginia Axline's "Dibs" used in his work with her.

I am rather sure, too, that I always had an unarticulated restlessness with Rogers' exclusive emphasis at that time on the technique of reflection of feeling. My temperament had pushed me much to a direct and personal form of address. I must have been troubled with the injunction that to respect the client and not moralize with him, I had to largely suppress my own imagery, let alone my temperament. Later on, as the pretense of all schools of therapy to attain a value-free mode of commentary to the person broke down, I understood better my early restlessness with Rogerian teaching. I crow a little now when I read Rogers' latest description of his work with people, but also remember how much all of us have been encouraged to authenticity by social changes heavily headlined as the cultural revolution.

After a year and a half at Chicago, I accepted Havighurst's offer to become his assistant, a privilege that I occasionally wish I had pursued much longer. I was in a hurry, however, and soon passed my prelims, developed a dissertation plan, and completed it in another year. I had not yet been able to integrate social psychological ways of thinking and my clinical interests. Even while maintaining my contacts with the Counseling Center, the research for my doctorate was in the field of group dynamics, then just beginning to take hold under the auspices of Kurt Lewin and what came to be known as the Bethel Bunch.

I developed a measure of group interaction. It was an extensive schedule and rather cumbersome compared to Bales' method, which he created just about the same time. But no sooner had I received my doctorate than I suppressed my interest in social psychology and in teaching. George Klein, whom I met in the Army, encouraged me to apply for a straight clinical position at the Menninger Clinic. Why I was in such a hurry to leave Chicago remains a mystery. Shirley and I had become aware of marital difficulties by then, but they seemed ordinary in the context of the cooperative way we managed for her to get her master's in social work at the time I received my doctorate.

Topeka Days

In February 1948, Topeka was the center of the post-war boom in the production of mental health professionals. Under the leadership of Drs. Will and Karl Menninger, the Clinic was the largest training facility for psychiatrists in the world. Like every visitor, I was impressed and awed by the famous clinic, begun in the early twenties by their father, Dr. C. F., who was still an active presence among the patients.

Psychology at the Menninger Clinic was not a second-class profession. David Rapaport, Sybille Escalona, Margaret Brenman, Robert Holt, George Klein, Lester Luborsky, and Roy Schaeffer had made psychology the leader in research and the equal of the medical analysts in the development of psychoanalytic ego psychology. Psychologists were accepted there for analytic training. After I had demonstrated proficiency as a diagnostic tester, I became a member of a diagnostic team but also began work as a therapist.

What impressed me most, however, was the open-mindedness among the leaders that encouraged the use of therapeutic orientations other than the psychoanalytic. Paul Bergman, a lay anaylst, was experimenting with Rogerian methods, and disciples of Wilhelm Reich were invited to join the staff. In staff discussions, particularly about hospitalized patients, the central emphasis was on the therapist's attitude toward his patients. The relevance of nurses, aides, and occupational therapists in the treatment of people was always underlined. I was again in the middle of a pioneering program and this time in the Corn Belt, in a town of 100,000, where I also experienced an intense cosmopolitan culture.

The years at the Menninger Clinic were the last in my career in which I worked closely with mental health workers. Whenever I become regretful in not being a part of a large institution, I think of the Menninger Clinic where I learned much about clinical work with all sorts of people. Whenever I argue for a variety of humanistic, subjective, and artistic experiences as most helpful in the coming of age of a therapist, I wonder if I can talk this way because the Menninger years of engagement in the daily tumult in the lives of addicts, deluded people, suicidal ones, gave me the confidence to speak.

Marital Breakdown and Psychoanalysis

Shirley was a social worker at the Clinic until shortly before Rena was born in August 1949. Though I was able to function in my work I began to feel unavoidably anxious. I could no longer deny that something was quite wrong in our marriage even though I learned much later that becoming a parent was a common enough trauma.

So I began therapy with Dr. Ellen S., and when she left for New York City, I resolved to follow her. The connection between the job I would seek in New York and my vocational interests seemed hardly important compared to the continuation of my analysis. In September of 1950 I thus unthoughtfully began a nine-year position at Sarah Lawrence College.

It has become fashionable for disillusioned defectors from causes to publicly confess and accuse the gods that failed. The history of psychoanalysis has been in large part a contrapuntal struggle between defenders of the faith and the heretics. I realize that in confessing my own defection I am a conformist. Yet I take pleasure not only in seeing myself among the heretics but in the fact that I now stand apart from all movements, perhaps in defensive pride to counter the considerable loneliness which membership in a movement ameliorates. I also think that we all benefit from patients' views of their therapeutic experience and there just has not been enough of these from professionals as patients. Many years ago we heard from a group of six prominent psychologists about their experience as analysands, and much too little since.[3]

I could go on and on about my years on the couch, but among the reasons that limit my fire is that I still find it difficult to laugh. The only possible joke I see in it is that E. S. was a great knitter and needlepoint artist, and though she completed many a garment and many a pillow cover, she never responded to my comments, so that as much as I knew I loved her, she still reminded me of Madame De Farge. It was a long ride in that tumbril pursuing the holy grail of the unconscious, followed by blurred years to recuperate from a broken, unrequited devotion.

I confess, however, that it was she who finally ended the ride. Declaring me unable to free associate because of my ego's adhesions to the past and an anal sadistic refusal to give her the pleasure of the release of my complexes, she set a terminal date, and stuck to it, when once, upset when rejected by a woman, I asked her to resume the engagement. I should be thankful to her for finally breaking my addiction, yet I cannot, since it was exploited for so many years and reasons. Not, however, for monetary gain, even though the habit cost me approximately thirty thousand dollars. I blanch at that incredible self-indulgence.

The system and E. S. as a person held me in awe and anxiety. The awe I think grew out of a need to submit to the most prestigious powers (my father?) and to the noblest, most intellectually sophisticated belief system in clinical work, let alone among modern meta-

[3] "Symposium: Psychoanalysis as Seen by Analyzed Psychologists." *Journal of Abnormal Psychology,* 1940, *35*(1 and 2).

physics. Who wasn't fascinated by Freud's erection in the thirties and forties? And should I count myself as a non male chauvinist pig in devoting myself to a woman years before women's liberation? These issues she and I never dealt with. Now, my patients might complain that I badger them excessively to look me in the eye and to challenge my assumptions and prejudices. When they thank me, I counter with my appreciation for their help and for all others who speak honestly to them. They appear dependent; I point that out. As soon as they feel they are my children, I promote them to colleague.

I was anxious most of those years. There was my unsatisfactory marriage to a dominating woman. I was passive, no doubt, and aggressive, no doubt, and my romance with my parents needed inspection. And the work at Sarah Lawrence was stumbling along, probably be cause I shouldn't have been there. Though I was enamored of the educational philosophy of the college (we taught students, not subjects) and possibly the attractive young ladies, I more often felt abrasive toward the upper-class sensibilities and good fortune of most of the students.

I was engaged in other part-time endeavors. I learned to work with teachers, parents, and their children as a school psychologist. And for four years I was the psychologist at the Morningside Mental Hygiene Clinic. This and Clark's Northside Clinic were the only interracial agencies serving the Harlem area. However, whenever I raised with my analyst my discontent about giving most of my professional energies to an institution with which I felt out of sorts, I was greeted with a variant of the psychoanalytic view about childhood fantasies. She once even reassured me that my not being challenged in my work at the college was useful in the sense that it provided a kind of sanitarium setting for the work she and I were doing. What an insult toward my colleagues and students! It is this quality of contempt for the meanings of one's realized existence that I recall with greatest irritation toward her and psychoanalysis. Reductionism (not historical analysis) is the bone disease of analysis, whose major symptom is an inward denigration of the importance of other people's work in other walks of life. How can we not see that our job is not only to save something of the present from the past but to consider the future as an unfolding of ourselves and the community of men? Freudians try, through reducing the untold meanings of our experience to a master revelation of buried complexes, to achieve a cure, once and for all. Paradoxically, the current vogue in therapeutic propaganda, albeit highly critical of analysis and grossly anti-intellectual, is offering the possibility of master revelations through primal screams, strips, touches, and whatever produces a circus of ecstasy.

There is one obvious quality in the current agitation for various kinds of encountering, however, which appeals to me: irreverence of the accepted norms. In present social concepts, the psychoanalysis I experienced stood fully on the side of law and order. The phrase used then was acting out. What that now means to me was an almost complete loss of proportion as to what acts are worthy of scrutinizing as immoral.

Once, in an argument, I threw my wife on the floor and my analyst noted the acting out as obscuring my awareness of my murderous wish. Any demonstration of anger or gluttony or sexuality could be grist for such a mill. I kept trying to pacify myself in order to experience the truth to be found in verbalized memories and fantasies. It just couldn't be my style. I'm six feet tall, a mesomorph with much restless physicality which got throttled during the process. I have a passionate temper, sometimes quickly and loudly aroused. Others think I am furious when I am only speaking loudly. No wonder I felt anxious for, in Freud's original idea, I suffered from dammed-up energy.

Perhaps she was right in saying I was trying to kill my father with each outburst and petty meanness. I tried to undo in analysis everything I learned to value about my father's ideology, and to change something one must demonstrate loudly and develop plans for action which can make a powerful opponent willing to negotiate on equal terms.

One further matter which has special reference to me and yet reflects on important questions in all our therapies. I have often speculated that what may have certified my bondage to her was the fear of going blind. The psychosomatic possibility regarding the illness in my eye which led to its loss was not to be ignored. Indeed, it was occasionally suggested that I might have gone only half as far as Oedipus himself. I have thus learned to be exceedingly circumspect in helping a person with physical disability and bodily pain who in his search for relief may play into any fantasies I have about being a magician. Anytime I formulate a psychosomatic hypothesis, I make sure the person considers this as a possible move of mine to dominate his life. Rather than interpret symbolic meanings of a person's bodily pains, I would rather talk with him outside the regular hours about the rest of his life and help him find an adequate physician.

Enough of the collected grievances which even when placed in a theoretical context smack of some self-pity and self-justification. Who hasn't gotten stuck in some process and felt afterward the waste of it? And perhaps I should even be thankful for those years in thrall which were followed, according to the best stories of positive outcome of therapy, by increasingly happy and "career productive" decades. After the divorce and three years of enjoying my freedom, learning from some casual and a few involved affairs, I met Luciana, fell passionately in love, got married, had two lovely daughters, wrote two books and some papers, and actualized myself as a therapist.

My Selves in the Office and Out

Anyone who sits in one place and has people from various walks of life come to sit with him and tell him their stories is a fortunate person. Without moving about in the world, I not only partake in the lives of ordinary teachers, parents, and students but find myself with civil rights advocates, organizers for the rights of disadvantaged children, couples forming communes, gay activists, movie and candlestick makers, computer technologists, and even some professional colleagues from whom I get the latest gossip. I intrude myself to make sure the person knows what he is offering me besides a fee.

Such vicarious pleasures do much to help me accommodate to the lives I never can live. Yet these unsolicited, unintended gifts also provide the context for the continuous rearousal and reinterpretation of my own anguish. Some people whom I recall with sorrow have helped me know fear and a few even terror. As the person becomes less impressed with my presence as a totem pole and more related to the conditions which give life to my efforts to help, he often enough shows me something fresh about ourselves.

Once I gained this perspective—that the person gives me in his ways as much as I give him—I learned to speak in the language of negotiation. For us to evolve an adequate contract through which our respective interests converge, the person and I must continuously monitor our respective vested interests that are in conflict. He and I review our thrusts for power and for love which thwart the other. If we fail to comprehend each other, it is our relationship that fails and not his personality or my character. No relationship, I insist, should imply that it contains wisdom that is unavailable elsewhere. I distrust any idea and sentiment, as understandable and enjoyable as they may be when sharing them with another person, as soon as they become labeled and part of a system. This includes the encounter movement, when it is presented as a way of therapy and not as a set of values which as variously expressed reflect change of attitudes toward what is private and what is public.

I suppose I could be labeled as having a high need for auton- omy. Though I would accept that as a designation encompassing my relative lack of investment in any professional organization, I think I am also ready to become dependent on another person who appears ready to do so with me. Thus from the beginning moments of meeting a patient I am ready to consider sharing with him my lives outside the office. In turn, I do not hesitate to act and converse with people I meet in nonprofessional contexts in the same ways I do with those who pay me for my time and services. Psychotherapy thus be- comes a way of life between any two persons who agree to converse in a self-critical and open-hearted fashion. Most people with whom I become so involved are met in my office, which I consider to be only a matter of the times we live in. It is apparently still easier for many to begin the process of self-revelation with another when the concen- tration of attention is on themselves, and they also feel safer to do so because they pay the person for his presumed professional talent to guide them through troubled hours with others without undue distress.

So, we choose one another, and hopefully the unknown reasons will sooner than later become clearer to each other. Sometimes they do in a rather sudden, even explosive way which may result in rapid good- bys. These occurrences are much to be preferred to holding on out of fear of not facing one's problems. (The possibility that I am promiscu- ous and fickle in being with another is certainly to be considered.) I have been accused of threatening to break off when things don't go my way and I am vulnerable to this charge if only because I have become able to affirm the other's right to leave as well. Undoubtedly, of much increasing significance, in addition to what may be an over-compensation for my personal experiences as an analysand, is the con-sciousness of aging and time passing.

I was told in early childhood that I almost died in infancy. Thoughts of wasted time and the brevity of life are daily preoccupa-tions. Though my appetites and pleasures balance what could become a morbid trend in my "rage, rage against the dying of the light," as Dylan Thomas has phrased this feeling, it is likely that my readiness to break with persons, no matter what the anguish, is influenced by this consciousness of death. More and more I hear myself defining a difference between others and myself as due to differences in age. And as any views of life can become self-fulfilling, I am increasingly persuaded that social and personal change is very real and very con-tingent on the times and contexts in which we come of age.

I suppose I am wishing myself a very long life so that in future decades I can reread what I have now written and realize how differ-ently I then made sense of my times. This will satisfy my wish for change and increasing diversity. Yet above all, I hope that I will find myself with more people who struggle to coordinate their lives as citizens and their public reputation, large or small, with their lives in intimacy and shared joy and suffering.

Selected Writings

The Healing Partnership: The Patient as Colleague in Psychotherapy. New York: Harper and Row, 1967.

When Parents Divorce: A New Approach to New Relations. New York: Pantheon, 1969.

"On N+1 Person Groups." In A. Burton (ed.), *Encounter: Theory and Practice of Encounter Groups.* San Francisco: Jossey-Bass, 1969.

VIII

The Therapist Has a Small Pain

Arthur Burton

There is a natural repugnance in man which militates against revealing the innermost details of his life. For a professional this places Pelion on Ossa, and perhaps explains why this book is a first of its kind. Indeed, we have all been trained to guard ourselves against disclosure, and even the best of personal analysis does not release us from this covenant. But, as we know, every need has its counterneed, and telling "one's story" is its own compulsion, as the popularity of autobiography demonstrates.

Psychotherapists have to listen so much that we at times wonder when our turn to talk will come. But psychotherapy, treatmentwise, is not so one-sided as it appears. The therapist's "third ear" is

186

always busily at work constructing his own existence as well as that of his client. Unfortunately, most of this therapeutic inner life is covert and shadowy, possibly even felt to be antitherapeutic, so that very little of it ever comes to light. The underlife of the psychotherapist is apt to remain down under! A psychotherapist who attains authenticity has automatically closed the gap between his real and therapeutic selves.

This chapter—like all others in this book—is a product of conflict: the conflict between disclosure, on the one hand, and clamming-up or analyzing, on the other. How to keep from presenting oneself in the best possible light, or contra, in the worst possible way, and yet preserve the objectivity which is the scientific mandate is the problem in writing such an autobiography. But is objectivity the proper word for the depiction of an inner life? It suffices, I suppose, that the objective intention is there; but no autobiography is ever seriously objective for it would then perhaps not be worth reading. I have partially solved this dilemma for myself by asking one of my longer-term clients to describe how she experiences me in therapy. By placing this side by side with how I experience myself, I may then bring some reasonable control to my vanity in this report.

This is not the place, nor is there actually publishing space, to give a complete documented history of oneself. I have instead selected those aspects of my life which I believe led me to become a psychotherapist and which allowed me to function in this way. I call the essay "The Therapist Has a Small Pain" because the important retrospective experiences seem all traumas of a sort—which they apparently are to all in this book—but traumas which paradoxically lead to fulfillment and joy, to being an identified person.

Being Jewish

I was born and am a Jew. My father came from a small "shtetl" in Moldavia, and my mother from that part of the ancient Austrian Empire of Franz Josef which Isaac Bashevis Singer describes so beautifully in his inimitable stories. Our home was kept in the orthodox tradition, and while my brother and I—the two offspring of this union—rebelled against it, its symbols, rituals, history, and identifications have always loomed very large in us. One knows this, in a sense, by one's identification with what happened at Dachau and Auschwitz. In 1971, when I visited the Jewish Memorial in the Warsaw Ghetto which commemorates the Jewish resistance to Hitler there, I felt fully a Jew, perhaps even symbolically dead and reborn, along with the six million others. I felt both a special sadness and an elation which can only come from being a Jew and accepting it.

To my way of thinking it is no happenstance that a majority of psychotherapists are Jews or that Sigmund Freud was himself one. Healing has a particular appeal for us, as Maimonides once pointed out, and mental healing is even more attractive than the physical variety. Is it because the Jew has a greater access to his neurotic suffering, or is it, as Mary McCarthy believes, that he is more sensual than others and psychotherapy feeds his sensuality in a rather brilliant and approved way? Does his very nurturing mother mandate him to offer healing nurturance to others in turn, or are the cabalistic, demonic, or Talmudic collective aspects of him more deeply rooted, needing to be expressed in this modern way? Or do all of these factors, and still others, apply in some matrix of unknown proportions? Can it be that millennial suffering, out-group membership, sanctity, unlimited self-doubt, extolled intellect, etc., sensitize one by tormenting rage to reduce the identical feelings in others? The rabbis of yore were at once gifted therapists and men of the law, the Torah, and they did their work well. Have we merely changed form? Body and mind seem closer together in the Jewish personality, and sickness is taken more seriously than by others—possibly too seriously, for every Jewish child grows up very much aware of his aches and pains. To cure is to have status and to be sanctified.

It seems that Freud was more touched by suffering than was Jung. That is, Freud identified with and experienced the suffering of his patients while Jung more observed and felt it in the breach. Psychoanalysis in the early days was lived and was not merely a profession. The internecine warfare of the old Vienna Circle was not just a staking out of a professional claim to creativity but a defense of a certain moral and interpersonal style of life.

Strangely enough, formal Judaism has not been particularly entranced with Sigmund Freud as one of its own, sometimes even denies that he was a famous son, but regularly and uniformly sends its offspring to his Institutes to be trained in his methods. Jewish mothers react peculiarly to their sons' offers to become psychoanalysts. They often game play as though it will not or should not happen. But underneath they recognize that this is the new Western form of doctor and will therefore fully justify their symbolic motherhood status in Vilna or Lodz where it still counts. Talk is a central Jewish avocation and to cure through talk a kind of miracle. The word is sacred and will ever be.

I belong to this historical collective and one which does not shrink away from Eros and Thanatos but embraces them with perhaps even a vicious fervor. Its origins are more than four millennia old and its archetypes operate regularly in each one of us and are not so easily denied. Among its verities are that life must not be wasted, that the quality of life must be maintained at the highest possible level, and that connubial or family centeredness is the *raison d'etre* of existence. Illness limits all of this, therefore becomes obscene, and deprives the Jewish person and family of its growth possibilities.

On a personal level, becoming a believing Jew is a dynamic mastery situation. On a social level, Jewishness is a working through of affect, sensuality, power, ritual, control, identity, self-hatred, spirituality, and the feeling of being chosen. It is also a coming to terms with the socially disagreeable. As a Jew one becomes more familiar with the pull of the regressive pregenital, with the harshness of reality, with the weaknesses of fantasy, and with the power of the intellect and reason. These lead in turn by unverbalizable processes to confidence and pride, to innovation and creation, to letting-be and going ahead. The limitations, joy, and suffering encountered in psychotherapy are familiar ground for the Jewish person for he is apt to have been there already. Strength is a function of weakness, of social deficit, and is the phoenix of a new constellation of ancient events now turned to growth and action.

The Word and the Deed

There is a basic and unbridgeable hiatus between the *word* and the *deed*. It rarely happens in the fortunes of men that one becomes a master of both. Mishima[1] perhaps portrays the conflict most

[1] *Sun and Steel* (Trans. by J. Bester) (London: Secker & Warburg, 1971).

poignantly of all, and he was finally forced to resolve it by seppuko—
the ultimate self-act of death. Psychotherapists become masters of the
word, but beneath it all I believe they have the basic understanding
that the deed or act is the true essence of man.

Freud reified the wish into a system of psychology by assuming
the equivalence of the wish and the act—the fantasy and the deed—
but empirical psychoanalysis often breaks down precisely at this point.
Insight is merely a prelude to action—is not the action itself. A wish
can never be its operational resultant. The paradox of a psychoanalyst
who is also a sports champion is a resolution of the word-deed dilemma
beyond possibility. At any rate, Mishima expresses his ontic longing in
the following way:

> *Refusing utterly to recognize the conditions of my own exis-*
> *tence, I had set about acquiring a different existence, had laid down*
> *the conditions for that existence, the steps it was necessary to take to*
> *acquire another existence involved flinging myself bodily on the side*
> *of the phantom evoked and radiated by words; it meant changing*
> *from a being that created words to one that was created by words; it*
> *meant, quite simply, using subtle and elaborate procedures in order*
> *to secure the momentary shadow of existence. It was logical, indeed,*
> *that I should have succeeded in existing only at one solitary, selected*
> *moment of my short army life. The basis of my happiness, obviously,*
> *lay in my having transformed myself, albeit only for a moment, into a*
> *phantom cast by far-off words from the past. By now, though, it was*
> *not words that endorsed my existence. This type of existence that de-*
> *rived from rejecting the endorsement of existence by words had to be*
> *endorsed by something different. That "something different" was mus-*
> *cle [p. 61].*

At about the age of five, at the time of the great World War I
flu epidemic, I became ill with a respiratory infection, possibly of the
same order, which when I recovered left me with a bronchial disability subsequently diagnosed as asthma. It was to hound me relent-
lessly thenceforth. This breathing difficulty changed the stream of life,
either as a result of the tissue damage involved or because the concomitant psychological aspects forced me to cater to it. My mind continually soared but my body kept me regularly tied. The world's
foremost allergists, internal medicine men, psychoanalysts and others
could never subsequently really free me from its ravages. It also set the
word in opposition to the deed in an impossible dilemma.

The dynamics of bronchial asthma, as we now know, make for a tighter and more secure world for the asthmatic. Feeling and sensation become ever more intense; the moment itself is sanctified, and the maternal relationship more poignant and life saving. The function of a personal analysis in such a person—precisely me—is to reduce the sensitivity and deathliness, but not beyond the point where the interpersonal is not valued as the supreme creative act of all. Proust,[2] who was also an asthmatic, possibly best of all demonstrates in his musings the relationship of the inner to the outer, of passivity to molar activity, and of the word to the deed. Laing, similarly an asthmatic, reveals the same word magic and actional stratification in more modern form. The inner world of the asthmatic eventually becomes a most florid one, and the compensations, while often real, are almost always in the direction of the word. But that being done, a sense of wanting still remains, and that wanting is the world of the deed. For Mishima, being a Samurai is more authentic than being a great novelist, and he finally killed himself publicly because of it, and then in Samurai dress. This was his final deed.

In coping with this problem as a youth, I went out of my way to make friends with athletes and coaches and both envied and despised them. But I did became manager of our high school football team and played tennis and golf in mediocre fashion. My best friend was the end on the football team, and he later distinguished himself at the University of Southern California, a national football power. I was jealous at the time of my brother who lettered on the swimming team. I never could make that inner circle of the champions, but the realization that I never would was slow in coming and I resisted it. I hated my body, ignored it as much as it would let me, and dreamed of the conquering deeds I would some day do.

As a young adult I purchased my first Porsche and driving fast became the thing. I participated in races close at hand, did a lot more fantasizing, and the car itself became the deed. I felt good and powerful driving it and was equal to all. But even here I could not drive with those few men who coordinate time, space, and equipment into that special act of creation which is "thunder down the home stretch." Alas, I could never be Sterling Moss.

[2] M. Proust, *A la Recherche du Temps Perdu* (trans. by C. K. Scott Moncrieff) (New York: Random House, 1927).

I began to travel vigorously and visited all the countries of the world, with the exception of Africa yet to come. But even here I could not refrain from writing articles for newspapers—from inserting the written word to describe my feelings where none was required. The speed and ascension of airplanes appealed to me, I felt good in them, and to fly in the Concorde or Supersonic Tupelov is my present dream. And some of my best writing has been done in airplanes.

In all of this, I am sad to say that the rift between the word and the deed did not change one iota. I am what I write and nothing else. I remain a man of the word, and I now mostly accept what I could not before accept—that Freud, Sartre, and Dostoevsky are more significant for me than Lindbergh, Bannister, or Parnelli Jones. A creative idea can alter the human condition, but no muscle extends beyond its sheath. The sword historically swoons in face of the word! I am now at home with the deep understanding that the wish, word, and symbol are the most powerful things in the world and that I am a kind of master of them. Complexes are not to be cured by swords but by words, and truth is always a conceptual matter.

Family Life

I grew up in a home in which tranquil periods of any sub-stantial duration were rare; perpetual churning, with its raw feelings, was the currency of the love expressed. In some curious way, intensity became the substitute for quality of emotion—and the greater the intensity, the more beautiful the experience. It was a matriarchal society and my father was securely lodged at the extreme end of the pecking order. I felt considerable pity for him and some helplessness. He was a failure in his own eyes, but more so in the eyes of my mother, who never let him forget it. In more than a half century after emi-grating from Europe, he never, for example, really developed fluency in the English language. He failed in business on several occasions and, finally, found consolation in being relegated to the lowest of occupa-tional ranks. But he worked very hard at what he did, received very few rewards for it, and became hostilely reconciled to permanent fail-ure. He was regularly opposed to education beyond that of elementary school, pointing out that at thirteen he had run away to London, Buenos Aires, and finally New York. (The Handlins have recently

offered a similar point of view, which is that the young today are having increasing difficulty leaving the nest, and there is something to be
said for what my father and others did then.) When he died last year
at eighty-three, I could not mourn deeply for him, even felt not much
loss, but was glad that he died painlessly in a coma.

My mother was an attractive woman who married "beneath
her," not for love but to command. She exercised total power, adopted
one crazy food notion after another, cozened, loved, and comforted
but at a price, went to school, also self-taught herself, and became very
successful commercially. While she claimed the direct opposite, she
manifestly enjoyed the stresses and strains which she induced in the
family structure. Obviously, in the face of my father's inadequacies,
and as the first-born male child (my brother came a year later) I
was caught in that family power matrix which nominated me—certainly not by acclamation—to fill in for my father. John Warkentin
once said that where the father is sexually adequate, perhaps even
powerful, then a child cannot be used as a substitute in this way.
Mine apparently was not. My mother downgraded sexuality at the
same time she found it in every nook and cranny of the world. She
was obsessed by it but obviously could not cope with it. As a result,
all of us were sensitized to an area of life which should have come
more naturally and spontaneously. Is this now why I listen daily to the
deepest sexual secrets of man?

Even today I regard a beautiful woman with a special awe that
should perhaps be reserved for a poem, or I see her body as an organic structure to be used for purposes of sexual union and nothing
else. There was a danger here of homosexuality but I could never find
it attractive or useful. I have been married to the same woman for
twenty-eight years and am more in love than ever. A friend of mine,
a marital counselor, once said that he thought most husbands he
counseled were clods. I am inclined to agree. Most of my clients are
women, a not unusual fact in our profession, but perhaps even more
so in my case. I like the smell, touch, and femininity of women and
cultivate them assiduously. It would be a strange world without them.

Yet not all was family negative with me. From my mother I
learned to appreciate, shall I say, Beluga caviar, the dignity and grace
of the Vienna of Franz Josef, the sonority of a Mozart piano concerto
or the profundity of a Bach fugue, the world of books, the love of

people big and little, the rare joy of Napoleon cognac. But, more than these, I became compelled to be successful—and work turned into joy. Even today, I would rather write than do anything else. I have long ago stopped shrinking away from my creative ideas, learned to put a proper value on them, and to fight down to the wire for them against any and all opposition.

But all of this is prelude. What is important for my psychotherapeutic career is that my family left me with what I call a riddle-residue. By this I mean that I was imprinted with the responsibility for the psychological welfare of our family—yes, its happiness—and to do this I had unconsciously to become a trained professional with deeper insight. The research of Henry,[3] Burton,[4] and others reveals that psychotherapists do not come from particularly happy families. In his problem family the healer receives a charge which mandates him to become a psychotherapist and thus solve not only the family situation but all others. Every client, in a sense, then becomes a part of his unconscious load, and the therapeutic relationship assumes a family quality of some moment for him. Transference is therefore not an imaginative construction but a living reality. And a personal analysis never fully resolves the family romance and satisfactorily negates the charge to become a therapist.

I believe that my family indirectly set me upon such quest and that my sensitive and humanistic involvement with my clients is backed by my specific family experiences, which certainly lacked humanism in proper depth. I have always met every new client with a special relish and expectation, with a sense of challenge like that of a knight on his way to the Crusades, so that psychotherapy is perhaps an over-determined matter. And I do not give up easily in therapy because the stakes are in a sense my own life.

I believe we become psychotherapists by unconscious choice long before the elective decision is made. We may, indeed, have little choice in the matter. Families assign healership roles to their members, but of course few of such role-holders become professionals. The therapist's family function may continue for years on both recognized and

[3] Henry, Sims, Spray, *The Fifth Profession.*
[4] "The adoration of the patient and its disillusionment," *American Journal of Psychoanalysis,* 1970, *29,* 194–204.

unrecognized levels, which would help account for the wide popularity of encounter groups where everybody can be a healer and be healed at the same time. (But such encounter healers evade the final responsibility of self by assiduously avoiding patienthood, which is a prerequisite to the final evolvement of authenticity. Only the ego and rarely the id are put on the line in encounter groups.)

The three facets of my development discussed above—being a Jew, the word/deed dilemma, and family imprinting—account for perhaps three-fourths of my involvement in psychotherapy. The remaining one-fourth, I would guess, is stimulated by a search for beauty, a philosophy of existence which places man at the center of worldly events, and the need for the power, prestige, and monetary advantage with which Western society rewards the healer. I could not on any basis be fulfilled as an engineer, banker, or even as a surgeon, for there is not much room in these professions for the beauty and tragedy of being man.

Several years ago the editor of the journal *Voices* asked a number of us to describe how we as therapists maintained our growing edge. The question is how do we maintain ourselves as therapists at the highest level of creativity, motivation, and involvement. In this connection I have recently offered the suggestion of an "annual satisfaction check-up" for psychotherapists,[5] to bring to awareness and counteract the gnawing inhibitions and personal frustration which regularly arise in our work. In this age of convenient electronic playback, no other profession practices so clandestinely as do we; and no other offers greater opportunities for personal grandiosity or permits one's own psychopathology to be so easily superimposed on its clientele. The implication, and possibly the documentation,[6] that psychotherapists seriously act out with clients is, I believe, quite true. But this actuality does not necessarily represent idiosyncrasy or peccadillo or psychopathology. It is in a sense indigenous to a healing encounter of great intimacy, and the damage, in face of the regular and consistent opportunity, is surprisingly small. We do not as the surgeon often does offer to electively remove the uterus; we do not, as the plastic surgeon does,

---

[5] A. Burton, *Interpersonal Psychotherapy* (Englewood Cliffs, N.J.: Prentice-Hall, 1972).

[6] M. Shepard, *The Love Treatment* (New York: Wyden, 1971).

provide new beauty of bust and face for vanity purposes only; we do not offer a heart transplant when the recipient body is regularly in a rejecting mood; and we do not promise a new life in the hereafter in return for a certain behavior and control in the present one. What we do do is to share our self with another self for the purpose of finding a higher level of fulfillment for both. Indeed, no other profession gives as much in the way of feeling and receives so little back as does ours. Does a fee make up for hours of anguish, despair, and pain? The reward instead comes in the challenge of re-creating a person who is a nonperson, by a jousting with the devil in unconscious form, and by helping the client come closer to *homo natura* and thus to himself. But this is not the whole story. It is rather that I am at home with clients and really come into my own with them. I am my fulfilled self and I feel good about them and with them.

Here, then, is what I said about myself in that earlier article.[7]

There are two things which cause me great pain: (1) when my Muse refuses to answer to me anymore; and (2) when I become from time to time ineffective in psychotherapy. Both events occur without apparent rhyme or reason and are, I believe, indigenous to the creative process itself. The recent suicide of a famous psychotherapist, who was also a personal friend, made all of these matters more intense. Over the years I have systematically nursed the growth aspects of my being, so as to maintain my effectiveness as a therapist and as a writer. In an uneven way, I have used the following approaches.

1. After more than twenty-five years in the practice of psychotherapy, I have come to the place where I accept only those clients for a therapeutic relationship where there is not only some promise that I can help them, but who offer something to me for my own growth. I do not know exactly what this potentiality in the client is, but my selective intuition has been more often right than wrong. I now tend to get restive with the client who offers me nothing in the way of growth and I give it considerable thought before accepting the client. This aspect of my work has probably been the most helpful in moving me forward and I feel genuine regret for anyone who must—for one reason or another—work with almost everyone who applies.

2. I have been strongly influenced by the existentialist and humanistic approach to man, and studies reveal that the life-force and existential thrust of the therapist is critical in the kind of treatment he

[7] A. Burton, "To seek and encounter critical people." *Voices,* 1969, *5,* 26–28.

*does. While these theoretical approaches have sometimes been described
as pessimistic, I find rather that they exalt life. In the past ten years I
have made it a point to seek out the critical people with these view-
points and to encounter them personally. Thus it has been my privilege
to talk with Ludwig Binswanger, Manfred Bleuler, Masako Murakami,
Juan Lopez-Ibor, C. G. Jung, Medard Boss, Gabriel Marcel, Karl
Jaspers, Eugene Minkowski, Igor Caruso, Carl Rogers, O. H. Mowrer,
Viktor Frankl, and others. Something "brushes off" in these wonderful
meetings and I become enlivened and purposeful. Each is followed by
a spate of new ideas, feelings, and publications. . . .*

    *3. I have vigorously and enthusiastically sought loving experi-
ences most often contradicted by my super-ego. This has from time to
time gotten me into some difficulties, but none from which I could not
extricate myself. Without risk-taking of this sort I would probably be
a pretty dull person. It has also been an opportunity for giving more
of myself in unique ways, and I have not regretted it.*

    *4. In more recent years I have experimented with the encounter
group approach. This in many ways has contradicted what I have
been taught as a psychotherapist, and it was not easy to make the
adjustment. But I have in this way gotten to know the "soul" of today's youth, which was impossible in other ways. We recently met at
a coffee shop under attack by the police and the experience was most
bracing, if not frightening, in the sense of challenging the community's
mores.*

    *5. I travel every chance I get and note with delight that my
favorite writers, for example, Nikos Kazantzakis, Lawrence Durrell,
Albert Camus, as well as C. G. Jung, did too. In these peregrinations
I often attend psychoanalytic and psychological meetings, but these are
secondary. Most important of all, I leave our culture behind and once
again come closer to nature, unspoiled people, and indigenous folk-
ways."*

Indoctrination to Psychotherapy

    I was early inculcated in the classical idea that a training
psychoanalysis was the royal road to the understanding of self. In actuality, even though I was involved in two separate courses of analytic
therapy, I found the results wanting. Not that there were not important benefits. Not that it didn't help me become a better therapist. But
I expected a great deal more than I got. Most analysands leave their
analysis with feelings of incompleteness or frustration. What did I
expect? And did I have a right to such expectations?

    I am firm in the belief that a fulfilled or well-analyzed person needs to know more about his logos than he does his id, more about his values and meanings than his pregenital character structure, more about the affectional than the instinctual side of his nature. I do not by this demean either the importance of the instinctual forces or the person's character armor, but simply say that even a full knowledge of them is not enough. My analysts were content to help uncover my pregenital character structure, my oedipal needs, my somatizing propensities, and other equally important defenses, but they ignored my overriding love of life and the deep feelings I have for all people. They offered me little in the way of ideals of growth or mental health, and in retrospect I now know that they themselves were somewhat afraid of total freedom and had little to offer anyone in this area. They had found a safe refuge in Freudian doctrine, propagated it, and then rationalized the healing results. It was only after I talked personally to Jung, taught at his Institute, that I began to feel there could be something more in psychotherapy. Intimate contacts at the same time with Binswanger, Minkowski, and Boss changed not only the stream of my therapeutic efforts but my feelings about myself. I became an existential humanistic psychologist and I set forth to critically amend Freudian psychology.

What I truly know about myself comes not so much from my patient status as from my deep explorations with clients, from sustained reflection and reading, and from experiencing life as a whole. There can be no dissimulation with clients, particularly those who are psychotic, for the alternative is becoming an inauthentic psychotherapist, or perhaps having a psychotic episode in turn. Clients bring out the best and worst in one; but, above all, they reveal the self as it truly is. The Kingdom of I[8] must fall in becoming an authentic psychotherapist.

And, strangely enough, it is the failures rather than the successes which reveal one's ego. Graham Greene discovered this, somewhat to his chagrin, when he recently summarized his life.[9] Without being grandiose, I believe my failures in therapy have been rare but when they did come they tended to be explosive and shook me up badly.

[8] I first found this phrase in Romain Gary, *White Dog* (New York: Bantam Books, 1971).
[9] *A Sort of Life* (New York: Simon and Schuster, 1971).

And I have learned from them, sometimes in a bitter way, but always learned.

I have a furious intolerance of sickness in any form, and it is inconceivable to me that a client would resist the cure—would be satisfied with a crippled existence. Freud, of course, pointed this up more than half a century ago. The fact is that most people will accept less than full freedom, less than what is possible for them. That they will play it safe at the drop of a hat comes as a shock to me again and again. I understand it intellectually, but emotionally I am impatient with it. The supreme injunction of man—the thing fundamentally contained in the Mosaic law—is that man should live his life fully, and this is what psychotherapy is all about. If it did not offer a model in this way, psychotherapy would merely end up as a technical expression like all others in the twentieth century.

Life Themes

My writings have a number of themes which periodically recur and are actually aspects of myself. Examining some of these may help to throw light upon me as a person.

Eros. Over the years my conviction has grown in psychotherapy that Eros, or its equivalent, is the leaven of existence. By this I mean not only the sexual libido, but Agape, mother love, and the positive or loving feeling aspect of all interpersonal relationships. I find Eros everywhere: in the drug scene, in the Jesus freak, in the activist black, in marriage, in all human relationships; and in the psychotherapeutic ambience particularly it reigns supreme. The concept of Eros has not been reduced one whit in importance since Freud formulated it—only its social valuation has wavered from time to time. Even the ethologists who explain infrahuman behavior in terms of reflexes, imprinting, ritualization, and so on, are hard put to omit Eros entirely. In psychopathology more symptoms are reactions to a real or imagined loss of love than we have heretofore allowed ourselves to perceive. All people have headaches, but only a few allow their headaches—no matter how intense—to change the stream of their lives. Eros serves in part to hold Thanatos in check, to provide existential hope, and life without it is closer to death. The definition of the neurosis may yet turn out to be the terror of Thanatos, and in these circumstances the correct prescription is love.

Whatever way psychotherapy is phrased, or is convenient to phrase, it involves not only increasing the supplies of Eros but providing it in a more soluble form. Doing this with proper éclat and timing is what makes the psychotherapist. But the Eros of therapy is more poetic than sensual, more symbolic than reflexive, more historic than contemporaneous, and more maternal than phallic. It has something to do with that first blinding fusion which ties infant and mother with basic trust. In psychotherapy these trust situations—or their deficits—are reestablished, possibly recapitulated, and for a time they become the central focus of existence. The most convincing demonstration of this is the chronic schizophrenic who is mostly refractory to any other therapeutic approach. But so few of us have either the interest, the time, the patience, or the courage to offer Eros to them, so they are considered untreatable. But for those healers who have attempted it, the power of Eros in human change is unquestioned.

The Body. Because Eros has been given so high a value here does not mean that the corporeal self must be denied. Indeed, all things work through the body, and without a body they end up as pure essences. No one can truly speak of love without having touched the love object. Poetic, brotherly, or Christian love always seems to be missing one dimension, and it may yet turn out to be olfaction. The neo-yogi practices of Lowen[10] and Schutz[11] which exaggerate the tangible body are all in the proper psychological direction.

The client is invariably afraid of his body, feels hatred for it, has difficulty locating its pleasurable orifices, becomes at times disembodied, and feels extraordinary pain or ecstasy through it as a form of communion. A neurotic is by definition a person who has lost his body; the therapeutic task is to return it to him. The particular American emphases on dieting, figure control, exercise, prostheses, and so on result precisely from our desire to recover a lost unity between body and mind. The extraordinary frequency of psychic depression at the climacteric is due to the fact that the body ultimately withers, and if

[10] A. Lowen, *The Betrayal of the Body* (New York: Collier, 1967). Also see his later works.
[11] W. Schutz, *Joy* (New York: Grove, 1967).

that exquisite body-mind unity has not earlier been found, then involutional depression is the outcome.

I have experienced a surprising psychotherapeutic thing. When during a long-term psychotherapy a client comes down with a fatal illness—cancer, heart disease—he precipitously discontinues psychotherapy at the moment his diagnosis is definitively established. One might expect, at the least, that therapy might help the client ease the pain of the coming death, and there is even some very slight evidence that spontaneous remission in the disease is helped along by an intense therapeutic relationship. But the client uniformly drops out. It appears therefore that when the psyche can no longer influence the body because the latter is going to die, the client has no hope of fulfillment and terminates not only psychotherapy but other intense love relationships as well.

The Logos.   The derivation of the word *logos* from the Greek root has a variety of semantic connotations. I use it here as an extension of Frankl's definition,[12] and logos, the "word," in modern form becomes (the nonChristian) *soul.* Soul, an important rock and hip concept, means an experience of deepest communion which transcends every ego boundary by the special nature of the experience itself. Poetry, drama, dance, sculpture, and similar art forms have logos as well. For the new generation, at least, to have logos is to be in communion with something very important, to have peace, freedom, and fulfillment, to be equal, to love Everyman, and to have meaning in life.

The logos functions as soul in dyadic psychotherapy, but this relation is generally overlooked .The various extant ego revisions of the Freudian system are all in this direction. The emphasis on the here and now, the diminished historical search, the therapeutic involvement of the family, the therapist as participant rather than screen, the recognition of the client as person, the use of creative media in therapy are all in the direction of therapy as logos; associational technique is beginning to take second place. That is, revisions from classicism are designed to help the client find a new meaning or logos in his life.

The humanistic propensities of therapist as man override his tactics, or the tactics merely become the tools of his propensities. The vehicle is a certain readiness to understand, feel, and be, and the client

[12] V. E. Frankl, *Man's Search for Meaning.* (Boston: Beacon, 1962).

reaction is instant recognition. The more authentic the therapist, the more he has these almost indefinable qualities, and the greater his suffering and joy and general experience, the greater his logos. These are the fundamental distinctions which make him human and responsive in place of merely scientifically objective. Of course, the logos sounds a bit mystical, but the logos principle is the personal experience of all healers and cannot just be wished away. Its presence often accounts for the different treatment outcomes produced by two equally trained healers.

Aggression. In my own life I have not known how aggressive to be, and I do not know how aggressive my clients should ultimately become. We have all been reared in the fiction that aggression is primitive, dangerous, and sinful. Yet the child soon sees parents act aggressively toward each other, his societies everlastingly make war, the business and industry he joins aggressively destroy competition without compunction, murder and suicide abound in his cities, and finally sexuality turns out to be a form of aggression. It takes little in the way of sustained hunger, incarceration, or sexual deprivation, for example, to bring primitive aggression out in man.

Extreme passivity in today's activist world, if not a variant of personality pathology, may in some quarters at least be considered a poorer quality of social adjustment. To revolt was after all the final philosophical message of Camus. Whether such revolt is personal or collective, or both, is a matter of some indifference in the face of the philosophical findings of life.

Psychotherapy helps passive people become more aggressive. But just how much aggression is the fine point. Should one applaud when the client can finally throw an ashtray at the psychotherapist? But I fully concur with Spitz that aggression is the carrier wave of humanity. It has the function of perpetuating the species: ethology fully demonstrates that the ritualizations of aggression are the woof in the fabric of culture, and without them we might not have a civilization. It is necessary to be aggressive to be fully alive, and the "flower children" are surely wrong in their primary phenomenology of passivity, as was, I believe, Gandhi. The question then becomes not only how to change the mythology of child rearing away from passive dependency, but how to both use and contain the demonic which is the root of man's aggressive achievements and disabilities. Man's development of weapons has reached the point where limited aggression in war is no longer possible. This means that human aggression outlets in war are no longer feasible, that human aggression must either be totally suppressed in some way yet unknown or be expressed in ever wider social forms in approved ways. One reason that so much psychotherapy involves sexuality is that sexuality represents a displaced and favorable social aggression. Make sex, don't make war!

Psychotherapy can in this sense be defined as applied aggression. One learns to aggress in a way one has missed along the way but under better auspices. Appropriate aggression is a beautiful thing, for it motors interpersonal relationships, feeds creation, and provides the necessary tension for existence. The newer confrontation techniques have been healthy in that they have released aggression and energy relatively quickly and in this way motored more affectional feelings.

My Genesis

I was born March 10, 1914, in Brooklyn, New York, and have almost no recollections of that part of Greater New York, even of the Bronx, where I spent my first six years. Both are now the worst slums in the world, and I have returned on at least one occasion to stand and see whether my memory would reinstate the early experiences I repressed. I feel hostile to my birthplace as though it gave me nothing but pain. I remember living high in a tenement, an anthill of people, and trying to find solace in a back courtyard into which garbage was irregularly thrown. Perhaps this is always why in now booking a room in a hotel, I pick one on the seashore, and the room must face the surf. I myself later threw my father's shoes into that pit, which caused a row which even now—five decades later—shimmers with vibrancy. I remember the snow, of being fascinated by it but of not being allowed to play in it, of being carried through it and upstairs with an asthmatic attack. Later, of playing "doctor" with the daughter of my father's friend, and of being caught at it. She was, I vaguely recall, a beauty and this game was my first great "incompleted activity" which gave rise to tension, perhaps to that great and insatiable curiosity of mine. Alas, I never saw her again.

A physician suggested that I be taken to Arizona or California and that the alternative might be early death. We relocated in Los

Angeles and most of my growing up was done there. In those days Los Angeles was still something of a large pueblo and had culture, glamour, and purpose. I particularly came to love the Spanish/Mexican culture which it represented, so that today the ancient Garden of the Hesperides can be found in Spain and nowhere else for me. I have a fantasy that I will some day be a grandee of Spain, perhaps in a new incarnation.

Los Angeles abounded with fine colleges and universities, and after two years at Los Angeles Junior College, where I discovered psychology under the auspices of an unusually gifted teacher, whose name I no longer remember, I went on to U.C.L.A. for an A.B. and an M.A. Clinical psychology there under Knight Dunlap, Roy Dorcus, and Grace Fernald was either the treatment of aphasia or working with nonreaders. I selected the latter and wrote a master's thesis on it.

I tried the University of Southern California, across town, but couldn't get interested in Milton Metfessel's birds reared in isolation, in fact thought it all silly (something I know better now); picked up a school psychologist's certificate; and then got accepted by the psychology department of the University of California in Berkeley. I was attracted by the warmth, humanity, and knowledge of Edward Chace Tolman and wanted to be one of his "bright" students—a group that has, it seems, made him famous. (I must say he was the worst undergraduate lecturer of record but was simply great in graduate seminars.) He agreed to take me on but worried that he could not place me academically at degree time because I was Jewish. He then later gently suggested a major in clinical for this reason.

Well, it seems Jean Wolker McFarlane, who headed the clinical program, did not think I was good training material—she didn't say so, but she assiduously avoided me—so I affiliated with Harold E. Jones in child development and Olga Bridgman in abnormal. My thesis was on a Lewinian topic, then very much the rage.

Berkeley was an exciting place in those days. It was most hospitable to the new field of clinical psychology and I was privileged to sit in on courses or lectures by Eric Erikson, Bruno Klopfer, Nevitt Sanford, and many others who first tried their wings there.

I received the Ph.D. two years after arriving but then eschewed an academic job because for both healthy and unhealthy reasons I wanted to return to Los Angeles. I there became the director of a new counseling agency. In later years I gradually worked my way back into academic life but have always felt a little alien totally away from the client. I am now on the point of renouncing academia completely again and feel not the slightest twinge of regret in doing so. It has been a vast disappointment to me in many ways and I am sympathetic with Carl Rogers' feeling in this regard.

Mature Years

In my later lifetime, C. G. Jung and Ludwig Binswanger had an important influence upon me and I spent time with both. Jung diverted me from Freud—just enough to allow Binswanger to make an existential phenomenological humanist out of me—opened up the true vistas of the mind to my understanding, and gave psyche and logos a proper place in my psychotherapy. Binswanger first explained to me what the incomprehensible "Case of Ellen West" was all about. From this I began to see schizophrenia not as a disease but as an existential process of the greatest moment. But, above all, the depth, sincerity, and authenticity of the two men swayed me like little else.

First Book

One's first book, even an anthology, is an experience that must be classed with the significant ones of a lifetime. No book which follows ever has the same impact. And *Case Histories in Clinical and Abnormal Psychology,* the first, was not only accepted by prestigious Harper & Bros. on my own recognizance, but until its publication almost no case history material existed for the student, a sad commentary on the clinical psychology of the time. It happened this way. Robert E. Harris, professor of medical psychology at the University of California School of Medicine in San Francisco, had invited us to a cocktail party. At about the third martini, we mutually decried the unavailability of case materials. "Let's do one," we said. I went home, made up an outline, showed it to him, found a publisher, and was thereby imprinted in a publishing career forever and ever.

Marriage

I delayed marriage until I was thirty, rejecting one candidate after another on either fantasy or real grounds. Women were—and still are—a puzzle to me and I really didn't know then what you did with them on a full-time basis! I was inclined to give either too much affection or too little—and then became angry when I couldn't find the proper proportion. I was also inclined to put my career above all else, because to make my mark seemed to have the greatest urgency to me, and I was thus often guilty of overlooking their needs.

This masochistic description makes me out a first-class bastard, but I wasn't really that. I was kind, generous, devoted, a good bread-winner, interesting, engaging, cultured, and I had gained a little knowledge of sex along the way. Life with me could be painful, but it was assuredly never dull. Mostly, the women couldn't keep up. I would, for example, impulsively say that we were leaving in two days for Dakar, or that I had to go tomorrow to Santiago de Compostella, and would go. I also tended earlier to some mild depressions, and no one in such a state of being is a very lovely person.

Edith Hamilton was my age when we met. Kind, gentle, under-standing, and with a sufficient balance of humor to handle all situations. Her background differed so greatly from mine that any reason-able marriage counselor would have forbidden the marriage at once. Still, we have been married twenty-eight years, and it has never been so fine as it is at the moment. Fire and brimstone and passion have now turned into love, respect, and friendship. We care for each other. There has been one issue, Vicki Ann Burton, age twenty-three, who is a fine schoolteacher but unconsciously working hard to become a psychologist. She is of course the apple of our eye and someday, I am certain, will tell her own story as she has uniquely experienced it.

Medical Center

Private practice does not come easy to a clinical psychologist. Even if he is a licensed practitioner, as he is in California, under the State Board of Medical Examiners, he is discriminated against in many ways regardless of his therapeutic ability. For example, some insurance companies will not pay a claim for psychological services at all; others will pay it only if a diagnosis is first made by a psychiatrist; and Medi-Cal, under a recent crash economy program in California, eliminated psychologists from the program entirely. Physicians refer reluctantly to psychologists, most frequently when the referral is for a child, for marital counseling, or for psychological testing. In my experience psychologists refer cases to psychiatrists with much greater frequency than the other way around, and any psychologist worth his salt regularly refers clients to internists and others for medical clearance, medical complications, and so on.

In most of my intramural professional life I was dependent upon psychiatrists for a number of things. I felt that they had not only the legal responsibility for the client but the clinical one as well. I believed I was there solely to assist the psychiatrist in formulating his diagnoses, carry out the treatment prescribed, train paramedical personnel according to his goals, and so on. For this role I of course received certain concessions. I could select my own cases for psychotherapy, more or less had immunity from close supervision, and regularly received the "blessing" which is the higher watermark of medical approval. There were social rewards as well, in the form of dialogues, cocktail parties, and so forth. While I did some private practice independently along with in-patient work, it did not occur to me that I could fully stand on my own feet as a psychotherapist and that I was buying psychiatric favor at a great cost to myself. I woke up in the following way.

In a famous medical center, the department of psychiatry was chaired by a man who was not only a noted psychiatrist but a member of a psychoanalytic institute as well. His list of publications was extensive, and the Ground Rounds he led on Wednesday mornings are still in my memory among the most important of my clinical experiences. Personally, he was affable, direct, given to quick mood changes, a fine host, and most often made you feel a member of a special family, that is, *his* team.

It so happened that at a critical social point in the community resolution of the functions of clinical psychologists in California, he wrote an ill-advised article in an influential Western medical journal which was received by every M.D. in the state, pleading for a limited or nontherapeutic role for clinical psychologists, even those with a Ph.D. and intern training. His extensive staff of psychologists, up in arms, urged him to recant or to modify his position, for not only were their duties in the medical school called into question, but they began to receive pressure from angry colleagues who urged reprisals against him. An any rate, his chief psychologist resigned and I was asked to take his place—along with a professorship—which I did. What impelled me to step squarely into this hornet's nest? I wasn't particularly

distinguished for my ego strength, but I guess I had made a reputation
for working well with psychiatrists. But underneath, my unconscious
was certainly preparing my crucifixion.

The medical center was without question the finest place I
have ever practiced my psychological skills. The psychology staff was
exceptionally qualified, consulting psychoanalysts abounded in great
numbers, and the medical students and the psychiatric residents themselves were a joy. But the chairman and I immediately did battle. I
basically wanted to kowtow and please him. I felt that it would be a
feather in my cap, for my profession that is, if I could get him to recant, or partly so, and I believed I had some kind of magic within me
which would enable me to do it. On a personal level we were fond
of each other, but professionally and publicly we could not admit this.
He soon found himself in a conceptual position on psychology from
which he could not retreat, at least not publicly. But he did retreat
privately, allowing psychotherapy and other practices to go on in his
department without appearing to notice them. The issue—but not the
feelings—slowly abated and things became better. They were well on
their way to becoming good when I decided to leave, for reasons not
exactly clear to me. I told him about my decision and he urged me
to stay. But I left after six months, with very mixed feelings.

In some curious way, I thereafter became freed of the psychiatrists. I no longer needed their support, began publishing with exceptional vigor, frequently challenged them clinically, became a small
expert on schizophrenia, and accepted private practice as my model
of professional freedom. And so it remains today. Interestingly enough,
my writings are better known to psychiatrists and psychoanalysts than
to psychologists, and I offer papers at psychiatric conferences three
times as often as I do at psychological ones. The Fifth World Congress
of Psychiatry at Mexico City, from which I have just returned, is a
good example.

Mental Hospital

I spent more than a decade and a half of my life as the chief
psychologist of a state mental hospital which held more than four
thousand patients. As I look back at this experience I break out in a
cold sweat. Not that it did not have its delights and learning oppor-

tunities, but it confirmed for me Freud's deep feeling that man is basically primitive and sadistic, even within a framework dedicated to mercy. How do you regularly write people off—and how do you do it in the face of a personal and public oath to spend your life alleviating their suffering?

The limitations of the mental hospital have by now been sufficiently documented elsewhere. I want only to point up the process by which often well-meaning personnel achieve such poor results. That the mental hospital has its own iatros is uncontested, but that it may overall do more harm than it does good can perhaps be debated. I have in the past called it the cheapest long-term social board-and-room known to man, and I believe its economics are precisely this. The term *hospital* fools no one who works in it. Only the family has its guilt relieved by placing its relatives in an ambience with a history of careful and devoted medical care: the hospital. Every staff member trades on the currency of medicine; that is, he sells medical cliches at the same time he jousts with demonology on a social science model.

The maltreated ones are not the patients but the staff, strange as this may seem. Self-hatred among the staff is rampant; success in one's own eyes in the mental hospital becomes no longer possible; and the similarities between staff and patient become too close for comfort. Obviously, since very few psychoanalytically trained people now work in such settings, personal shortcomings are easily displaced on the patients because self-reflection can lead only to either attacking the administration, which can be fatal, or attacking oneself. Eventually one will have to leave; but the rewards are just enough to keep one firmly fixed in the post, and afraid. When I first came to this particular state hospital, I was furnished with any amount of filet mignon, garden vegetables, a patient to wash my car, and even a house to live in. All of this at a few cents a pound, but with the understanding that it was one of the written and unwritten perquisites of having to work in such a setting. Then the retirement system involved in the employment was extolled: "Work with us and we will amply take care of you in your old age." But creative thought and innovation became a form of administrative sickness. Such things were quickly quashed, and the final result was a staff who valued security above all. Emphasis was on keeping order, obeying rituals, and maintaining a firm distance from the clientele.

Of course, the beautiful aspect of the hospital resided with the patients. Despite their often impossible burden, I found in them a deep humanity, a resolute humor, a desire for truth, and an uncompromising stand against contemporary family and culture which often made psychosis more acceptable than social hypocrisy. I know that I may here be accused of romanticism. But romance has a better prognosis and is generally better for people anyway, so I do not mind. And I have Rorschached and examined thousands of such clients and I believe I know whereof I speak. The demon in a sense has always been more engaging to me than the saint.

In retrospect, I found that the staff, with some few exceptions, did not really believe in the cure—that one can be permanently relieved of a mental illness. They saw mental illness as a taint, like the Mark of Cain, and felt that the patient should continue to bear it because in some way he had earned it. Furthermore, it was believed contagious so that the world at large had to be protected from the host. Electric convulsive treatment, lobotomy, stereotoxic surgery, and similar treatments all arose to confirm the poor prognosis in their minds. "Desperation" treatment confirms a desperate situation in the mind of the staff and the patient, and psychotherapy is fought in the mental hospital not because of personnel shortages but because it introduces hope where none is wanted. Psychologists in the mental hospital, I found, were more hopeful people than those medically trained. As a consequence, they were perpetually in hot water with the administration.

There is probably no worse administrator in the world than I am. I really made a complete hash of it, for I was fighting for the patient when, as a member of the administration, I should have been fighting for control and the hospital culture. Then I had periods of nihilism where I withdrew into scholarship—and finally I had to drive my Porsche too fast to give me some kind of balance. But, as the next section reveals, I discovered schizophrenia and its cure there. Harold Kelman said to me when I left to become a full-time professor, "Art, if you do not continue to treat people, you will lose your Muse."

This was a sagacious observation, for I found that students could never replace clients, that is, unless they too became clients. I become impatient with the normal. They bored me by their simplicity —by their routine appetites, fantasies, and satisfactions. But the neurotic or psychotic has a rich depth of feeling and personality, a basic understanding of and hunger for existence, a courageous proximity to Thanatos, which no nonclient can match. Bizarre? Possibly. But it was my choice to treat these people, and my happiest moments have been in doing so. All of this the mental hospital taught me—or rather showed me—and I am eternally grateful. In all my years on the wards I never once felt afraid, but walking through Central Park in New York City at night sent a chill up and down my spine.

Understanding Schizophrenia

Within psychotherapy itself there is sufficient scope so that one may encounter life—and even oneself—on any level of convolution and complexity. Without doubt schizophrenia represents the farthest extreme, which not even Freud dared to challenge and Jung gave up after one book. It is precisely this area of treatment that a small number of brave or foolhardy psychotherapists elected to enter. For about two decades I have been one of these.

There is indeed no scientific effort which brings less reward than treating schizophrenia. It was no happenstance that the mental hospital was indirectly founded to tuck them safely out of sight. And even when a psychotherapy is successfully done with a chronic regressed schizophrenic, the results are so incomplete, so circumscribed, and so disappointing to both as to make this therapy a form of psychological masochism. Why then did I find in this kind of person the supreme challenge? Even though I no longer work in in-patient hospital settings, I still believe this is the greatest professional experience of all. And others—say, Don Jackson—have said the same from out of their deep personal experience.

Schizophrenia represents the bizarre and sublime in one neat package. At one moment, the greatest poetic and existential truths flow from their mouths; in the next, one is back to Dante's final circle of hell. The diversity of man is never greater than here, and it must be said that this condition has a kind of perverse beauty. To solve this riddle is truly to understand ultraindividual differences, and perhaps the secret of life as well. In the evolution of the personality, the organization factor has certainly gone awry in that structure we call schizophrenia—and it needs to be put back together again. Temporality, spatiality, causality, subject-predicate are all reversed or reduced in valuative power. What we hold dear the schizophrenic despises, and even feels nausea about. Social activists notwithstanding, he is the true dissenter of culture, and his honesty goes way beyond anything known to college youth or revolutionaries. Indeed, I have challenged some of my more violent students to become schizophrenic as proof of their good faith, but they do not want to belong to a nonsociety such as this. Schizophrenia is not so much an organic disease, as we would conveniently like to believe, as a life-cumulative existence of a special sort, a rag bag of bits and pieces of images, icons, affects, percepts, and habits. There is nothing as such to cure in it; rather one must demonstrate to them that alternative life possibilities lead more directly to fulfillment and to a change in their human situation.

Curiosity as a part of creativity knows no bounds. For some of us, if it is necessary to become a healer, then it also becomes necessary to heal schizophrenia. But the wise ones give up after one, two, or three lessons; for the rest, the quest is not so easily stilled. Healing schizophrenia is subduing the demon *par excellence*. It is also being in league with him. The alchemical problem is not the historical one of changing base metal into gold, but of converting schizophrenia to health. This is indeed the modern version of this medieval problem.

Of all my treatment cases those schizophrenics I have worked with more rather than less successfully[13] have given me the greatest professional satisfaction. They remain most vividly in my memory and I am still not separated from them. But not a single one can be called a friend or even an acquaintance, and from not one have I had the feeling of being loved. This seems a bit hard. And one does not do psychotherapy with schizophrenics: one lives it. If one lives a relationship, then one has a right to at least infrequently receive a token of that relationship. Or is this sentimental thinking?

I have puzzled about my interest in schizophrenia and concluded that should the causes of schizophrenia ever be discovered, I might lose interest in the problem. I have, I suppose, to do the impossible, and I cannot tolerate the failure of intimacy which schizophrenia represents. I unreasonably want everyone to be fulfilled and happy, particularly my clients. The fact that the schizophrenic initially

[13] "The Quest for the Golden Mean," in A. Burton (ed.), *Psychotherapy of the Psychoses* (New York: Basic Books, 1961).

refuses my overtures makes me all the more determined to help him. This goes along with a general trait of mine reported by relatives and friends: I refuse to give up, whatever the odds, for I believe that there is always some other way a thing can be done, that one has only to want to do it badly enough and to persist. I believe in myself, my capacities, and, unfortunately, even in some situations where even Atlas would fail. But I wouldn't have it any other way. This attitude calls for crossing swords more than I like; but it is the way things are. For this reason, I was deeply hurt when Carl Rogers gave up his work with schizophrenics in Wisconsin after a few years.

Experience of Self

How then do I experience myself and how do I come through to clients? Here the shoals of Scylla and Charybdis await us, with vanity on one shore and piety on the other. A psychiatric friend recently objected when I wanted to call my last book "a primer." He said I was incapable of writing anything that was a primer. I have a tendency to complicate things, and my prose is often heavy with images and metaphors—the complex and involved is the most mysterious and gives me the greatest satisfaction. No pure symbols exist, only clusters, aggregates, and compounds of symbols, and psychotherapy is the analysis of complex symbols on the way to the mandala: the elemental of life. I read detective stories for relaxation and Agatha Christie appalls me by her simplitude whereas Georges Simenon delights by his convolutions. I look first for the Gestalten, for the wholes, the cosmic verities, and only then am I content to reduce them to their molecular building blocks.

I am too romantic for my own good. By this I mean that I even tend to cloak shit with a poetic wonder. On the Island of Rhodes, I felt fully at home in the old castles of the Knights Hospitaller of St. John, and pageantry of any kind sets my processes aquiver. I believe in dignity, splendor, and overriding human causes. Man, in my belief, cannot be reduced to one of Lorenz's geese or even Goodal's chimpanzees. Science suffers from its divorce from the romantic, which is why I prefer to read Dostoevski or Solzhenitsyn to Skinner or Reich.

A graduate course in aesthetics at U.C.L.A. confirmed my then latent opinion that everything natural and human has a certain beauty about it. I go thousands of miles to see the beautiful, but I also find it everywhere. And beauty is a part of every authentic person. At first clients cannot experience a tree, a river, a mountain, or even a Renoir. But as treatment proceeds, these things come to be a more regular part of their lives. Indeed, should it not occur I might consider the treatment a failure.

Beauty is not necessarily the Aphrodite of Cnidus, the Parthenon of Phidias, the fugues of Bach, or even the legendary Helen of Troy herself. But beauty is that concatenation of form and substance which unifies inner and outer into a blazing harmony of peace, freedom, and contentment. It is the peak experience with all conflict removed. Authenticity demands beauty and makes it possible in turn. Some, such as Goya and Faulkner, have been attracted to the ugly, the misshapen, and the bizarre, which have their own beauty, I suppose. But in the writings, say, of Kazantzakis and Camus, beauty is the proper justification for being—both inside and outside.

A client once gave an instant summation of me as "direct and sensual." She was certainly on the right track. I have many times wished that I could dissimulate more, play pastimes and games, and take a greater part in that comedy of manners which makes up the fabric of our social life. But I cannot. I have a streak of honesty in me which forces me to tell the truth. Of course, I have learned the proper timing of it in therapy, am even a kind of master of it, but I know that truth is relative. Our clients do not want logic, rationality, and justice, if it means they have to give up fantasies and covert needs. The fun world is not of such logical order, and only when clients are forced to by despair and suffering will they look truth in the face. Freud had this same difficulty with truth, and it got him into a lot of trouble.

Sensuality requires no apologies, and I do not apologize for mine. Flesh does not contradict spirit. A person who has never received stroking has no basis for higher-level feelings and impulses. The hypothalmus needs a constant bombardment of stimuli, and sensuality simply reflects the quality of that stimulation. Casanova is a somewhat comic modern figure, but he may have been a happy man, and he did make many ladies happy. His *Memoirs* reveal him to be a sensitive and often disciplined artist as well. Asceticism, as Judeo-Christian salvation, was never more than dramatic self-personification, and it was basically estranged from existence. The current strain about the marriage of priests reveals that the imaginal and ceremonial wedlock to the godhead may serve institutional religion but not always the person himself.

I have a strong need for justice: it matters that all of us share in the gift of life. I am for liberty, equality, and fraternity and work for them in all areas of my living. But I expect the person to find and fight for his own justice. The Hassidic tradition which finally led European Jews to the gas chambers of Auschwitz like lambs because it was "the Lord's will" sets my teeth on edge. Justice is a higher-order concept of man, and as such man must derive it for himself. Cynicism, copping out, passivity, and default may lead to nihilism and rebellion but never to justice.

Adjectives have been found to be a good way of describing a personality. Some which apply to me are: ambitious, concerned, intuitive, loving, introvertive, sensitive, logical, sensual, affective, tough, fair, demanding, conscientious, poetic, credulous, persistent, and impatient.

If we now turn to how I am experienced by others, here is the report of a client who is in longer-term therapy with me.

How a Client Experiences Me

My husband discovered Arthur Burton through an article in the journal *Voices*. We have both been in individual therapy with him for a year. Dr. Burton is a man of medium size with a face whose age I can never determine. He has often a shrewd expression; it can also be ironic, humorous, or loving. He usually smokes a cigar. Although I once hugged him when I was very happy, and crawled into his lap when I was desperate, a certain formality in his manner has always maintained the requisite objectivity. Each time I walk into his office I experience the sensation that he is utterly tabula rasa, with no expectations as to how I'll be. His commitment is both detached and involved.

I liked Dr. Burton the first time I saw him, but it wasn't for the usual reasons that I like people. He wasn't at all effusive; on the contrary, he was almost entirely silent. But he did say something, after I'd delivered to him my confusion, that was terribly reassuring to me. He said, "You know, all life is—" (he paused) "I don't want to sound trite—a stream or river or flow of energy or whatever you want to call it; you won't always be feeling as badly as you are now." I had a weird sense that he knew what I was going through, and was also reminded of the process of life within myself.

A very important factor in my therapy was the following. Two years ago I had been in therapy with a nationally known man who was opposed to conflict analysis and to whom I had an extremely strong father transference. I was soon trapped in the task of trying to please this man, which largely meant never letting him see the craziest part of me: for most of my life I'd been repeating wishful little jingles I'd made up, the theme of which was that I was well-loved and that everything was all right. I had been very involved in music and was internally compelled to repeat these jingles to any form of music I ever heard. Also, whatever I said or thought was accompanied by a simultaneous internal translation of it into French and/or Italian. I had pretty much accepted that I would have these rituals all of my life and that I could never divulge them to anyone. When I first saw Dr. Burton I was extremely tense and my "words," as I called them, were eating up most of my life. One night, after a month in therapy, I forced myself to write down these phrases in my diary, so that I could tell them to Burton the next day. In his office I announced, "I'm going to tell you about my secret which I've never told anyone." He smiled at me in an understanding and "I expected this" sort of way, and I knew it was all right. He said, "From the very first I noticed an air of transliterative preoccupation about you." He now had my secret; so it was no longer a secret. It was oddly comforting to me to know that he'd guessed it all along; most of all, that he could stand my craziness. The "words" almost completely died off from that day on.

As I think of Burton's style, it appears to fall into two categories: the indirect and direct approach. Both ways were a form of confrontation, both I often loathed, yet each was useful. (Even though the last year has involved more conscious pain for me than I've ever had, it never seriously occurred to me to leave therapy. I guess that the reason is because I wanted to change myself more than anything in the world, even though it clearly meant an adventure I would hate most of the time.) Burton is a master at the philosophical conundrum and also at the mot juste statement. These statements, such as "Fat girls can't be passionate, can they?", in this case delivered in a tone of semi-irony, totally pulled my defense rug out from under my feet. What the hell did he mean? My original reaction was always to clam up in wounded fury after an abortive attempt to figure out what he intended. In like manner, he would suddenly relate an incident to me of a friend of his or of a well-known person. What was the connection with me? At first I thought this Koan master was intent only on befuddling me; but as my therapy progressed and I trusted him more I saw that they were meant, rather, to elucidate. The catch was that I had to think for myself and overcome a resistance or two along the way.

I recall one other time that was devastatingly powerful for me: I had a beautiful Peruvian necklace of the sun and moon which I had worn virtually every single day for two months in therapy. On this day Burton referred to it as my "amulet." This one word forced me into bitter tears of recognition. It laid bare to me the extent to which I had used magic to organize my life and kept away the unknown. Burton asked one day if I would give up my amulet to him. I didn't know how symbolically he meant this, but one day at a time when I began feeling a lot stronger, I impulsively gave the necklace over to him. He gave it to me at the end of the session, but for me the meaning of my gesture was the act of faith that I could give to him a whole aspect of my personality and not get it back.

I now see that Burton's style was intended as a challenge both in the sense of a difficult task for me to work on and as a confrontation. He "dared" me to maintain my defenses which had come so close to destroying me. He chided: "After all, all I can offer you is a little reality." An agonizing reality he once offered me was in connection with a fantasy I had long had as a witch. This was an unshakable image, both terrifying and comforting in its power. While I was talking of it one day he said, "OK, why don't you cast a spell on me right now?" There was a moment of panic in which I didn't know whether or not he was serious, and then I saw that the panic was that I didn't have any spells at all, least of all one that could dupe this man. One of my big demons was exorcised with that challenge. I must add here that my previous therapist had become enchanted with the array of archetypes and images that I applied to myself and was apparently unaware of the source of conflict they were to me. Burton recognized my great ambivalence in experiencing myself as a witch; that is to say, he took it seriously, yet was not enchanted by it. This attitude of his increasingly gave me the sense that he was on my side as I wrestled with the unholy angel of my unconscious. This has been a major experience of mine in therapy: that the two of us were allied against my demons.

There have been two occasions this year when I felt on the verge of a breakdown. I was not delusional, but I was terrified and furious and felt like giving up entirely. At these times Burton was both supportive and challenging. Primarily, he did not become tangled within the morass of my emotions and made it clear that he was there to help but that I would do the work of extrication myself. They occurred in February and in May and had to do with having to take a look at how much I was not the woman I thought I was. The second time was so fierce that I had to leave my husband and move to my own apartment, so that I could reassess everything I'd been doing and hopefully find a new self. I was completely raw but realized that somehow I had to find within myself the energy for getting born again. A main intention was to punish Burton for all the pain I was feeling (he was causing), and to make him mother me in my infantile state. I pushed, but he wouldn't capitulate. One day in the thick of it I told him that all I wanted to do then was rant and rave at him. Matter of factly and without irony he told me that that kind of behavior belonged on a psychiatric ward; if I wanted to act that way, I could go to one. But if I wanted to talk about how I was feeling I could do it in his office. That session was a silent one for me and when I came home I cursed Burton for not taking care of me, for not giving me every drop of milk I needed then. I wished to God that I was in gestalt therapy where, it seemed to me, I could rant and rave all I wanted and perhaps even get group support. But that day was a turning point for me because I discovered some rationality and began turning my fury against my sickness and self-destruction. I told the infant in me to shut up and take whatever milk I had to give it.

Burton's therapy sometimes consisted of remarks he made to me about myself that were not riddles and often involved his personal reaction to me. I was not used to anyone being really straightforward with me, especially in a critical sense. My first day in therapy he gave me not only the words of comfort I mentioned, but told me that I was a "special person," that I had a great deal of creativity as well as conflict and that I might as well use that conflict to metamorphose it to the level of art. My first therapist had also told me that I was a special person, but I felt more and more that it was his way of being on the make for me. It blew my mind to have this second doctor say it to me and I almost left his office that first day. Burton told me that I was free to go and I saw that he meant it. I was indignant, but remained. From that first day, Burton brought out my two areas of greatest conflict. Was I really a special person, was I a witch? Was I always going to be "possessed," by demons or creativity? And secondly, this direct, and, it felt to me, loving statement about me was too close; it impinged upon me too much and stirred up the scary feelings I had about my father. Was he going to compound that scene for me, as my first therapist had done?

There are two things I want to say here about the way in which Burton helped me with the complex of feelings I had about my father: one positive and one negative. The former is that he has enabled me to become aware of the extent of sexual feeling my father and I had for each other, yet has also enabled me to separate myself from this so that I love my father in a more human and less erotic way. He has also shown me that he does not experience me as my father did. He has consistently pushed me to respond more to him (Burton) as a person; this has been an integral part of my therapy because I had had such a great fear of letting men in, in an emotional way. However, there is one negative thing I have never "forgiven" him for, since to me it transgressed the unorthodoxy I admire so much in Burton. One day as we were talking of my lack of openness to men, my wish-fear that they'd see me as a sexual object, he said, "You know, you don't turn me on. There are women clients I have who cause me to have an erection; I would like it if one day you could do that to me." Rationally, I understand he was referring to my daring to be more attractive to men; but at an emotional level it freaks me out to think of him getting an erection as we talked in his office.

Burton has told me that I bored him, that I was beautiful, that I had nothing to give him, that he would be sorry if I killed myself but not broken up. He has told me that I could call him at any time of night or day; he meant it and I often called him when I felt I couldn't cope. All these things, at their given moment, helped me. He has even referred to me as a schizophrenic, because of the elaborate defense system I was building up. At first I got really furious when he dared to call me that. That is a very scary word and it had never occurred to me before I went to him that my need to protect myself was so extreme. One day when I got openly angry at him for calling me that word, he countered, "Every time I use it, a look of comfort goes across your face." "Goddamn it," I thought, "if that's how I'm making myself feel good, no thanks. I'll have to find some new way."

The story of my therapy is that I had to find other ways of making myself feel good. Some of my friends have told me that Burton put me through too much pain this year and that my therapy could have gone in a more gentle manner. He has told me that I was one of the most challenging cases he has had, since my unconscious was so powerful and even though I appeared rational and coping. But it was even more than that for me: For most of my life I've received a great deal of admiration from people, for being emotionally honest and happy and nice and creative. So my secret was more than just my "words"; it was that I was killing myself in a psychological way, that I was a furious, unfed child. I can't see how realizing this could have been any less painful than it was.

Burton, after exactly a year of therapy, has now been urging me to evolve as fully and creatively as I can. I am just beginning to hate him less for the pushing and reap more rewards from the doing. I am fantastically happy (some of the time) to experience myself as a different person. I am thankful and slightly disbelieving that I couldn't trick Burton into letting me off the hook of my unconscious.

Final Reflections

If I consider the major professional areas of my life—teaching, research and writing, encounter groups, international travel to conferences, and the psychotherapies—then the last ranks as supreme in the panoply of things I do. Because I feel so effective in this setting, and all the indications are that I am helpful for most people, I have at times wondered whether I had a separate and distinct ego for psychotherapy. I like myself best when healing, and people like me best when healing. This has sometimes created a dilemma which Steinzor (in this book) resolves in a superior way—by carrying over the healer into one's social life and making no distinction between healer and client or healer and nonclient. Encounter group people seem to do this as a regular thing.

I am sad to say that it does not work for me. I cannot maintain the heights away from the therapeutic hour, and I feel it an imposition to attract, interact, and hold friends through a clinical persona. Therapy certainly is life but a different kind of life. I would not want my life to be only a therapeutic scene, and I am not so certain that my clients want me extratherapeutically, even though they may think they do. Perhaps one phase subsidizes the other and this subsidization is necessary to live both phases. But, of course, there is only one me, and I consider it a most felicitous thing that psychotherapy puts me in contact with highly talented and creative people, allows me to be with them for the common welfare, rewards me in a brilliant economic way, and permits me to be in touch with the best in myself.

Concluding an autobiography is almost as difficult as commencing one. All those I have read have ended on a somewhat incomplete note as thought the writer were waiting for something more. That something may be Thanatos, which is of course the final ending of all. But one has many autobiographies, and my definitive statement has yet to be written. My interest in psychotherapy continues unabated and my best books are yet to be written. I firmly believe that Freud's message about man was the correct one and that it merely needs to be brought in tune with the times. He was the one who discovered the true psychic individuality of man in both his demonic and loving forms. And while he had little use for civilization, seeing it as taking more than a fair toll of man for what it offered him, he always extolled the individual and sought to give him a freedom from both his personal and cultural restraints. Our clients still seek that same freedom.

Selected Writings

Psychotherapy of the Psychoses. New York: Basic Books, 1961 (with collaborators).

Modern Humanistic Psychotherapy. San Francisco: Jossey-Bass, 1968.

Encounter: The Theory and Practice of Encounter Groups. San Francisco: Jossey-Bass, 1970 (with collaborators).

Interpersonal Psychotherapy. Englewood Cliffs, N.J.: Prentice-Hall, 1972.

IX

Search for Love

Reuben Fine

In titling this autobiographical study I wanted to focus on the central theme of my life as far back as I can remember. For the last thirty years, my dominant passion has been psychoanalysis. But the course of development has led me to a clarification of what psychoanalysis is, both as a philosophical system and a psychological approach. It is the study of love in all its manifestations.

Early Years

In the light of what I know now my early years were tragically traumatic. My father left home before I was two, and mother never remarried, in fact never even showed the slightest interest in any other man. Her dominant motive was to take revenge on my father, whom she always referred to as "that bastard." One of the great triumphs of her life was to have him jailed for nonpayment of alimony, when I was about ten. She used to say of this event: Revenge is sweet. One sister, two years older, and I grew up in the shadow of this protracted battle.

Looking back, it is easy to see that I was always concerned with overcoming the differences between my parents. At an early age I memorized Robert Browning's little poem:

> *He liveth best*
> *Who loveth best*
> *All things both great and small;*
> *For the great God*
> *Who madeth us*
> *He made and loveth all.*

Poetry (until the time when I began to write it much later in life) was never any strong interest, so this poem must have had special meaning.

On the surface at least my love for my mother was very strong. She presented herself as a long-suffering, self-sacrificing Jewish mother and consciously urged upon me the duty of taking proper care of her as soon as I was in a position to do so. Obviously, this set the stage for the many later rescue fantasies which cost me so much heartache. The diappearance of an uncle from the scene when I was eight removed the only male figure with whom I could identify (father had almost totally disappeared) so that the relationship with my mother remained quite intense for a long time.

School quickly became a welcome outlet from the misery at home. From the first grade on, when stars were literally passed out to bright children, I remained a star student. Intellectual achievement became one of the guiding principles of my life, and has always remained so.

Since I went to school in the 1920s, when the IQ had just been discovered, I was pushed through at a rapid rate, having a high IQ. At fourteen I was out of high school, at eighteen out of college. Naturally, my emotional growth had not kept up with the intellectual, so a considerable imbalance resulted. Mine was the sorrowful adolescence, torn by loneliness and sexual conflicts, described by innumerable writers.

There was one bright spot which made my Sturm und Drang period somewhat different from that of others—an unusual ability at chess. At sixteen I was already one of the best players in the country and at seventeen one of the best in the world. From then on school became secondary; chess offered too much immediate gratification, even though I always knew that I would some day come back to an academic career.

The depression (my graduation from college came in 1933) made matters considerably worse, since there were few jobs around. I became an international grandmaster and toured the world playing matches.

In some way my first marriage, in 1937, broke my interest in chess, and in 1938 I returned to New York and to philosophy, which had intrigued me so much during the last two years of college. Morris Raphael Cohen was then the great intellectual luminary at City College and I had avidly listened to all his lectures. The next few years contain some of my happiest memories. For as much time as I could spare from making a living, I studied philosophy at Columbia University, particularly with John Herman Randall, of whom the students used to say: "You can throttle Aristotle, but you can't hold a candle to John Herman Randall."

Randall is perhaps best known to those who never studied with him as the author of *The Making of the Modern Mind,* probably the most widely used text in the intellectual history of modern man. As a person Randall was, like Cohen, an extraordinarily impressive scholar. No facet of human learning seemed to have escaped his searching inquiry. To him philosophy was an adventure in the history of ideas, not a static collection of systems, and I have always thought of it in that way. His views and teaching have strongly shaped my attitude toward the many philosophical systems that exist in psychotherapy.

World War II interrupted my carefree study of philosophy. My military time was spent in intelligence work of various kinds in wartime Washington, but the horrors of the war impressed themselves on me deeply. Most members of my parents' families, and much of my wife's family (she was Dutch), were murdered by the Nazis, along with the other millions. To this day I am horrified by the thoughtless rebels of the younger generation who choose Hitler or Stalin as heroes.

Analysis

My first encounter with analysis was a lecture by A. A. Brill at City College when I was an undergraduate. What he said I do not know, but I do remember his flashing eyes and the forcefulness of his personality. Stimulated by him, I visited some lectures on abnormal personality at Columbia, which were then open to anybody who wished to attend.

Some years later an analyst who had been trained by Freud, Dr. Louis London, offered to take me on as a free patient, as his contribution to the theory of psychoanalysis. (That was still being done in 1936.) He had consulted with Dr. William Alanson White, who had assured him that the unraveling of what makes a man a chess master would be an important contribution to analytic theory. The only hitch was that before he could see me for free, he had to wait for a wealthy patient who could pay thirty to fifty dollars an hour. Although this benefactor did not appear, and I never became London's patient, he explained a lot about analysis to me. I recall particularly the sense of liberation and freedom to write which, he explained, had resulted from his analysis, an experience similar to mine at a later date.

So it was not until I got to Washington that serious analysis began. The initial encounter with an analyst, Dr. Benjamin Weininger, was occasioned by my marital difficulties. He recommended analysis and I readily acquiesced. Weininger was the most extraordinary personal experience I ever had. He was then one of the leaders of the Washington Psychoanalytic Society, along with Sullivan, Fromm-Reichmann, Fromm, and others. At that time, however, there was still no talk of a Sullivanian school. The William Alanson White Psychiatric Institute started courses around 1942, and I began attending them shortly thereafter. But it was still a pretty open affair.

Unlike Sullivan, with whom he was very close, Weininger wrote very little. But everybody considered him a great analyst. Frieda Fromm-Reichmann once told me that he was an authentic genius as a therapist. He seemed to have an uncanny knack for hitting the right spots, and my analysis progressed by leaps and bounds.

At first the analysis was conducted along classically Freudian lines, but then Weininger began to introduce a number of philosophical ideas. He was one of the innovators who brought Buddhism to the attention of the psychoanalysts in this country. Although his philosophical approach was most congenial to me, I came to see that my response to it was a resistance to deeper understanding. Eventually the problems had to be worked out by the familiar analytic technique of understanding and outgrowing my childhood conflicts.

Sullivan, whom I came to know fairly well in this period, was regarded by everybody as one of the great seminal teachers of his time. He was particularly remarkable as a therapist for schizophrenics, whom all others thought of as virtually hopeless. From the earliest days of my training with Sullivan I have thought of the unwillingness to treat schizophrenics because they are so "sick" as a countertransference. Of Sullivan's system I have come to think much less in the course of time, especially after my intellectual study of Freud.

Toward the end of my time in Washington (1944) I decided to become an analyst. Which degree should I pursue: medicine or psychology? Since I was then thirty-one years old, an M.D. degree meant postponing work with psychiatric patients for at least seven or eight years while the doctorate in clinical psychology offered immediate therapeutic experience.

The choice of psychology was made with many misgivings. First of all I knew from my previous work in the philosophy of science that behaviorist psychologists, in the vast majority in the universities, were hopelessly confused about the nature of science and the proper scientific approach to human beings. Second, even my slight contact with the field had shown me that most psychologists were opposed to any truly dynamic approach to people, although that was also true of most psychiatrists.

Fortunately, I was able to find a program at the University of Southern California which allowed me to enter clinical work almost immediately. The first graduating class in clinical psychology in 1948 comprised Edwin Shneidman, Joseph Shoben, Edith Lord, and myself, all of whom have since made their mark in the field in one way or another.

Armed with a Ph.D. I returned to New York in 1948 to pursue further training in psychoanalysis. For the next five years I studied with a number of the leading men of that time: Bunker (with whom I reentered analysis), Roheim, Theordor Reik, van Ophuijsen, Bychowski, Rosen Wolf, and many others. Hospital work, teaching, private practice, personal analysis, controls—all took up so much time and energy that it was not surprising that my marriage began to founder. In spite of all the conflicts, these were exciting years. I have come to agree with Kris' formulation of the "formative decade"—it hardly seems possible to become a competent therapist in less than ten years.

In the beginning, and partly because of the many therapeutic experiments that had been done in Washington in the early forties, I was rather hesitant in my analytic approach. The guilt about not being good enough to "mother" entered into my feelings about patients, and I kept asking myself, "Am I really helping them sufficiently?" As so often happens, this doubt was made worse by getting truly difficult referrals. Several times teachers and supervisors chided me for taking on such patients. Yet I persisted and even helped people who would otherwise have been considered hopeless.

In the early fifties many of the improvisational ideas being put forth appealed to my adventurous spirit, and I would try them out on selected patients. Nothing ever seemed to work except psychoanalysis— and the deepening understanding of countertransference. If I have come around, in the clarification of my own thinking, to the most intense concentration on analysis, it is only because repeated frustrations with other concepts and techniques have taught me that nothing else really works.

Reanalysis with Henry Alden Bunker in 1951 led me to an intensive reexamination of Freud. Bunker was one of the earliest Freudians; he had been president of the New York Psychoanalytic Society and had even translated one of Freud's works (*The Problem of Anxiety*). Upon rereading Freud I made the unhappy (later happy) discovery that most of what had been said about him, by *both* culturalists and Freudians, was in fact wrong. My intellectual background led me to go back to the primary sources, and there began a most delightful excursion into the history of psychoanalysis, psychiatry, and psychology which has stood me in good stead. Eventually, this led to the secure conviction that Freud was by far the greatest mind the field has ever known. But his views have to be clarified, and this I eventually tried to do in a book.[1]

The shift from Sullivan to Freud also led to a rethinking of Sullivan's views. Here I made the surprising discovery that those who proclaimed adherence to Sullivan most loudly were scarcely familiar with what he had said. They are as neo-Sullivanian as many of the contemporary "Freudians" are neo-Freudian. Such occurrences are re-

[1] *Freud: A Critical Revaluation of His Theories* (New York: McKay, 1962).

markably similar to many events in the history of philosophy, where great teachers are often taken up as leaders by their followers, who distort their ideas, sometimes beyond recognition. Jacques Barzun once wrote a book in which he showed that Darwin was not a Darwinian, Marx was not a Marxist, and Wagner was not a Wagnerian. In the same vein Freud once told Reik: "I am not a Freudian." Yet all this had to be understood as a psychologist, not rejected out of hand. Man's inordinate insecurity, even if he is an analyst, and his need to circumvent this insecurity by fastening on a teacher or guru were the answer. By this I mean transference, in ordinary psychoanalytic language. And just as our patients often do not hear what we say, followers often do not know what the leader has said.

Inevitably my position as a lay analyst led me into a variety of political activities. Here I cannot say that I have been remarkably successful, nor that I have particularly enjoyed the fray. But since throughout my career the lay analyst has so often been threatened with extinction, either by the physician or the psychologist, I necessarily had to join up with those who were defending against the threat. I have been active in one analytic organization and have started two others in the course of time. My preference is to work independently in my own Institute.

So much for a sketchy account of the main events of my life. In what follows I will stick to the topic of healer maturity, the main question of this book, knowing at the same time that the ideas set forth are as truly autobiographical as the accidental and transitory experiences that have actually occurred.

Love the Universal

The unifying thread in my life, both personal and intellectual, has been love. Through analysis I was able to find love and through practicing it I was able to teach others how to love. The proper elucidation of the nature of love is thus, to my mind, *the* problem to be faced by all the sciences concerned with man. Insofar as they do so, they further human knowledge; when they do not, they are trivial or simply talk gibberish. The emphasis on love necessarily leads to a total reevaluation of everything that we know, just as my own personal search for love has led me to examine everything I was ever taught.

To begin with, the most immediate question we face is the "patient" and his "therapy." Advisedly, both these terms are put into quotation marks because they have to be completely redefined. A "patient," conventionally, is somebody who is "sick" and comes for "help." But his coming is self-determined, his sickness is not a sickness, and the help is listening. Can anything be more paradoxical? "The patient is not a patient, the doctor is not a doctor," Freud once said. And Sullivan taught us that those who are in therapy are in while those who are not are not; the difference is zero. And Randall once said of the Sophists of fifth-century Athens that they questioned the way of life of their contemporaries, much as if someone today were to ask a graduate of a business school whether a few more dollars would make him happy? Increasingly, it became clear to me that psychotherapy is a philosophical pursuit.

But if psychotherapy is a branch of philosophy, what kind of philosophy is it? Certainly it resembled none I had ever encountered in the academies. Gradually, I realized that psychoanalysis offered the first significant answer to the age-old question of how man can find happiness—significant because it was the first to ascertain that man holds on to his unhappiness by remaining unconscious of his true motives. "Know thyself," said the Delphic oracle; but it remained for Freud to show how.

Yet the patient comes with a medical bias: he is "sick." How is this to be converted into a philosophical orientation, a realization that he is suffering from a disturbance in his love life? In analytic language, this conversion involved a shift from a symptom emphasis to a character approach. Some could make this shift; others could not.

I came to see that there is, on the one hand, a certain self-selection process among patients and, on the other, a necessary quantum of reeducation by the analyst. People who turn to analysts are those who feel love as a problem or who are ready to see it as one when it is pointed out to them. Those who maintained their attention on the symptom left treatment at an early stage; those who were willing to explore their love lives stayed.

Normality and Schizophrenia

All this confirmed what Freud had taught—that everybody needs analysis and that normality is analyzability, not a surface conformity to societal demands or the ability to "get along." This had been my point of view from the very beginning, but it brought increasing conflict with many of the practices common in the field, such as sending a patient to a "psychiatrist" for a "diagnostic interview" to decide whether he is "sick enough" to have "treatment." Although such talk is everyday parlance in our field, it is nevertheless the sheerest nonsense.

The only real question in the beginning is whether the patient will accept treatment, and if so, on what terms. Acceptance of treatment is more important than the specific terms. Here a conflict arises with certain classical analysts who insist that only if the patient comes five times per week (or four, or sometimes three) can he be said to be in analysis. If love is the goal, no rigid formalism can lead to it. To such an unbending dogmatism Freud himself was strongly opposed.

Inevitably the question of diagnostic categories enters the picture. Freud offered many diagnostic proposals, but most of them have not stood the test of time. Sullivan, in his lectures, was entirely opposed to diagnosis, although his posthumously edited material presents a somewhat different picture. My attitude toward diagnosis has undergone a number of changes. Initially, there seemed to be something to it, especially since as an expert in psychological tests I could distinguish different degrees of pathology as well as different life styles. Yet the practical use of diagnosis always gave me the feeling that the people involved in it did not know what they were doing. It dawned on me that diagnosis must serve some psychological function for the diagnostician. If it has no patient intellectual value, it must somehow fit in with his defensive schema. As another defense mechanism, diagnosis must be part of the therapist's countertransference toward the patient. This recognition shed much light for me on what was going on in the field.

From the very beginning of my study with the important practitioners at Chestnut Lodge (Sullivan, Fromm-Reichmann, Weininger, Bullard, Rioch, and others) schizophrenia was the condition in the forefront of our discussions. Sullivan, in his grandiloquent manner, spoke of the "disease which I at times have called schizophrenia." Yet he also insisted, even more than Freud, that there was a continuum from the normal to the psychotic.

While agreeing with this formulation today, I would go much further. The clinical schizophrenic is a person with a deep sense of despair about ever achieving any meaningful gratification with another human being. He is at the furthest remove possible from love. But the diagnosis of schizophrenia is the defense mechanism of the profession. I most emphatically disagree with the usual cliche that the schizophrenic is the "mystery man of psychiatry." The evidence is overwhelming that this condition, like all other human personality traits, is the result of early familial experiences. That constitutional factors play a part as they do in personality in general is certainly true; but what that part is remains an unknown quantity. We have to go back to the nuclear family.

The use of the term schizophrenia as a professional defense mechanism helps the psychiatrist cover up his own personal problems, conceal the enormous hatreds that rage in society, and block awareness of the revolutionary implications of the whole science. This term may also be used, from the practical point of view, to maintain a steady practice, since many patients labeled "schizophrenic" pose such obstacles to treatment that they rarely get better. On top of that, for therapists who are not too sure of their ground, as is true of a great many, a diagnosis of schizophrenia can be a convenient alibi: if the patient does not get better, he was too "sick"; if he does, a miracle has been accomplished.

With love as the central concept in place of diagnosis, the question of treatability or untreatability takes on an entirely different cast. My position now is that the patient must be made aware of his love problem as soon as possible; his reaction to this awareness will be the main determinant in how much change will be brought about. The masochistic neurotic looms so large in our clinical practice not because he is "sicker," but because he is more willing to look into himself than is his sadistic counterpart. Ackerman's concept of the family scapegoat has been especially useful here. The family scapegoat comes to treatment but the family bully stays away in our present cultural context.

Once more these considerations force a reexamination of what is meant by a "patient." If people are convinced that they are not sufficiently loving, they will come for help. But that is a far cry from any of the traditional formulations of the major disciplines. Above all it reveals that *psychoanalysis creates its own patient population*. The implications of this statement for history and for understanding our culture will be elaborated below.

A query can be interposed here: if love is the goal, why can it not be taught directly? That has been the practice in Christianity and other religions, and many philosophical systems as well. The answer lies in the unconscious. Man's capacity to deny and rationalize even his most barbarous deeds is much too strong. Philosophical wisdom can only be achieved through a psychological voyage. Yet at the same time the psychological voyage without a formulated goal becomes an empty exercise. Both psychology and philosophy are essential to the person.

Therapeutic Process

If the patient is one who goes on a voyage of self-discovery toward the goal of love, what then is the therapeutic process about? Here reality necessarily enters the picture. No one should delude himself into thinking that the therapeutic process is anything but extraordinarily difficult.

In the beginning of my practice I still cherished the hope that somehow I could shorten the process which had been so long and painful for me. This hope was soon shattered. The patients had to spend long weary hours talking of their mothers, fathers, childhood, sexual conflicts, hostilities and so on. There was no hiding place, and there was no short cut. This is Freud's momentous contribution. Therapy involves making the unconscious conscious. In this uncovering transference and resistance play a central role. In theory nothing has changed since Freud's day. An epochal step forward in the understanding of the human mind remains there for all time.

While the basic outline of analysis is astoundingly simple, its practice is astoundingly difficult. Make the unconscious conscious. Yes, indeed! The first patient wants to know why I prefer another girl in the group (all this fantasy buttressed by much misinterpretation). The second is curious as to why I am so interested in her sex life. The third demands to know how I can say that happiness can be found in life when I do not offer it directly. The fourth, a high school student with multiple problems, insists that he is forced to come here by his father and will not talk until I tell him he is free to leave. And so it goes.

Whatever the philosophy or aspiration of the therapist, most of his time is taken up with everyday realities, which are all too often forgotten, to be replaced by the everyday reality of the next session. The analyst deals with millions of trivialities. And yet somehow, through all of these, there looms a larger goal, the transformation of a human life. It is only this goal which keeps the analysis going.

It took me a long time to accept this reality of the analytic life. My own background had familiarized me with abstract and philosophical ideas to such an extent that I began with the illusion that they could easily be transmitted to others. Actually, in my own analyses I had discarded the philosophical trappings and dealt with my own everyday realities. But surely, I thought, it would be different with others, especially those whose backgrounds had not been as traumatic as mine. Not so. I came to appreciate the truth of Freud's remark that every human being has to liberate himself from his mother. There is no other way. At best we can concentrate on this as *the* problem; everything else wastes time.

Love is intimately tied up with sexuality; in any clinical discussion the two can scarcely be separated. Yet they have to be. In view of the developments in ego psychology, the whole attitude toward sexuality had to be clarified. At first I took an ego approach, working with the character resistances rather than the direct sexual material. But, as someone has said, whatever the theoretical orientation of the practitioner, children are all Freudians. At that time my own children were growing up (a boy and a girl) and they left no doubt about their intimate knowledge of the Freudian scheme of sexual development, which they had not learned from books. Since then I have always told students who fight the traditional description of psychosexuality: "Don't argue, have a few children." In my therapeutic work with children the sexual material was equally manifest.

I soon came to see that the chance to reveal sexual secrets is one of the great advantages the analytic situation holds for the patient. And every patient had some kind of secret. No matter how liberal they appeared to be in their sex lives there was always some material held back. This material and the reasons for holding it back become an integral part of every analysis.

Talking about sex has a way of getting people excited and it is no different for the analyst. The need to defend against this excitement is excessively great on the part of many analysts. My experience was that if I could find the patient alluring it did more good than harm; if I could not find some sexual interest in the patient, the analysis came to grief. This is similar to the parent-child situation. The child suffers much more from a parent who is cold and distant than from one who is warm and loving, even if that warmth occasionally spills over into too much physical contact.

Inevitably the emphasis on making the unconscious conscious brings up the question of alternative techniques, especially those connected with touching and body contact. I have never been able to see how these could be of any help to the patient. Most practitioners I have observed who go in for these techniques belong to a "lunatic fringe" characterized by a gross distortion of what Freud and other analysts have said, an unawareness of transference and resistance, and a considerable amount of intellectual dishonesty. Analytically, they substitute foreplay for intercourse, even when they actually have intercourse with their patients. For what they offer is a quick excitement rather than a more measured gratification. And as a rule the transference consequences are disastrous. Occasionally the outcome is inconsequential; almost never is it helpful. Sometimes the patient confuses the excitement derived from sex play (in whatever form) with real help. Here, too, the training and integrity of the therapist must help him work through the fantasies rather than exploit the frustration.

Approaches to Psychology

As a theoretician I have come to believe that the implications of psychotherapy for psychological theory are of incalculable import. They are in fact so enormous that the whole structure of psychological science has to be revamped to account for them. A good part of the professional difficulties in the field derived from the confusion about the nature of psychology and psychiatry. Psychology is the basic science, the study of man. But as a scientific study of man it has to be pursued clinically, in accordance with the data available. The insistence on experimentation in the study of personality is one of those colossal errors in the history of ideas for which mankind has paid dearly. The experimental psychologist has the clinician in a double bind: he pursues useless research via experimental designs (ignoring the fact that none of this research ever led anywhere and that it is theoretically incapable of doing so) while preventing the clinician from pursuing useful clinical research. The proper study of man is still man, but he must be studied directly. This is what psychoanalysis is as a dynamic psychology: the direct observation of man in his most vital concerns. Psychiatry, apart from its dynamic aspect—which is psychoanalysis—is a confused mixture of speculation, hostility, medicine of unknown value, and pure hokum. Yet in the present scene the psychiatrist stands much higher on the social and professional scales.

This gigantic professional error is due more to the ignorance and intransigence of psychology than to the claims of psychiatry (though these are often meretriciously self-seeking, especially in the case of the drugs). For the most part practiced by individuals with an academic orientation, psychology has been afraid to get involved with the most significant human experiences. In many cases such involvement would mean literally dismissal from the university, as happened to a professor at Illinois who was fired after he openly recommended premarital sexuality. As psychoanalysts in private practice we are much freer, for we can openly recommend both premarital and extramarital sex without fear of the consequences. It is no accident that psychology is in danger of falling apart in its main professional structure, especially the American Psychological Association. For any reorganization to be meaningful it must be effected on a sound theoretical basis.

My background in philosophy has been kept alive through the search for a satisfactory approach to psychology, a main preoccupation for the past few years. Instead of overemphasis on the cognitive functions, psychology must resolutely set itself to study the problem of happiness. How have men sought happiness in the past? How do they seek it now? How successful are they? These and similar questions are the ones that are really worthy of a science, not the critical flicker fusion frequency or the conditioning of the eyelid reflex, for these are mechanical details which are secondary to man's principal affairs. In this search for happiness love has always played a central role and in all probability always will, so that here again psychology and philosophy overlap.

All the social sciences study man in some aspect of his functioning. The artificial divisions into psychology, economics, history, linguistics, and so on are purely arbitrary, for more crucial is the functioning human being. The German term *Geisteswissenschaft* is more appropriate than the English equivalent, and perhaps the best word is the humanities. Psychology is crucial to all areas of the humanities and in turn can derive much valuable material from them. But the experimental model, except for certain minor areas of cognition, has to be abandoned in its entirety. Let us be brutally frank about the situation: the experimental study of personality has been and is scientific idiocy. Let us make sure that the experimentalists do not hide again behind a mystical aura of science which when looked at more carefully, *in the light of what science really has been and is,* is sheer poppycock. It is no accident that Skinner in his latest book steers behaviorist technology into a road which could easily lead to a form of fascism (just reinforce people to like to do what they are told to do), while psychoanalysis comes back over and over again to democracy and basic humanistic values.

Once psychology is rewritten to become the core of all the humanities, as psychoanalysis has attempted to do, it will be a far cry from what it is today. Then the student will study such questions as what makes people work (economics), why social classes keep their distance (sociology), why and how the language of the conqueror takes over (linguistics), how obedience is taught in cooperative cultures (anthropology), and how the tragic history of the blacks explains their present low level of intellectual achievement (history). The student will not be able to say, as so many do today, that the introductory course in psychology is really biology. He will realize instead that he is studying man in his essential functioning, using whatever empirical information and conceptual tools are available.

Psychoanalytic Values

The values that have dominated my life are those derived from the main tradition of Western European humanism: truth, love, achievement, reliance on reason in place of authority, and a search for happiness on earth rather than in heaven. No man can really practice as intimate a discipline as psychoanalysis without conveying his values to the patients, nor do I see any particular virtue in concealing them. What must be avoided is the seductive opportunity to become the almighty authority who forces his values on others. Patients nowadays tell me that I come across to them as very sincere, without the trappings of showmanship, which assures me that I am on the right track with them. Few patients who see an analyst over a period of time will be unable to observe certain very real qualities in him, over and above the transference manifestations.

The healing encounter has been one of the major growth opportunities of my life. In my most recent book, *The Healing of the Mind*, I have tried to convey to others how this could be done. To help in this process, the analyst must always be aware of his counter-transferences and be able to use them constructively. Just as there are always transferences (in the broad sense of the word) there are always countertransferences. It has always seemed to me that when analysts say they have no countertransferences they are defending themselves against some strong feeling about the patient. I am always involved in one way or another in the lives of all my patients.

Neither transference nor countertransference is inherently bad (the opposite view derives from a misunderstanding). Positive transference, found in most successful patients, determines the success of the procedure; if there is too much negativism, the patient simply leaves. Likewise, positive countertransference has a strong effect on the outcome. I have time and again observed that patients seem to respond merely to the interest shown in them, even when everything else seems hopeless. Just now I am working with an attractive young girl who bawls me out unmercifully almost every hour, calling me immature, a quack, cold, a sex manaic, and so on, yet at the end of the hour she gives me a deep, longing look and says softly, "See you next time." She has been to two previous therapists, neither of whom seemed to care very much about what happened to her. I care, and it carries over.

Not that the analyst is so omnipotent. Merely caring for patients is no guarantee that they will recognize it and respond. Many, caught up in difficult transferences, do not, and leave treatment. But most stay. But not caring for the patient is a sure way of stifling whatever progress has been made or can be made.

Yet this kind of therapeutic caring is by no means easy, and it has in fact taken me many years to reach a point where it is manageable. Patients make abusive remarks, suddenly decamp, make all kinds of demands, some of them quite outrageous (one college student demanded that I pay the tuition which his father would not give him, and when I refused, he broke an ashtray in the office), and behave in other ways which are ordinarily not endearing. The analyst must learn to take all this hostility and still continue to care for the more decent values which the patient is struggling to bring to the fore. When a patient comes for the first time I often construct a vision of what life might be like for him (or her), and in the course of time gradually convey this vision to the patient. The Greek word *theoria,* from which our word theory derives, actually means vision. This dynamic use of countertransference is the *theoria* on which my entire technique is based.

Another value of the countertransference approach is that it opens the analyst so that he can learn from the patient. I have always inveighed against the medical model which sees the healing encounter as a doctor-patient relationship and is the kiss of death. The model should rather be that of a teacher-pupil or philosopher-follower relation. In this model the pupil is often not too distant from the teacher in many areas of his functioning, and from these the teacher can learn. For example, we deal with many persons who in spite of neurotic difficulties are still able to function quite adequately at certain tasks. Many patients do in fact work more effectively in the real world than do their analysts. How they manage this can be used to advantage by the analyst.

Even in the interpersonal realm many patients can be teachers as well as pupils. Sexually, many young people have experimented more than have their elders, and they can show the analyst how he can reach new sources of pleasure that he had never thought of before. My own sex life has been quite free for many years, so this applied to me chiefly in the beginning of my practice. Even homosexuals can teach a heterosexual man to be less afraid of men.

Analysis cannot be conducted in the abstract; it needs a foil. While many have formulated the goal of analysis as continued self-analysis, few have carried this out. The analyst is in a better position to do so, because he is barred from acting out with the patient whom he is trying to help. Properly considered, he therefore has no choice other than continued analysis of his reactions to the patient. Every patient will remind the analyst in greater or lesser degree of personal figures from his past, and close observation of his reactions to the patient will work out the meaning of those people in his life. Here, too, as in the patient's analysis, the process will be tedious and time-consuming, yet all the more rewarding in the long run.

While I have no great admiration for Jung, either as a human being or as a thinker, one remark he made has stuck in my mind: "Often conflicts are outgrown, rather than resolved." In my own life this has frequently been the case. Conflicts have faded away over a period of years. Sometimes they flare up again briefly, then disappear. This process has required extensive self-analysis in which my own analytic work with patients has provided much of the material.

The experiencing of countertransference has also led me to a deepening awareness of human relationships. Conflict is inherent in the human condition no matter how well analyzed the person is. But it can consistently be reduced, and the pursuit of this consistent reduction is what makes for real growth and maturity.

The healing encounter cannot, in my experience, become the model for other human relationships, except perhaps for the parental to a limited degree. Love in ordinary life should involve a maximum degree of participation, gratification and enjoyment, which must necessarily be kept to a minimum in therapy.

My model in analysis is the classical one of releasing the id, which I formulate as expansion of the libido. It seems to me that ego psychology, as formulated by Hartmann and others, wanders too far from the libidinal gratification which remains the *sine qua non* of healthy living. The ego itself is not inherently a new concept in Freud's later formulations; it existed in one form or another from the very beginning. But the superego is radically new. I see anxiety as related on the one hand to libidinal desire and on the other to superego punishment. Hence analysis becomes necessarily superego analysis. My views have been described more extensively in *The Healing of the Mind* and in a forthcoming work, *An Inquiry Into the Process of Psychoanalysis,* so I shall not go into them further here.

Sensitivity Training

Do I have any use for sensitivity training and encounter groups in my technical armamentarium? I do group analysis, so in one sense the answer is yes. But in another, deeper sense, the answer is no. First because the very terms *sensitivity* and *encounter* embody the typical kind of intellectual dishonesty which is so prevalent in the field. If they have any adequate basis, they are group therapy; why then use another name? If they do not have a really adequate basis, why use them at all?

Certain questions are all too often sidestepped in the realm of psychotherapy by a process of misleading labeling. The term *behavior therapy,* for example, seems to imply that analysts do not concern themselves with behavior. This is of course entirely untrue. "Client-centered counseling" carries with it the implication that analysis is analyst-centered, which is absurd. What Gestalt therapy is supposed to mean is a mystery which I do not pursue with any diligence, for I always regarded Perls as a high priest of the lunatic fringe.

There are two real issues in encounter and sensitivity training: first, does a brief encounter of a day, or a week, have any lasting value; and, second, should physical contact be allowed or encouraged in therapy? With regard to the first, the evidence to me is ample that if there is no follow-up to the brief encounter, it has only some stimulus value which is soon undone; if there is a follow-up, that becomes more important than the encounter.

As far as physical contact during therapy is concerned, most of what goes on I would characterize as foreplay or aggression. Some of it, such as hugging, kissing, touching, is direct foreplay; some of it is aggression, as for example pinning a helpless victim to the floor. The question then is: should the analyst, or other group members, engage in foreplay or violence with the patient? To put the question in this way naturally makes the answer clear. The patient has to steer toward a real experience of intercourse, in both the literal and figurative senses, since intercourse does have a double meaning in ordinary language—sexual and social. Excessive reliance on foreplay, particularly when accompanied by a loud claim that this is "liberation," weakens the drive to intercourse and to real resolution of the person's problems. Once a friend of mine, an excellent analyst, was asked whether he had sex with his patients. He replied: "If they don't need it, why should I interfere? And if they do need it, why should I be the guinea pig?"

Further, the encounter-sensitivity movement has a dangerous tendency to violence. There are already a number of groups where patients are encouraged to hit one another and some lawsuits for damages have resulted. I abhor violence in all its forms and feel that this tendency in encounter groups should be quickly eliminated. The profession is sowing the seeds of its destruction with this madness which, besides, is totally devoid of any meaningful theoretical rationale. Love cannot be reached through the pursuit of hatred.

These are times that try men's souls. Everywhere we hear the cry: in a society as disordered as ours is, how can we take the time for individual therapy? With such objection I would make most emphatic disagreement. We need more therapy, not less. I share with all other thinking men of our time a deep concern for the moral and physical rot that is everywhere around us; but I do not believe that there is any easy solution.

Many psychologists wish to abandon psychology altogether, and some turn to politics. That is their privilege. One psychologist, the distinguished former secretary of HEW, and now head of Common Cause, has already done so. I wish him every success. But politics involves a maneuvering for power which requires techniques of its own and in which the psychologist is as much a layman as anybody else. Once a politician, all his expertise as a psychologist goes down the drain. Some years ago I was on a program with a woman, a professor of psychology at a leading university. She stated that if she were a black in our present-day society she would shrink from no act of violence, no matter how extreme, to enforce her rights. Such a statement is truly horrifying, especially since she did not even consider the consequences of what she was saying.

Furthermore, the history of the world is a history of bloodthirsty quarrels which have literally sent mlilions of people to their graves. It has been estimated that in the present century *500 million* people have died violent deaths as a result of war and its effects. More violence is certainly not going to help.

We have, in our psychotherapeutic techniques, a uniquely novel instrument for changing the human psyche. In spite of constant disparagement and intense opposition, psychotherapy has shown enormous growth. Why throw away something new and good and revive something old and useless?

With age my convictions have become increasingly radical. I believe very strongly that the psychotherapy movement, properly handled, can have a noteworthy impact on the future of human civilization. But to do that we must be clear about our knowledge, our goals, and our techniques.

The encounter group should be viewed as means of education, not misrepresented as therapy, and should be led by really qualified persons. As an educational process it can be secondary to therapy, or an adjunct to it, but it cannot replace therapy.

It is necessary to reform the fields of psychology and psychiatry along the lines I have tried to indicate above. Psychology, the basic science of man, deals with how man can achieve happiness and with how he has tried to do so in the past. All our knowledge reveals that regardless of political or economic system the release of violence is destructive to the human race. As psychologists we know all too well from our clinical work how devastating the effects of violence can be on the individual. Let us emphasize this knowledge and its implementation.

It seems to me that at present there is a bankruptcy of ideas among American and liberal intellectuals in general. This bankruptcy derives from their unfamiliarity with psychology or their identification with psychological reactionaries such as Skinner and other behaviorists. Love is essential to the world, and we know a lot about where it comes from, how it can be molded, how it can be developed, and how it can be passed on from one generation to the next. Secured in this knowledge and all of its dynamic consequences, psychology can really become the ideology behind a significant social revolution. To be part of such a revolution belongs to my self-actualization as a therapist.

Selected Writings

Psychoanalytic Observations on Chess and Chess Masters. New York: Psychoanalysis, 1956.

Freud: A Critical Reevaluation of His Theories. New York: McKay, 1962.

"Interpretation: The Patient's Response." In E. Hammer (ed.), *Interpretation.* New York: Grune and Stratton, 1968.

The Technique of Psychoanalytic Psychotherapy. New York: McKay, 1970.

Healing of the Mind. New York: McKay, 1971.

X

Paradox of Being Alien and Intimate

John Warkentin

This is a difficult chapter for me to write. I find trouble starting it and continuing with the writing of it. I want to say mainly, though, that all people, and that means all therapists, have within a "sickness" and a "wellness" that is part of our being. It is this sickness and this wellness in my history that I am dealing with in this paper as well as in my practice.

I have lost interest in "doing psychotherapy." The word *therapy* refers to healing, correcting a defect, or otherwise looking for pathology and then fixing it. Now I am more interested in growth. My concern with myself, and therefore with the people I see in my office, is to encourage all our human potential. But my spurts of initiative gradually dwindle. I need two essential ingredients to rekindle my

243

growth: stressful, anxiety-provoking experiences and simultaneous security of support in a strong intimate relationship. Without these essentials I am likely to go comfort-seeking.[1]

Psychotherapists[2] are people who have learned an unusual respect for emotional pain and emotional satisfaction. They are willing to suffer through crucial endings in their way of living. They have been reborn more than once, in keeping with the comment of e. e. cummings "We can never be born enough." Getting born is always dangerous. Thank God that we cannot remember our first birth, except by way of our permanent fear of death as we face times of rebirth in the scope of our years.

I was conceived on a train traveling from Russia to Germany. My Mennonite parents had married the day before without ever having had a single date. They were leaving their comfortable rural life in order for my father to do graduate work at the Baptist Seminary in Hamburg. Europe was getting ready for the First World War when I was born on June 18, 1913. A year later we became enemy aliens under daily police surveillance. So my parents moved to the small village of Wilhelmsdorf located on an island in a swamp in South Germany, where a part of Napoleon's army long ago sank on their way to Russia. My father taught in the local boys' school. All my early memories there were uneasy. Part of the time we did not have enough to eat and would glean the grain fields after they were harvested so that we could make a few loaves of good bread. We could hear the cannon booming on the western front. German soldiers, some wounded, escaped the war by setting up camps near our village, and they looked threatening to me. In retrospect, it seems likely that they were heavily armed army deserters who were probably indeed dangerous.

I had three playmates. One was Dora, whom I was never permitted to see again after taking down her pants behind a bush at age two and a half (about that time I had a ruptured gut and spent many weeks in the hospital away from home). The second friend was Ernst; he was run over by a truck. My third friend was Fritz, and he taught

---

[1] This paragraph (and some others in this chapter) were taken from the author's editorials published in *VOICES*, 1965–1970.
[2] This term will have to serve in designating our work because no better word is available.

me some things about sex so that my parents disapproved of the friendship.

My first day in school was frightening: I was still "the Russian enemy." In second grade everything got worse; I was farmed out to a foster family and wet the bed every night and got punished every morning. My three younger siblings were kept at home. For my third and fourth grades, the family had moved to a village near Frankfurt, Germany, and by now I was an irritating, unpleasant kid who often got beaten up by other boys as well as at home. At age nine I ran away on a bicycle for one day, got home late that night, fearful of the next big whipping, and had my first severe asthma attack.

By the time I was ten years old, the whole family was depressed and miserable. For five years we had been getting periodic grim news of the disappearance or death by violence of most of our relatives in Russia. My parents lost the vague hope that they might somehow recover some of their family property. On borrowed money our family of six migrated to the United States to Newton, Kansas. It was a very unhappy trip; I worried constantly about going to a strange land where I could not speak the language, and all of us seemed to have a continuous foreboding of catastrophes to come.

In Kansas I was by far the oldest boy in the first grade, and on my first day in school knew only two English words, "yes" and "no." The war against the Huns was still on, in 1923, and the larger "patriotic" boys regularly beat me up during recess. When I cried to my parents about it, they urged me to be nice to the other children, "just be a good boy," and "Mennonites do not fight." I got over the nonviolent Mennonite tradition by age thirteen and after that I was known as "a mean kid," so that nobody bothered me. I was alone.

As the lonely years dragged on I had some awareness of deserving the Shitty Childhood Award (I learned to call it that only recently). My memory for ages ten to sixteen is very uncertain. I blamed my parents. By now, in the security of my present living, I see all those "bad" first thirty-two years of my life as very fortunate in the making of a psychotherapist. No psychotherapist I have known came out of happy, comfortable early years.

Making a therapist out of me began with an unwanted conception and developed through years of physical and emotional privation. A "patient" with an orphan syndrome has a familiar feel to me because I felt like an orphan. My conscious memories of parental rejections, which included being farmed out to a foster home at age six, now give me a warm tolerance for those who struggle with similar histories. A paranoid person reminds me of the frightening rumors I heard as a child: "They say that the French are coming." Incidentally, people who go through an emotional rebirth experience with me seem always to have a phase of paranoid fearfulness during their times of greatest change.

As I now (at age fifty-eight) try to learn from my childhood, I am impressed with the great importance of sexuality as life-preserving. For many people sex seems to be more important than God, or even life itself. I was reminded of this by a minister who saw me for consultation because his church board was considering asking for his resignation; he had preached a sermon to the effect that there were greater sins than adultery, for example, murder.

Going back to my own childhood history, to Dora at age two and a half, I visited southern Germany and Wilhelmsdorf in 1957. I found Dora's old uncle. I introduced myself, including my status as a "university professor" in the United States, and asked if he would give me the married name and address of Dora. He abruptly refused, obviously remembering me as a "bad boy." He reminded me that forty years of living could not erase a sexual sin committed at age two and a half.

Perhaps the greatest pain I ever experience with those who come to my office has to do with loneliness. It feels so familiar when they describe their hunger for personal loving and then explain how they deliberately reject any person who tries to get close to them. That is how I was. The isolation of an emotional cripple makes further rejections almost certain. It is good to know that there really is no such thing as unbearable emotional pain. I like to tell the story of a very shy teen-age boy who had had only a few dates because he was too awkward. As he developed a little more courage he resolved that he could tolerate some rejections and started walking along downtown propositioning all the pretty girls who came along. He mentioned this to a friend who said, "Gosh, didn't you get slapped?" and the young man answered, "Sure, over and over, but oh boy, when it worked!"

My pioneering parents deserve credit for endowing me with

a desire for educational achievement. Perhaps it was because my mother only got to the fourth grade, at which time she was kept at home to care for her psychotic mother. I found it easy to love my mother, because she was also "crazy." Father never managed to get her into a psychiatric hospital, although one time we got as far as the driveway of Menninger's Clinic in Topeka. My concern for education also came from my father, who got his Ph.D. from Chicago University at the age of forty-nine. His thesis was on "The Devil in German Literature." In any case, by the age of thirteen I was determined to be a doctor. This was puberty for me and the beginning of a lifelong interest in sex. Eventually, I got a master's degree in psychology at Brown University and a Ph.D. at the University of Rochester.

My interest in people goes back to my earliest memories. When I was five years old, my father took me by the hand one evening to take me on a long walk. (I found that same path through the woods on my visit in 1957). I was very surprised because my father ordinarily never touched me except to whip me. When we arrived back home, a doctor was there and told me that I now had a baby brother. This was a complete surprise to me and I later asked mother where she had been keeping the baby before it was born. She said that it had been "under her heart." She never would tell me how the baby got there or how he got out. From my mother's tension in regard to the baby, and the many angry scenes between my parents, I knew at an early age that the most important "facts of life" are sexual and that these determine our destiny more than any other factors.

I spent a lot of time with my fantasies regarding what makes people tick. My first introduction to a systematic learning of psychology was an attractive young woman teacher in high school who seemed to pick me out as her favorite student. Later, at Bethel College, Dr. Peter Schellenberg taught psychology and made me his paid assistant. His interest was entirely clinical and it was exciting to learn from him. I expected a similar climate at Brown University when I went there for graduate study but was corrected in my initial conference with the chairman, Dr. Leonard Carmichael. He explained that I would spend two hours every morning cleaning up the cat colony; then I would devote my daytime hours to scientific research on animals and my evenings surveying the literature at the library. When he moved to Rochester a year later, I went along to continue my research on the

visual acuity of animals and assisted Dr. K. U. Smith in his study of
the cat's visual cortex. In Rochester I managed to get away for one
day a week to do psychological testing at the nearby Boys' Industrial
School. I also attended conferences of the psychiatric staff at the medical school and was a co-author of a paper describing the connections
between homosexuality and paranoia. The most absorbing clinical
experiences during my two years at Rochester were in the Guidance
Clinic headed by Dr. Carl Rogers. Here I once more found the kind of
psychology that really interested me. Rogers was a wonderful teacher
and friend; he often invited his staff and students into his home. I
remember myself as a rather uneasy person at that time and once
when Rogers had us over and suggested we all model something with
clay, I just made all of my clay into a cube in order to not give myself
away. It took another ten years before I could accept my paranoia and
my voyeurism. In Rochester, Rogers was gradually developing his "nondirective" or "client-centered" therapy and his whole staff were en-
thusiastic about it. However, although Rogers had departed from the
orthodox analytic method, he maintained the distinction between
"healthy" and "sick" psychodynamics. This prevailing good-bad dichotomy plagued me for many more years until one great hour with
one of my therapists when I realized that I was not a good person,
and that I was not a bad person either.

After finishing my doctorate in 1938, I married Linda Brown.
We had had a long five years of courtship. At this time I also had the
first opportunity of my life to earn a living wage and became a regular
staff member in Rogers' clinic. I was not so nondirective as he would
have liked. I still think I could have worked happily there for some
years if it had not been for the conflict between psychologists and
psychiatrists in Rochester at that time.

Rather abruptly I decided to give up all my new comforts and
put in the five years at hard labor to go through medical school at
Northwestern University. Dr. A. C. Ivy, professor of physiology, had
told me some years earlier that he would hire me as an instructor if I
"knew enough." I went to see him and he thought I did; in addition,
he made Linda his chief secretary. Those were good years, except that
I became suddenly hypothyroid within a month of coming to Chicago
and only sheeps' thyroid tablets kept me going in the upper third of
the class. Graduation from medical school permanently cured my hypo-

thyroidism. Going to medical school had meant a return to pork-and-beans living. But it was worth it.

Since my biological father shared so little of his inner life with me, I made much of the surrogates. From Carmichael I learned the value of understatement and a sharp tongue. From Ivy, and his well-worn face, I got the warmth of saying with kindness when a student was flunking, "You need to learn some more." My research at Northwestern was once again in an area of my personal dynamics: hunger. I established that white rats who are given a choice of diets will be healthier than matched littermates who are fed the famous Osborn and Mendel diet. I also established that thyroidectomized rats will eat more protein than normal to take advantage of the specific dynamic action of proteins. Finally, I helped establish that there are reflex centers in the belly of a dog (and presumably in people) which can operate satisfactorily with no connection to the central nervous system. In the course of my surgery on dogs, I managed to produce one male animal in which I had severed all the sympathetic nerves to the hypogastric area so that he lived for the next year with an absolutely permanent erection. I even got a diploma as a dog surgeon!

My internship in the hospital next door to Northwestern was strenuous; I had a bad peptic ulcer syndrome and lived mostly on boiled chicken and milk-and-cream. But finances were getting easier because of the large royalties from the *Physicians' Handbook*, which I wrote and finished when I was a junior in medical school.

On July 1, 1943, I started a surgical residency, and two days later the first of our four children was born, Marilyn Jean (she now has her Ph.D. in biology and is teaching at the University of Illinois). The Second World War had started and the draft board was after me. I entered the Army Medical Corps in September 1943. The young clerk at the Induction Station saw that I had a Ph.D. in psychology on my papers and told me that I was now a "psychiatrist." Her observation determined my work for the next ten years.

I learned a great deal in the Army. At Carlisle Barracks I found that I could easily walk twenty-five miles in a day. Walter Reed General Hospital had some unusual patients. At Welch Convalescent Hospital I was made sanitary officer to stop an epidemic of diarrhea. The cause was detergent on the dishes. The next official order was that I would become a group therapist with combat veterans (I never mentioned my German birth). At Oak Ridge General Hospital we had a nine-bed ward staffed by too many nurses, attendants, social workers (two), and psychiatrists (five). Oak Ridge was called "Dogpatch" and the "Manhattan District" ran it. It had a population of 75,000, but the people at the bus depot at Knoxville, Tennessee, just twenty miles away, claimed that they had never heard of it.

At Oak Ridge I met Dr. Carl A. Whitaker. We liked each other and worked together for the next twenty years. At Welch Convalescent Hospital I had experimented with groups of three up to groups of 150 people and had found the ideal group therapy setting to consist of eight people meeting for one to two hours. Carl and I learned to lead groups together. The hour following a group session we regularly set aside to review it and to make notes on what we had learned. We also experimented with office interviews in which both of us were present, and again regularly spent the following hour to evaluate the experience. We called this "multiple therapy." Neither of us had ever heard of more than one therapist interviewing a patient together, even though both of us were familiar with the medical practice of having a consultant on difficult cases. The logical next step was for us to see a married couple together, and, after that, to see parents with children present. We were very surprised at the hostile reception we received at a meeting of the American Psychiatric Association when we reported our experiences in multiple therapy or what is now more often called "co-therapy."

After the war, Carl Whitaker and I came to Emory University Medical School to implement the psychiatric teaching program which Dr. Lawrence Woolley had begun. Dean Gene Stead had become interested in promoting psychotherapy. However, he left Emory just before we arrived, in the fall of 1946, and the program we had outlined did not materialize. Nevertheless, we had seven years of teaching there with all the medical students in group therapy during their first two years. During their junior and senior years the students had much clinical experience in interviewing psychiatric patients and they got magnificent results. From 1946 to 1949 I was also chief of neuropsychiatry at Lawson V. A. Hospital. During my last year there I successfully ran the wards without electric shock and without using drugs of any kind. This was most unusual in the V. A. system.

In the meantime, the American Board of Psychiatry disallowed

some of my residency credits and I consequently spent three lonely
months at the Menninger Clinic in 1951. Then I had three happy
months of residency at the Pennsylvania Hospital where I was able to
work with Dr. J. Edward Taylor. We wrote a paper together on the
effectiveness of physical cuddling of supposedly hopeless schizophrenics.
That fall I took the American Boards in Psychiatry and passed them,
which I considered to be an answer to prayer since the Board had a
reputation for flunking psychotherapists.

Teaching has always been one of the pleasant challenges of life
to me, even though as a child I vowed never to do what my father did.
Despite my fondness for teaching, the day I was notified of having
passed the Boards I prepared to go into full-time private practice in
psychotherapy. I was then forty. That was in June 1953 and I have
never regretted this move. I still teach, and some of my happiest
working hours are with younger colleagues who join me in "technique
seminars," the sort of thing that used to be called supervision.

During my early years, up to age thirty-three, I had planned
to die at age forty. In a way I did. I changed my life style in a big
way and gave up several of my secret hopes. I gave up the idea of
being famous and settled on being an ordinary psychotherapist. This
included not being financially comfortable and not living on the North
Side of Atlanta but working long hours with little leisure time. (I was
through with the fantasy that my breaks were still coming and sooner
or later "all would be well.") At this time I stopped looking for the
"end of the rainbow" and accepted a pedestrian kind of living. I was
suppressing my creativity, but it emerged despite myself and I eventually became editor of *Voices* and again enjoyed being creative.

The years in private practice since 1953 have been good years.
I have always had the good fortune to associate in my practice with
valued colleagues who were both loving people and good therapists.
We have enjoyed practicing together in a remodeled home on Peach-
tree Road in Atlanta. The practicing in an old home gives a feeling
of casual warmth to us and our patients which we previously did not
have in a modern office building.

My family life has consistently been the most significant factor
in my office performance. Linda and I did well together during the
grim years of getting through medical school. We then developed personal difficulties with the luxury of an army lieutenant's salary. Even

before our second child (Jim) was born, she wanted to die rather than live with me. With the birth of another daughter and another son (Pamela and Bill), and many hours of therapy for both of us, Linda and I accomplished a coming together which brought us pain and also very much joy. The next fifteen years were the most wonderful years of my life until now. I had a certainty of my own person and an enthusiasm in working which was unexpectedly satisfying. In retrospect, I realize that I had expected to go through life moderately depressed but did not do that.

In the 1960s, I felt that all the bad years were over. Increasingly, I felt the keen edge of my own creativeness and the wholehearted enthusiasm of expressing it in interviews with "patients" and in my writing. It was in the fullness of this joy of working that I accepted the editorship of *Voices, The Art and Science of Psychotherapy,* a new journal about the person of the therapist which the American Academy of Psychotherapists had been planning since 1956. With Tom Leland as associate editor, our first issue came out in the fall of 1965. This journal was almost like a fifth child to me, and also to Linda.

But something went wrong about October 1966; Linda developed lower abdominal tumors which turned out to be cancerous. That fall I had returned from a Los Angeles workshop more full of myself than ever, and Linda felt excluded. She was expected to die in early 1967. In answer to prayer, we had three more wonderful years together, interspersed with awful months while she was in the hospital. She finally decided to die on February 26, 1970. Much like my early years, these last three years with Linda were like a series of dreams which I cannot quite remember.

Tom Leland and I gave up the editorship of *Voices* largely because I simply could not bring enough initiative to that effort during Linda's illness. Strangely enough, my functioning in the office seemed to be hindered very little. It was as if my whole person was actively functional at the office even on days when I had had little sleep and was too depressed to drive my car safely across town. I wondered if this was a hysterical dissociation, my life with vitality in the office and my depression outside of it. In retrospect, it now seems more like psychotic dissociation. In any case, I maintained my financial income in the face of staggering medical costs. As I write these words and remember these things I still get depressed and my penis shrinks up short.

For twenty years Linda and I had been traveling the North Georgia mountains over weekends looking for a retreat spot which we might buy. We found it in the fall of 1965 near Clayton, Georgia, and called it "Cloudland Mountain." We moved a house trailer onto it with a caterpillar tractor and piped water up from a spring despite the assurance of local people that this would be impossible. In January 1968 we began the construction of a house which would be both a home and a conference center for therapists. During the building of the road up the mountain, three bulldozers went over the side and were damaged; further attestation to the comments of people that this would not be a possible feat. However, it was also testimony to our determination to build a dream center. It is still in process of being completed; hopefully it will be done in the next year or so. Meanwhile it is usable for interviews, group marathon sessions, and just plain enjoyment as a hideaway.

After Linda died I was desperately lonely, with all the old hunger of an orphan syndrome. Office relationships were not enough to feed me. I often looked with curiosity at bridge abutments along the highways, debating suicide at one hundred miles an hour. I dated some after a few months but was too depressed to be very interesting or entertaining. My fear during 1970 was that I might marry in order to fulfill a need; some men marry what they need and I did not want to do just that. I finally decided in the 1971 AAP workshop at Stone Mountain, Georgia, that I would never get married again. Paradoxically, after this I really fell in love with a psychotherapist colleague of many years, Dr. Elizabeth Valerius.

Liz and I had a grand church wedding at Thanksgiving time in 1971. Both of us entered this union with misgivings and with much determination to stay together whether we eventually might love each other or not. She was up against the problem of being married at all, and I was up against the problem of getting divorced from my wife of thirty-five years. Since Liz and I had worked well together professionally in previous years, we are now looking forward to further professional work together. (We are writing this chapter together.)

Both of us were surprised by the lively reactions of our patients to our marriage. Some were obviously jealous and resentful, mostly patients of the opposite sex. Others were very pleased, as if to say that we as "the therapists" would now be less provocative or demanding sexually. They also seemed to feel that if it could happen to us, it could happen to them. Most of our patients were just pleased that we were making a new start in life together and would probably be better therapists in the office because we were living a more satisfying life at home. It was noteworthy to both of us that a number of our patients became engaged, married, or just started seriously dating someone when we became engaged. Again we were impressed with the impact of the therapist's personal life on the lives of his patients.

Dr. Burton's request for this chapter came at an ideal time for me. During recent years I have been systematically and also haphazardly assessing my past, present, and future as husband, father, and therapist. This is the order of importance to me. My one great phobia since childhood has been that I would be an evil influence on others. I was afraid to have children for this reason. Now it is apparent that sometimes my presence makes life better for others. However, at this point of my starting a new life, my most active concern is to have fun for myself. Unless the joy of living is in me, I would be offering myself to others with an empty hand. This special kind of selfishness, that I should want a good life for myself, is to me a primary hallmark of the "mature person." The necessary concomitants include physical health, a willingness to postpone immediate satisfactions, a place to express my irritation and anger where it causes the least trouble, enough money for the necessities, and above all else an active sex life.

The only ready antidote to my periodic lifelong depressiveness has been sexual joy. In the scheme of my life style, such sexually satisfying living has been possible for me only in a committed relationship. When I live with the daily expectation of uniting with my beloved, then I am available freely to love others (without overt sexuality). My day in the office is usually made when my wife and I part company happily after breakfast. Then it is a rich opportunity to be in my office with persons who are cultivating an intimacy with me. At work and at home my lifelong desperate hunger for people is being more richly satisfied than ever before and it makes me want to live for a long time.

Going back through many years to my first interest in counseling I find it began at age six for me. My father was a teacher in Wilhelmsdorf. One day he brought a young boy to our house and to his bedroom where they talked. I was listening at the keyhole and gathered that something sexual was being discussed. I craved such an occasion for myself, that is, an intimate talk with my father, which I never had. (He died in 1948 and his last comment to me was "It's too bad that we never got acquainted.")

Later, at sixteen, I was in love for the first time with a girl of whom my parents disapproved. I made a Sunday afternoon appointment with a young minister to talk about this. I walked the three miles to his home in order to keep this meeting a secret from my parents, I "spilled my guts" to him, and walked home with a great sense of relief. As I got to the front door, my father opened it and said that the minister had called. He then asked me, "Why did you have to tell him all that?" It took me sixteen more years before I freely confided in another person. That Sunday catastrophe was the beginning of my departure from home, which I did after high school graduation about a year later. I was determined to get through college and graduate school without money from my parents, and I made it. Those were the early nineteen thirties, and I regularly earned ten cents per hour until President Roosevelt came into office and established a minimum wage of fifteen cents.

All of my history contributed to my moods and ways of being. Linda often complained that I was too moody, and she was unable to feel any closeness with me. I began looking for a therapist. The psychiatrists I had met in medical school were not the type of people I would wish to confide in, and besides they were busy using their new electric shock machines. The clinical psychologists I met were not of the caliber of Rogers. In 1945 I finally began regular interviews as a patient with a man who had managed to outlive much of his medical tradition, and for the first time since childhood I felt glad to be alive.

I had been suicidal many times in the preceding years. At age fourteen I was going to stick an icepick in my heart but was interrupted. In the years after that I often drove cars so recklessly that I wondered why God was keeping me alive. With the explosion of new life within me, beginning in 1945, it was altogether different, and if my depressions sometimes were more severe (so that on occasion I was afraid I would just stop breathing), they were of shorter duration. The times of exuberance made it worthwhile to survive the bad times. I had a sense of *inescapably growing* within myself and with others. I continue to feel this and have the certainty that I can always find Another who will be close to me when I am ready to interrupt my loneliness.

From 1945 to 1958 I continued "in therapy" (a term I no longer like) with four different male therapists. But I was never "fully analyzed." Meanwhile the workshops of the American Academy of Psychotherapists, and my own "patients" (especially in group therapy), periodically challenged me to new inner movement. After Linda died in 1970, saying again in effect that she would rather die than live with me, I once more began looking for a therapist. I was arranging to commute to another city for therapy, and perhaps go under an assumed name in order to be "just an ordinary patient," when my prospective therapist wrote that some of his group patients were already looking forward to seeing me because I was so famous. "God protect me from my friends!"

I was finally accepted as "an ordinary patient" by a woman therapist in the fall of 1971. I admire her. In my own practice I probably would have turned down a patient like me who came just a few weeks before a second marriage. What pushed me now was that Liz was hurting with a turmoil in me which involved ghosts from my past. In earlier years my effort as a patient in therapy was to get insurance against my becoming psychotic; then I had nightmares of being given "a little treatment" in a state hospital. Now I see myself as just a normal person who can become still more free to live in the present and to give and receive from those near him.

My concept of the therapist has changed over the years. Back in the early nineteen fifties I used to be very formal in my professional manner. Gradually I lost the various rules about "how to be a good therapist" and just settled for what might be practical. Persons who sat in utter silence with me through many interviews somehow seemed to be able to benefit. Others chose to be physically nude during their interviews and in this way achieved greater emotional nakedness with me. Still others came for special educational help, such as how to be better parents, or more successful sexually or financially, or even just to learn about human nature as a kind of hobby. Gradually I learned to accommodate myself to these many ways in which people use me and to accept their goals as being satisfactory for them. This last matter, about goals, was particularly difficult for me because I somehow wished for everybody who came to me that they might have the same kind of life which I was living. It is a relief finally to be shed of that sense of obligation.

Another difficult transition in past years was in working with other therapists as patients when they also brought some of their professional problems. To discuss their own patients with them is usually called supervision. Somehow it gradually worked out well not to labor over the technical distinctions and to deal together with whatever matter is in the forefront of the patient's consideration. However, given a choice, I still prefer to deal with professional problems rather intellectually in technique seminars and with personal matters in more intimate sessions. When we discuss professional issues, the goal is to improve the skill of the therapist; when we discuss personal matters, the goal is to modify the character structure of the person.

The future of psychotherapy, as I see it, is in the hands and breasts of women. The early history of our "profession" was in the hands of "father psychiatrists" such as Sigmund Freud, Adolf Meyer, Harry Stack Sullivan, Franz Alexander, and others. Gradually a split has developed during the past quarter century between the "fathers," who evaluate and offer prescriptions, versus the "mothers," who offer a personal relating to their patients. There are obviously sick people who are so disturbed that they require hospitalization and some form of control and physical treatment for their emotional condition. Such administrative management by fatherly psychiatrists should not be confused with a mothering psychotherapy relationship in which a non-diseased person can be born again and grow some more. This difference is evident in the atmosphere of the consultation. In my own office experience, no patient has ever been primarily interested in my genitals. But many have warmed themselves in my presence as a maternal person, dreamed of me as a woman with breasts, and felt nurtured enough to make a new start.

I now see myself in the following ways.

(1) I am a psychotherapist. Many of my sharp edges are worn off. The learning from my formal training and especially from the years of being taught by patients is now more available to me because I am becoming less arrogant. Psychotherapy is not yet established as a profession (and it may be many years before there are university departments with respected chairmen who are "psychotherapists"). In the meantime I fantasy myself as sitting at one end of a log with

a patient at the other end, and the process of our communication is psychotherapy to me. The only crucial items in this sharing on the log are the maturity of the so-called therapist and the willingness to learn of the so-called patient.

(2) There have always been days when I regretted having become a psychotherapist, or even being alive at all. I have resented the relatively low income. But I have never seriously considered any other profession. At age forty I still wondered what other way of life might be more satisfactory professionally. Now I am too old to change, and besides I am really happy with the contribution I make to people. I particularly like to see patients who have had several other therapists because they are likely to be more ready to learn.

(3) What Dr. Arthur Burton has called "a personal demon" in my case is my depressions. As best I know, all sincere therapists share this "monster" with me. My depressions have become manageable in two ways: (a) Sharing the details of my depressions with my therapist or with patients. I always seek a benefit from having suffered the pain of feeling worthless. (b) On occasions when the conflict was so great that I curled up in bed in the fetal position for many hours, my depressions repeatedly enabled me to make the troubling decisions that were necessary for my welfare. My depressions are not an illness to me. Colleagues have disagreed and have urged me to prevent my gloomy periods. But, if I could not escape from stress into depression, I think I would lose much of the joy which I have in my exuberant times.

(4) My definition of neurosis is: a large remnant of childhood attitudes plus too much pride. I think of psychosis as a neurosis plus a great determination to make the parents suffer for "what they did wrong." This means that I see all mental illness as a learned condition which can be unlearned in relationship to a mothernig therapist. I have no systematic theory of personality or emotional illness. However, I do recognize the dynamics of neurosis as a crippling condition in which a person is too proud to spill his guts in despair, while stubbornly refusing to risk new ways of being which differ from what he always thought (what he learned from his parents).

(5) I have never been bored. When I worked with clinically psychotic persons, such as diagnosed schizophrenics, it was a lively experience of seeing their psychodynamics in myself (just to a lesser

degree). Even though I have now limited my practice to normal people, the excitement is still there because they also have all the schizophrenic dynamics. There are really no superficial people. I consider myself very fortunate to be doing such interesting work, particularly when I can experience a degree of falling in love with a patient. This is not a threat to my marital commitment but rather is a further installment on the resolving of the romance with my parents and my siblings. When I can no longer fall in love with patients to some degree, I will be approaching the end of my vitality as a therapist.

(6) Psychotherapy is foreign to the social context of our culture. This troubles me as a person because I belong to my society. Yet by definition the patient and I meet in order to discuss the unacceptable aspects of his living. This intimacy is similar to that of marriage, and sometimes patients are more open with me than they are with their marital partner. In either case it is important to use the applicable primitive language, the four-letter words that carry the most feeling. For example, one of my failures was with a couple who insisted on seeing me only together, because she had had sexual intercourse with her two preceding therapists, and then she added that they would never be back if I used a "dirty word" with them. This prohibition was my warning that we could never be close at all, and I was unable to get past it. I still hurt with this couple.

(7) The crises in my life might not seem so to passers-by. This includes my being an alien in Germany and once again an alien in Kansas, to have another boy shake hands with me when I was ten years old and say warmly "I am glad to meet you," or at sixteen to have a college student tell me that I was the brightest person he had tested when I thought that I was stupid. These were crises to me. All of my sexual relationships were crises which still remain very much a part of my life. The authorities I defeated and those to whom I bowed are also still in my guts. All of these major turning points of my personal and professional living have identified my present place. To some degree I am being "lived by my unconscious," but the arena of that living is always clearly identified by my history. I have construed my own crises and used them. One thing I have learned: *I will love dearly any person whom I get to know intimately.* This assumption has worked well for me.

(8) My erroneous assumptions during my early years as a

therapist still haunt me. Formerly I presumed that male and female souls were similar. I even thought that all souls (or unconsciouses of people) were essentially the same size. These were errors. Men and women differ in their value systems. Men awaken to adult sexuality all at once; women do so in a series of new awakenings until after the menopause. These are great differences between the emotional functioning of the two sexes. Each has a specific devil, the male and the female, and the devil we each know will be less frightening than the devil whom we do not know. In therapy I hope to help people to know their own personal devil, to live with him and even to love him.

(9) "Getting rid of anger" is a refrain often heard in any therapist's office. A major discovery for me was that *anger is not a necessary feeling*. We simply need not fight every battle in sight. Our impulses are not necessarily significant. What we designate as anger could sometimes be the initiative of living in the face of obstacles. And if we can learn to offer affection to those who oppose our moods, the "anger" we feel may become the urge to achieve something satisfying. Ass-kissing may reap richer rewards than standing up for our rights.

(10) Complaining about parents is also standard practice in any psychotherapy. This is an early phase of emotional growth. None of us had extra-good parents or we would not be therapists. If we have had children, we certainly recognize that we as parents were less than perfect, even with all the advantages of our psychodynamic training and personal therapy. We do not serve our patients when we encourage them to pick on their parents, as I did in 1947 when I wrote a letter to mine stating that my emotional crippling was the result of their being such lousy lovers. They did the best they could, considering their own ancestors. They gave me enough so that I could achieve a much better life than they ever thought of having.

(11) I enjoy being just "John" to my family, friends, colleagues, and patients. The world is good to me now. I have enough reputation to attract people. My satisfactions are with my wife, and in my professional work I look particularly to groups and marathon meetings for further stimulation. The one great lack in my life has been the paucity of laughter, and this I continue to seek. As Martin Buxbaum said, "We were born crying; we must learn to laugh." Years ago I went only to those movies reputed to be funny. I continue to seek oc-

casions when the humor and paradoxes of life invite a smile or even a belly laugh. (The only term which Eskimos at the North Pole are said to have for sexual intercourse is "laughing together!")

(12) My value system and my ego ideals have gone through many changes during the years. I still cry on occasion without knowing the reason, and then feel relieved and cleansed. Periodically I make further progress in forgiving my parents so that I might "live long in the land which the Lord my God giveth me." My morality now is based on the question "How will I like myself?" This is the guide for my behavior, rather than the question of what is "right" or "wrong." When people ask me personal questions, I answer in the context of how can I be loving with them. I now see myself as becoming almost loving enough.

My summary of what is a good therapist includes being a good teacher, a sincere friend, a student of people, a lively person, and especially a good lover. In looking for office partners in past years I was primarily concerned with finding good therapists. My first concern was whether I had a good gut feeling about them. My second concern was whether they had had a significant experience as a patient in psychotherapy. Other questions included the quality of their doctoral training, intelligence, and physical attractiveness. It was also important to me to be able to be comfortable with them in our everyday working association. Thereafter, some personal questions included: Has this therapist forgiven his parents? How willing is he to be transparent? Has he done enough living to be nonjudgmental with people who are less mature than he? Has he a comfort with his primitive earthy feelings? Has he a good sex life? Does he have enough security within himself to be sincere and gentle in the face of a hostile group?

Good psychotherapists are people who respect emotional pain because they have had it. Pain can mellow and soften us. However, prolonged severe pain degrades a person and after that he should not be a psychotherapist. To the degree that I have outlived my childhood bitterness and pouting, to that degree I am now valuable as a therapist.

My value as a therapist is actually only equal to my value as a person who continues to become. My seasonal becoming has necessarily included times of cold withdrawal to allow for inner resting and restitution. Even more, I love to remember the warm times when my person bloomed with a new fullness to overflowing. These times of Spring were always in response to a new Friend. I feel with Rod McKuen:[3]

> *May your hand be full for always*
> *if only with another hand.*
> *May your heart be empty only*
> *long enough to give you cause*
> *to fill it up again with love.*
>
> *May your soul be lost by you*
> *only to be found by God.*

Selected Writings

Partners in Psychotherapy. *Voices,* 1967, Vol. 3.

The Usefulness of Crazyness. *Med. Times,* June, 1961. (With C. A. Whitaker, T. P. Malone, and R. E. Felder.)

Physical Contact in Multiple Therapy with Schizophrenic Patients. 2nd Int. Cong. of Psychiatry, Zurich, 1957. (With J. F. Taylor.)

Support through Non-Reassurance. *Am. J. Psychotherapy,* 1956, *10,* 709–715.

A Philosophical Basis for Brief Psychotherapy. *Psychiatric Quarterly,* 1949, *23,* 439–443. (With C. A. Whitaker and N. Johnson.)

[3] *The Carols of Christmas* (New York: Random House, 1963, p. 6).

XI

In Quest of the Professional Self

Rudolf Ekstein

It is now a good many years since I gave my aged father a copy of my first published book in one of those rare happy moments when one feels like the accepted and beloved child. He accepted it graciously and proudly and told me that while he did not think he would under- stand very much of it he nevertheless felt that he was its coauthor. I expressed puzzlement, and he told me how at the beginning of my high school years in Vienna, when I was about eleven years old, one of the teachers had called him in for a conference and had advised him to take me out of high school and to put me into a trade school. The teacher suggested that it must be sheer torture for me to be kept in high school, that I was unsuitable for it. My father told me that, since he had not followed the advice of the authority, he felt he was the coauthor of the book. That remark, all these many years later, about an experience of which I had not been directly aware at the time, made me think about that eleven-year-old boy, and I will try to describe how I remember him, how I saw him grow up and later move toward a profession.

My recollections about him are influenced, of course, by the task at hand. The biographer, whether he writes about somebody else or becomes an autobiographer, is somehow deeply attracted by his subject and will be involved with him. He loves the subject of his interest, and even when he can create some objective distance, his biographical or autobiographical comments will be related to the purpose which motivated him to make the observations. I think it was the late Siegfried Bernfeld to whom was ascribed the bon mot "The trouble with self-analysis lies in the countertransference." What is the trouble with autobiography? Is the autobiography an alibi? A self-justification? A monument for the future? Or perhaps a search toward self-actualization? Is such an autobiography to inspire others? Is it to hide or to reveal? Is it selected truth or a struggle with emerging conflict? And what is its true meaning if it is an invited statement about one's professional self-development? Can we prove that Friedrich Nietzsche was wrong when he suggested once—before Freud—that "if truth and vanity were in conflict, vanity will win"? But really I do not want to escape from the task of capturing something essential about that young boy.

As I Remember the Young Boy

Shortly before the teacher had talked to his father the child had spent a few weeks in the city hospital because of a chronic ear condition which would later cause partial deafness. He was lonely and frightened but glad that he had escaped serious surgery, although the physicians had not cured his infected ear. A special type of surgery, not known then, would free him from this difficulty much later during his adult life.

He was an only child, brought up by a kind Catholic woman, a simple and pious person who was deeply dedicated and he recalled later that she once told him: "You are a handsome little boy. You don't look Jewish at all." Thus, while she was also a reliable caretaker and stood by him while his father was away in military service, she really was remembered as a mother substitute, which indeed she was: an excellent, loving, and beloved substitute mother trying to make up for the loss of the real one. When his father came home from the war, the little boy started elementary school, which he finished in four years, and then entered high school, an education available for the few who could pass the entrance examination and whose parents were willing and able to pay the modest school fees. The pressure of the new school, his illness and hospitalization set him back. The teachers frightened him and the competition was much harder than that in elementary school. Of course, he did not know of his father's school conference, but he did everlastingly recall that during one of their Sunday walks his father told him that although he was aware of his low grades, he very much wanted him to continue school, and to try and make it. He would love to further his son's education toward an academic goal, but he would not bring up the subject again. Behind that last comment was hidden the seriousness of the school conference. The little boy lost a year, was set back, and then started again. There were many lonesome hours, feelings of shame and guilt, endless painful fantasies, and an ever-increasing determination to try once more. During the following year he had some of the same teachers and they could not quite believe the change that had taken place. He had taken hold of himself and within a few months moved toward the top of the class. The other day I found among my papers an essay that the young boy had written. He had chosen as his hero one of the Nibelungs: Hagen von Tronje. Hagen actually was one of the most disliked of the mythical figures. Many found him unattractive and evil, but the young boy defended him. In this school essay he suggested that Hagen von Tronje, one-eyed warrior, was the only faithful leader among the Nibelungs. He stood by his king and he did whatever he had to do to defend the weak king. The Huns finally destroyed the Nibelungs but Hagen von Tronje defended his king to the last. The young boy went on with his story, which up to that moment had been a recapitulation of the material he had studied, and he saw the Nibelungs rise once more in Valhalla together with the gods. Here Hagen von Tronje was honored and rewarded, and he was allowed to sit next to the highest deity, compensated for his faithfulness, for his endurance, for keeping his promise, and for fulfilling the expectations of his king. As he developed the story he turned Valhalla into the Christian heaven. Violent struggle became equanimity.

I am now tempted to analyze this story, to see whether we can understand this child's successful attempt to resolve his epigenetic crisis during prepuberty. But instead, I want to mention the cultural milieu at that time. The young boy had identified with the courageous underdog, who, even if defeated, would rise again. Little could he know at that time that one of the intellectual heroes with whom he would identify in late adolescence, Sigmund Freud, had early chosen as his hero Hannibal, the Carthaginian. *Hannibalem ante Portas,* the hero who never conquered Rome but threatened the Roman Empire, had become the ideal of Freud, whose discovery of psychoanalysis perhaps had then a similar fate. There was another later hero of that boy as he grew up, an intellectual and political hero who synthesized democratic socialism and Marxist theory with psychoanalytic thinking. That hero, Siegfried Bernfeld, had chosen as his own hero Sisyphus, who defied the gods, that eternal teacher who tried to bring knowledge to the people and who endlessly suffered but never gave up on his task. Do these heroes of antiquity describe the Jewish intellectual, who can never really become a part of his beloved Vienna, but who wants to make a contribution and finds he has chosen an impossible task?

Let us return to that young boy. He had now become a good student, and the very same teacher for whom he had written that essay on Hagen von Tronje asked him whether he wanted to tutor some of the students who could not keep up. Tutoring students in one's own class, as well as younger children, was a cultural tradition in Vienna and many young people worked their way through school by means of tutoring. But our young boy, now proud that he was chosen to teach, and not yet thirteen, made the decision that he wanted to do that even better than did his own teachers. That was his kind of revenge, and rather than suggest that he had identified with the aggressors, I recognize more his deep desire to understand children in trouble. He would be a teacher, he decided early, who would not only know his subject matter but would understand the learning child. Most often he worked with troubled children and thought he understood them.

Know that from then on his learning task in high school offered no particular problem. Much of his desire to teach grew out of a rebellious spirit which required that he teach better than his teachers and that he understand the children better. He identified particularly with the troubled child except that he wanted the troubled child to not accept his fate. It was a strange double identification. He accepted the goals of the teachers but struggled against their methods. Soon he felt, as did many others, that school could not be the center of his life and he found an outlet in the Socialist Youth Movement.

Youth Movement and University Years

This youth movement, rebellious in spirit, wanting to change the world, held ideals which combined social purpose—a society of peace, free of the struggle between competing classes—with a requirement that each member also achieve for himself, move toward a better self, an expanded mind. This mixture of individualism and social responsibility, of identification with the group and acceptance of self-development, was to characterize his search for ways of growth which would permit him to give expressions to both sides and which at times seemed to represent a dichotomy impossible to resolve. He remembered with fondness one of the early slogans of the socialist labor movement of that time: "We Socialists have led the Viennese workers from the gin bottle to the workers' symphony concert." This youth movement never gave up on society, never spoke about withdrawing from social life and escaping to nature. It filled the life of this growing adolescent with deep meaning never to be forgotten when he became an adult, in spite of the fact that he now lived in a society which was deeply divided, full of irreconcilable conflicts, and moving toward its own dissolution. The polarization of society involved every student, every high school teacher, every university teacher, and only a few were left who tried to remain above and beyond polarization. The struggle for self-perfection and the hope of making a social contribution seemed to be a utopian fantasy. Among the essays of this young man, now an adolescent of sixteen or seventeen, I found one about *The Nature of Utopia.* He spoke about his feeling that the utopias, unreachable goals, eternal longings never to be fulfilled, only approximated, nevertheless had to be the guide for him who wanted to be a decent person. Little did he know then what task he had set for himself, trying to maintain ideals in a social world which was to break asunder and which would take away from him the very social basis for the tasks set. He saw himself now as a youth leader—and an effective youth movement leader he was—who wanted to lead the young people into a better world, a more ideal world which would urge everyone to strive toward self-realization. Often he was confronted by more radical leaders who did not see the goal of education as leading people out and upward, but as indoctrinating them for political ends regardless of their individual fates and opportunities. He did not want youth to be mere tools of the state or of the party apparatus.

As he graduated from high school he had one more tense situation with his father. The first one when he was eleven or so had brought about his inner commitment to learning. The next confrontation dealt with the deeper goals and purposes of learning. He wanted to study psychology, to develop scientific insights, and not simply rely on his talent to identify with youngsters. The science of psychology would, he thought, open for him the inner world of the child, the inner world of the man. His father, on the other hand, thought that he should look for a practical profession. Perhaps he ought to become an engineer, or even a lawyer. The compromise was a meeting with a vocational guidance counselor, a member of a new profession about to become popular in Vienna. The man listened to father and son and I suppose he must have felt like King Solomon as he offered advice after a few minutes of listening. No, he had no particular tests which could possibly evaluate whether this young high school graduate would do better in engineering or in psychology. The tests dealt merely with mechanical skills. But the counselor suggested that irrespective of what the young man studied, he would finally find himself unemployed in an overcrowded labor market. Therefore, if the father could afford to help this young man go through an educational program he might as well do so to keep him busy for four or five years. Since it made no difference anyway, it might be best if the son were allowed to study whatever he wanted. This advice was the green light toward an education and toward unemployment.

That was the state of affairs during the last years of the First Republic. The search for meaning became intensified. University psychology at that time was not interested in the inner, the deeper and unconscious world of children; it represented more the usual academic tasks and therefore could not give a full answer to the questions this young man raised for himself. He was surrounded by the ideological struggle which went on at the university, a powerful struggle for the acceptance of basic philosophies, none of them truly accepted by all, all of them suspected of being outworn commodities on the intellectual market.

The youth movement's search for truth, for genuine purpose, that search for the ideal world and the perfect social system, was carried out most of the time outside the academic institutions. While he attended course after course he found the greatest personal meaning in that youth movement.

From Weltanschauung to the Philosophy of Meaning

Then, almost by chance, in the search for a way to examine the meaning of philosophy, he found his way to the *Wiener Kreis,* the leader of which was Moritz Schlick. It was indeed a radical philosophy, but only for a radical solution could he search at the time. Its purpose was to do away with all philosophical systems and to replace them with a method of philosophizing which tried to establish meaning by a study of language, of scientific systems, and philosophical schools, a method which is known here as the philosophy of science. The young man experienced these exciting years with his great teacher, deeply idealized, distant, not really allowing intimate contact, but nevertheless deeply touching him, as an inner revolution. He learned from and through his teacher how to think. At first this thinking was under the banner of debunking philosophical systems. He adopted the same kind of attitude that had characterized the Marxists' attempt to understand and debunk the existing social order. It was a deeply critical attitude, a rebellious attitude, even though represented by an aristocratic gentleman who seemed aloof from the social struggle of his time, above and beyond that struggle, searching for truth, as if it were possible to do that while sitting on the clouds high above the social conflict. That capacity for distance later became an important ingredient for the future therapist. It would enable him to listen to people, to their inner conflicts, without taking sides, to remain equidistant from the conflicting forces, in order to recognize their nature and to help develop a solution. At that time he began to discover how often a meaningless proposition, or even a philosophical system, went beyond the rules of language, beyond the logical possibility of verification or falsification. This early school of logical positivism, the early basis of the philosophy of science, insisted that only those propositions have meaning whose methods of verification or falsification can be defined.

This young man, trying to search for an identity, a lasting purpose, spent himself discovering how he could put different interests together to form a philosophy of his own and not be a blind follower. That is never an easy task. One loses friends and group affiliations, spends many lonesome hours in deep internal struggle often without clear direction. His conviction was to lead young people out into a better world and up toward a better use of themselves. He looked for a psychology which would permit that.

His search was for meaning in philosophy, that certain love of wisdom. So far he had found only a method which was attractive because with it he was able to overthrow all philosophical systems by suggesting that they were really a meaningless overstepping of language rules. Soon such philosophical analysis led him to a critique of the very social beliefs, those sociological models of change, the historical models which had guided him in trying to understand the world. He became self-critical as well. And as he got deeper and deeper into the philosophical tasks (this now having become his major academic effort), he also could not help but discover that this new philosophy was also an incomplete instrument. He then started to tackle the issue of what was the meaning of meaning; and he did so with the help of his teachers, who were at that time working with the same problems. It was obviously not enough to maintain a system of communication which permitted only scientific sentences (postulations) and theories which were open to verification or falsification, to confirmation or disconfirmation. The whole system of human communication had areas of meaning far beyond the ones that the scientist had in mind when he immersed himself in his research.

One summer, while working with children in a summer school, he discovered during long discussions with like-minded colleagues, and deep into the night while the children were asleep, Siegfried Bernfeld's volume on *Sisyphus or the Boundaries of Education*,[1] a powerful

---

[1] *Sisyphos oder die Grenzen der Erziehung* (Leipzig, Vienna: Internationaler Psychoanalytischer Verlag, 1925).

appeal to understand education both in terms of its sociological and its psychological meaning. It was an early and convincing attempt to synthesize Marxian understanding of the social world and Freudian understanding of the inner world. The social world Bernfeld suggested sets the outer limits of education, while the inner world of the child, his unconscious, sets the inner limits for the influence of the educator. It was this book which made the young man look for places where he could learn more about Freud than was possible through the reading of his works in the university library. The university was critical of Freud. Where was there a source of direct learning?

Only a few socialists of the time were friendly to Freudian work. Most early leaders found more comfort and support in the thinking of Alfred Adler. The young university student had taken some courses in the Adlerian Institute but was not sufficiently attracted by them. He then learned that very nearby—actually some fifteen minutes' walk from his home—was the Vienna Psychoanalytic Institute. That Institute had engaged in training pedagogues so that they would become psychoanalytic pedagogues, members of a new movement, small in number, but immensely effective. He was then twenty-three years old. He was interviewed by a Dr. Hoffer who wanted to know how he had become interested in psychoanalysis. The young man told him he had read the book by Bernfeld and the very next week he was accepted and entered the courses. Only years later would he find out that Bernfeld and Hoffer were lifelong friends. They had started psychoanalytic work with children right at the end of the First World War and were leaders of that movement.

Path to Psychoanalysis

I find it difficult now to continue in the third person and to distance myself from the young adult. The biographer of the little boy now has to become an autobiographer at the moment professional and psychoanalytic training start in earnest.

The year 1935 not only marked the beginning of my formal training but was also the first year of open and victorious fascism in Austria. The year before, the parliament had been dissolved; the socialist parties and their unions, as well as the youth movement, had been destroyed. Whatever continued now did so under illegal circumstances. The political dream had come to an end. The hope for external change had been destroyed, and the inner struggle—divided as it was between the belief in outer change and the belief in internal change—found its expression in the painful necessity of making choices. Of course, every young person goes through such decision making, although not always under the political pressure of such disturbed years.

Bernfeld's moving from youth movement to psychoanalysis now also became my Sisyphuslike task. I have collaborated on a book, *From Learning for Love to Love of Learning,* which describes the history of psychoanalytic pedagogy that for many of us has altered the history of our professional and scientific life.

The next three years before Hitler's invasion were unbelievably hectic. We continued, of course, with our social and political friends, endangered our careers by constantly being confronted by or confronting political police action, and hoped against our better judgment that the Republic might soon be restored. At the same time I recall how desperately we tried to finish our academic work. We counted the days leading toward the diploma and leading also toward the invasion we knew would come. One day, shortly after I had finished my thesis on *The Philosophy of Psychology,* Schlick, that great and beloved professor, was slain at the steps of the university, murdered by a confused fanatic. Schlick's ethics had been an appeal to kindness, but he became a victim of hate. I continued with Bühler, who kindly took over the supervision of my thesis, and I received ,my Ph.D. late in 1937, a few months before the invasion. The Bühlers became good and close friends of mine in later years, but at that time I recall one of the main questions he asked me at the *Strenges Rigorosum.* What objections do we have, he inquired, to psychoanalysis? I led, like others, a kind of double academic life. I went to the university for formal recognition and I went to the Psychoanalytic Institute in order to learn about the inner world of people. I solved the struggle between the wish for official status and the desire to be courageous and honest by quoting Bühler's objection to Freud in his classic volume *Die Krise der Psychologie.*[2] That did it. I now had my doctorate, the realization of my great ambition. I recalled the vocational counselor who pre-

---

[2] (Jena: Fischer, 1927. 3rd ed., 1965).

dicted unemployment after the graduation, although little did he or I know that it would not be unemployment but flight into exile which was to follow academic achievement.

During the years when I worked toward the high school teacher's diploma I had worked extensively with children in private tutoring, and had started to work under supervision with children with learning disturbances. It looked as though I had achieved a safe career, but a few months after the invasion I found myself on foreign soil, a refugee in search of ways to make a living, while maintaining the secret hope of restoring my career and moving toward psychoanalytic work.

During the analytic training period in Vienna, three intensive, inspiring, and unbelievable years of growth took place with such teachers as Bertha Bornstein, Edith Buxbaum, August Eichhorn, Anna Freud, Heinz Hartmann, Willi Hoffer, Ernst and Marianne Kris, Editha and Richard Sterba, Robert and Jenny Wälder, and many others. It had nevertheless become abundantly clear that there would be no psychoanalytic pedagogy in Austria. There would be no place for anyone in our school systems; in fact, some, such as Fritz Redl and Edith Buxbaum, had left even before the *Anschluss*. The identification with the analytic teachers led to a kind of transformation. We wanted to work with children, understand their inner world, influence them, but the educational zeal slowly turned into therapeutic interests. During that first phase, psychoanalytic pedagogy was not clearly differentiated from psychoanalytic psychotherapy, and the new goal for a good many of us was then to become a therapist, an analyst.

Of Obstacles and Opportunities

Many of the analysts went to England and America. The American Psychoanalytic Association, mindful of its close association with the American Psychiatric Association, closed the door to lay people. A new obstacle, not entirely negligible even in Vienna, with Freud endorsing and defending lay analysis, had grown to enormous proportions. But by now I had become used to running obstacle courses. I spent some of my early years in the United States in social work, in clinical psychology, in clinical teaching, and all these learning experiences have helped me to increase the interests and talents which had occupied me in Vienna when I tried to combine humanitarian and scientific interests.

After some years in institutional work, and later in private practice, I found my way to the Menninger Foundation in Topeka for ten years of intensive work as a training analyst, as director of child psychotherapy at the Southard School, and as a teacher of psychiatrists. I was also engaged in research concerning training issues as well as work with the psychotic and borderline conditions of childhood.

There was an opportunity to put together clinical interests, old philosophical and methodological interests, and the search for meaning on all levels; to follow the humanitarian impulse, that belief in the personal growth of every individual combined with increasing social responsibility, through which I could develop the notion of a psychoanalyst who is not simply living in an ivory tower, in a private practice heaven, but who sees himself as a part of society, responsible and responsive to that society, and at the same time strives untiringly toward a richer professional self.

I had by that time become a competent analyst, and as I look at my early publications I realize that they are dominated, to a large extent, by my interest in theory, my old search for logical clarification, and an attempt to synthesize different theoretical schools. The influence of the philosophy of science brought me to an early conviction that I would not really want to join the ideological warfare between the different psychoanalytic or psychological schools. I allowed myself to be somewhat above the struggle, like Schlick, and to gain some distance. Not that I did not go through the usual childhood disease of being overcommitted to one particular system, one particular model of the mind, one particular teacher, but I did not do too well with that phase. I aimed at synthesis between the different schools, although I had learned that philosophers have always aimed at synthesis and then usually came up with their own system which they assumed to be the best and the one final truth. In two papers, I tried to convey the nature of these theoretical differences which actually hide different technical commitments. But never did I really try to replace this or that psychological system with a more ideal one. I have not found it comfortable to develop *the* psychoanalytic system, or *the* psychoanalytic theory. Some theoreticians, of course, have gone that way and some always will. I was more impressed with the idea of understanding theory and its implications than with being dogmatically committed to an idealized system. It is perhaps my philosophical background which helped me to believe not in *the* psychoanalysis but in psychoanalyzing; not in *the* theory but in theorizing; not in *the* thought but in thinking.

The stress on activity of the mind instead of on the final result led me away from theoretical papers, almost a kind of inner conversion, and I immersed myself in writing primarily clinical papers. I was never satisfied with mere case descriptions but felt that every clinical paper should have a theoretical or technical point, even though I did not want these points to lead toward a final theoretical or technical commitment.

The experience at Menninger's initiated a phase away from a kind of theoretical idealism to clinical pragmatism. The clinical pragmatism was enhanced by the fact that we were not only training psychoanalysts but training all clinical professions. I was there introduced into the world of American psychiatry, having become acquainted earlier with American social work and clinical psychology. I saw in Topeka a kind of diluted utopia, a model organization of a psychiatric training system, in which all the behavioral sciences could work together but where psychoanalytic thinking would be an integral part of it all.

Toward Experimentation and Discovery

This experience led to two major contributions which should be mentioned here. The first one had to do with my old passion for teaching. Although I was not then teaching children, I was teaching professional people, and I became keenly interested in methods of teaching and methods of clinical supervision; there was ample opportunity for practice, experimentation, and research. Not only did I have the opportunity to teach all the clinical professions but I also began to train supervisors. Together with my former student Robert Wallerstein I had developed a system of practice and research in clinical supervision. The outgrowth was a book published in 1958 *The Teaching and Learning of Psychotherapy,* which has recently come out in a second revised edition.

Another outgrowth of my work in Topeka was the study of

therapeutic processes with psychotic children and children with border-line conditions. When I became the director of psychotherapy at the Southard School, I was soon puzzled to find that many of the things I had learned earlier were inapplicable to the very sick children there. The first case we followed, "The Space Child,"[3] treated by the un-forgettable, the late Dorothy Wright, opened a new world for me. In the beginning it was trial and error. Much of what I had learned in the past I had to forget. I had to live myself into the worlds of both the therapist and the child. It was as if we had to form a new kind of triple working alliance to reach this boy. I must mention that we treated him some ten years. There are few human beings I could truly say I know better than this child. Yet through these many years I never saw him, and only near the end of treatment did I actually have a short meeting with him. So intensive was the work that I often did not quite know whether Dorothy Wright treated him or whether I did. We lived through the agonies of a terrifying world. It was not only his inner world which was terrifying but his external fate as well —the mother who could not accept him and the father who committed suicide, both living in a neighboring state but actually living millions of miles away from him, as expressed in his space odyssey. He surely helped us to discover many aspects of endless inner space. I soon realized that I, too, should become engaged in treating such children, and I have believed ever since that only he can teach who can do, and who does: that the clinical teacher must also be a clinical practitioner.

This phase of work with psychotic children was also one of in-tensive collaboration with a variety of colleagues. I am forever grateful to them. They all are enumerated in my first volume on childhood psychosis, *Children of Time and Space, of Action and Impulse*. It is not merely my volume but theirs as well. They are the coauthors, and I trace the wish to be a teacher who does not remain forever the au-thority, a kind of father figure, but becomes the brother and collabo-rator of his students, back to my early youth movement experience. This is true for all my books and many of my papers. What I am say-ing is that I feel that inner guarantee for creative work, as far as I am concerned, lies in the opportunity to teach, to give, to mobilize, and to

[3] R. Ekstein and others. *Children of Time and Space, of Action and Impulse* (New York: Appleton-Century-Crofts, 1966), chapters 15 to 18.

lead people out toward higher levels of work, higher professional and scientific ambitions.

I did not always succeed. I did not always make friends. There is much that is painful that goes on within oneself, and between one-self and these colleagues, that sometimes cannot be resolved. I found this to be true in Topeka and also here at the Reiss-Davis Child Study Center. But I would not want to have it any other way. There must be a price to be paid for productive cooperative effort.

I have learned through these experiences that for me there are three conditions for creative work. The first is that one must have the capacity at times to do it alone. One must think alone, be with oneself. One must bear lonesomeness and sometimes move away from friends and colleagues. It is as though one can only grow if one lives in a monologue.

The second condition is that one cannot always continue alone, but needs a second person. I speak of one's personal analysis and one's working relationship with the psychoanalyst. I am personally deeply indebted to the late Edward Hitschmann for this experience of change and growth. And also much individual learning must be carried out in our field via individual supervision. While language in the first in-stance is like private language, the language in the second situation is an intimate language between two people. There is finally the lan-guage which requires one to be able to talk to, and with, many people. I am referring to the pluralogue. A good analyst, then, needs to be able to be with himself and his own thoughts, and he must stand loneliness and distance. But he also must be able to break the autistic-like barrier and be together with the other person. And if he is to become a teacher, he must step out into society and be capable of group association and group communication.

For this reason I have never felt completely happy in private practice alone, and I would not choose to be. I prefer to work in group situations, clinical situations, where there is an intimate integration between service, training, and research.

Philosophy and Society

It is a long way from the search for meaning in choosing ideal political systems to the search for meaning in different philosophical systems to the search for meaning of a neurotic or psychotic system, an elaborate dream, or a bizarre metaphorlike language construction of a sick child. It takes a long time to be able to differentiate between normal and psychotic play and to invent systems of communication about which none of us would have dreamed when in the past we sat in a philosophical seminar.

It is a long way from the beginning moment when one is guided by theoretical doctrine to those moments when one is willing to rely also on empathy, a feeling of oneself into the life of another person, when one is ready to allow countertransferences to become true parts of the game rather than experiences of which one is ashamed and which one does not fully master. There is no end to that way of learning except the end of life itself.

There is also no end to the obstacles in the way. As I write this, we live in a world of increased social upheaval. Many concerns of psychoanalysis in the inner workings of the individual mind are being attacked today, as incidentally they always were, by people who believe in mass solutions, instant answers, people who are interested in the manipulation of others, the sheer modification of behavior, and who define psychological science in mere external terms. Since we are again dominated by social crisis, we find people who see their task merely in crisis intervention and who have given up the deeper implications of psychological growth. These are issues which indeed will affect many younger people in the process of trying to develop professional identities. I do not worry about them. This is their struggle and perhaps they will solve it. Perhaps their solution will be different from that of the generation of people with whom I feel identified.

As I look at my professional and scientific life today and ask myself once more: *Quo Vadis?* I find much which gives me reason to be satisfied. Most of my clinical work is in adult analysis, part of it in training analysis. I teach in both of our local Institutes and many of the local training centers, as well as in our own clinic. I have been permitted to take my work to many groups and many people and have published in many of our standard journals. Some of the work, I am sure, has made an impact. The work of Schlick, of Freud, of Anna Freud, and the work of those near them has inspired me most and has offered me the guiding work ideals; a composite of these constitutes my professional ego ideal. But I have chosen as models for identification people who do not or never did really want mere followers. Part of the professional ego ideal I have chosen is independence of mind, that readiness to free oneself from incomplete insights that need renewal, amplification, and a deeper level of sophistication.

I have maintained from youth movement days a compassion and love for people in need of help and a willingness to be an active part of society regardless of how difficult that may be at times. I am sometimes torn between the old quests for effectiveness in social and individual change. Is it external change or internal change? Are we to follow a Marx or a Freud? Or is a synthesis possible and is society ready for such synthesis? I am also torn between collectivism and individualism, and I try to find a synthesis between monologue, dialogue, and pluralogue. When is one or the other applicable?

My most recent book, also on childhood psychosis, and again a collective work, is *The Challenge: Despair and Hope in the Conquest of Inner Space*. The title, as well as the writing of the book, did not come easily to me. I had been living in a period of success and reward. In 1970 I had been invited to Vienna to give the Freud lecture for that year. Just a year before, the two present political parties had united to open a Freud museum, and I was to return to my native land to help strengthen psychoanalysis and to honor Freud. Old friends were to be there, now representatives of the Austrian government, persecuted with me during Austria's fascist days. We were to celebrate the restoration of the old values. Anna Freud had proposed as the topic of my lecture "The Influence of Psychoanalysis on Education and School." This was a return to the interest which brought me to analysis some thirty-five years earlier. It was a great and a bitter moment. The triumph of that return was fused with the immense pain of learning that my old father had died back in America, our second home. He had read the draft of the paper, and I still wonder whether he remembered the teacher's advice given when I was eleven. (The book is dedicated to him who taught me to turn situations of adversity into activities of hope.)

Family

Can one really write a professional biography unless one also stresses personal factors? I know how much I owe my wife and my children in terms of personal satisfactions. I needed the love they gave me, the loyalty they maintained. I needed the deep opportunities they gave me to love them and see them grow and accompany me through life. I do not think they would have wanted life to have been different for us in our family, my American family. But it must have been difficult for them, for my wife Ruth, and for my children, Jean and Rudi, to live with a psychoanalyst like myself. They had to cope with my long working hours, my preoccupations with myself and the patients, the students, and the institutions, the need to work and to have a kind of secret intellectual life with a world of books and ideas. Sometimes I tried to share some of that with them, and perhaps quite a bit was shared. They were willing to let me have that private world although I often sensed their jealousy and envy. I wish I had told them more often and more fully how much they mean to me.

As I move from the parental role into the age of the grandparent I wonder what I anticipate for myself as a psychoanalyst, a teacher of psychoanalysis and psychotherapy, and a researcher in the clinical field. Perhaps I can best illustrate it if I refer to some thoughts expressed in a recent unpublished paper, "Psychoanalysis—Prologomena to Its Theory, Its Techniques and Issues of Training."

Of Things to Be and Things to Come

Psychoanalysis has occupied me through practically all of my adult life. As I observed its development, the various psychoanalytic schools focused on different aspects of the search for meaning. For this reason I have never looked at "my system" as a final one, a definite one which must win the struggle against all the other psychotherapeutic systems. It is not the result but the process which chiefly concerns the practicing analyst, the researcher, and the educator. The issue is not "to be" but "to become." Professional self-realization is never an end product, always a process, a becoming. What then would be the future of "my" system? I feel like Freud who suggested that whatever a man will leave behind is at best "the patchwork of my labors," and it will be up to others to continuously work on the synthesis of different psychotherapeutic attempts.

I do not mean to say that I am committed to eclecticism. An eclectic gathers a point from here and from there and feels that everybody is right. He gets along with everybody and everything, and he finds that everybody has a bit of the truth. I do not mean to be that all-accepting. Not all in today's marketplace of psychotherapy represents even part of the truth. By synthesis I mean the scientific task of collecting data, searching the evidence, and searching for methods of unifying systems and improving techniques of treatment, as well as throwing out wrong data, concepts, and methods. Unification is not meant to be a compromise but a synthesis. "Unity of science" is a work direction, not a goal, not an end point.

Where will psychoanalysis go? To a large degree the social effectiveness of psychoanalysis depends on the status of society. Many an insight of the past, a discovery in antiquity, an invention made during the Middle Ages or the Renaissance, even techniques developed in our time, have been lost or may get lost whenever there is social regression and violent change. It may well be that we might suffer a kind of temporary social regression in which all individual psychotherapy might suffer. One-to-one psychotherapy may even be pushed from the social scene for a while. Civil war and war time conditions are not conducive to the kind of effort that I have described in these pages. Such setbacks took place several times in the history of psychoanalysis, but always psychoanalysis recovered. Our society now has a variety of options and it is hard to predict which it might follow. If it follows the options of a free society, which include freedom and dignity and individualism integrated with social responsibility, psychoanalysis will have its secure place.

What will be its new direction? It has moved from instinct theory and from the theory of the unconscious to include other considerations as well. We moved toward the structural model, the study of ego and superego. We moved to ego psychology and object-relations theory. More and more we have moved away from mechanical models to humanistic models. While at first there was only drive, now there is also the will. While at first there was only the blind struggle between opposing forces, now there is also the consideration of adaptation, of problem solving, of synthesis on different levels of consciousness.

In research we have moved from the case study to process study. We now study not only transference but countertransference. More and more we have studied the psychoanalytic tool, the analyst himself, and we have developed better training and teaching techniques. We have moved from training for psychoanalysis to psycho-analytic training. We have moved from psychoanalysis in isolation, and in open warfare with academic psychology and medicine, to new islands of full collaboration. We have maintained our identity, yet we have created bridges to other behavioral scientists. Much of the original hostility on both sides has turned into mutual respect. Psychoanalytic thinking is used in other scientific disciplines, and we have learned that we, too, must be accessible, as well as have access, to the general information explosion.

All predictions in this field, due to the uncertainty of our world, are at best self-fulfilling prophecies or magical wish-fulfillment. Therefore, rather than being a seer, I would like to describe some healthy developments of which I would love to be a part. I should like to see psychoanalysis and psychotherapy develop a more open system of training. Psychoanalysis should overcome more fully the separation between medical practitioners and people who come from other fields and who are today admitted for psychoanalytic training only if they are research minded. We need talent from all fields. Some-times when one looks at the former interests of psychoanalysts, lay analysts as well as medical ones, and particularly notes those who have contributed to the field, one realizes that it may be statistics or English literature, physiology or pathology, art or pedagogy, economics or sociology, social work or clinical psychology, pediatrics or internal medicine, which makes the important contribution.

Furthermore, I hope we continue to give up the isolation of private training institutes, and that psychoanalysis will now be ready to return to the university fold. Psychoanalysis should have indepen-dent psychoanalytic departments in the universities, not dominated by any of the other disciplines but freely dedicated to the search for truth and the search for healthy application. Most of us who think along these lines have one foot in private practice, the other in clinical or teaching activity. Is it too much to ask for a utopian development that would put us back into the university, so that there could be new creative islands of growth?

Whenever a science becomes accepted, and analysis is certainly accepted today in America in spite of some of its setbacks, it risks becoming diluted. Ecclesia militans after having become ecclesia triumphans may become ecclesia dilutans. Unless there are islands of research, of constant questioning, of constant progress, psychoanalysis, like other activities, is in danger of becoming institutionalized. Can we create, however, psychoanalytic institutions which have built into them the task of scientific change? Can one see to it that the task of change, of constructive development, of endless renewal, becomes everybody's vested interest and a genuine part of our inner and institutional life?

I end my autobiography in identifying with Freud's cautious 1925 reflections on the future of psychoanalysis:

> By a process of development against which it would have been useless to struggle, the word "psychoanalysis" has itself become ambiguous. While it was originally the name of a particular therapeutic method, it has now also become the name of a science—the science of unconscious mental processes. By itself this science is seldom able to deal with a problem completely, but it seems destined to give valuable contributory help in the most varied regions of knowledge. This fear of application of psychoanalysis extends as far as that of psychology, to which it forms a complement of the greatest moment.
>
> Looking back then over the patchwork of my life's labors, I can say that I have made many beginnings and thrown out many suggestions. Something will come of them in the future, though I cannot myself tell whether it will be much or little. However, I can express a hope that I have opened up a pathway for an important advance in our knowledge.[4]

Selected Writings

With E. CARUTH, G. W. FRIEDMAN, A. MANDLEBAUM, J. WALLERSTEIN, AND D. G. WRIGHT. *Children of Time and Space, of Action and Impulse.* New York: Appleton-Century-Crofts, 1966.

With R. L. MOTTO. *From Learning for Love to Love of Learning: Essays on Psychoanalysis and Education.* New York: Brunner/Mazel, 1969.

"Psychoanalytic Reflections on the Emergence of the Teacher's Professional Identity." *Reiss-Davis Clinic Bulletin,* 1970, *1,* 5–16.

The Challenge: Despair and Hope in the Conquest of Inner Space. New York: Brunner/Mazel, 1971.

With R. S. WALLERSTEIN. *The Teaching and Learning of Psychotherapy.* New York: International Universities Press, 1971.

[4] "An Autobiographical Study." In *Freud's Collected Works,* standard edition, Vol. 20 (London: Hogarth Press, 1959), pp. 3–74.

XII

Letting Go and Going On

Werner M. Mendel

I write this material with the basic view that I can understand where I am partly in relation to where I have been and partly to where I am going. I am firmly committed to the existential circular view of time. The past and the future equally determine the present. The present is that moment in which we behave, in which we act and feel and think. The present is a moment of action which moves from the future to the past. Aristotelian time attempts to explain the present primarily in terms of how we got there from the past. My concept of time requires that I tell you not only what I have had happen to me before, but also what I hope, what I expect, and what I plan. To understand me you must see how the future and the past meet in the moment of my existence which is my Here and Now.

This, like any autobiographical sketch, suffers from problems of selective inattention and pinhole vision. Remembrances told are always filtered and rephrased. They are presented sequentially only as the result of retrospective distortions. Therefore, and for a variety of other reasons, I will not attempt to present my genesis in any orderly way nor will I purport to tell you that those things which I mention here are the most important. They are simply the events, the feelings, and the psychosocial circumstances, as I see them today through my retrospectoscope, which seem to have some relationship to where I am, here and now. To tell you where I am requires the distorted reporting of my own eyes which see with limited view my own system of values and motivations and the reader will have to extrapolate from that.

The Past

My past consists of a series of accidents. This is difficult for me to admit because I do not believe in accidents. I believe in a world in which I am the center and in which all things that happen to me are the result of something I do. I do not accept that I was thrown into the world, that I was walking down the street minding my own business when suddenly this or that fell upon me. I always have control over my position vis-a-vis accidental happenings. To a large measure, particularly in my adult life, the accidental happenings are my doing, my choice, and my exposure. Perhaps my attitude about personal responsibility even for accidents comes from my having participated in catastrophic world events. I anticipate that I will participate in further catastrophic world events in the next decades. I have never found that "accepting," "making the best of it," "adjusting to" has suited me. This philosophy of personal responsibility is also very much part of my treatment approach. I maintain that the individual is centrally responsible for himself, for his behavior, and for his decisions in both health and illness. I insist that I am in charge of my existence and that I always have some control. By this I do not mean that I am in charge of environmental factors which I cannot possibly control. But, finally, when all is said and done, I make the decisions and I develop my attitudes no matter where the brackets of my existence are placed by the internal or external environment.

I am an only child, born to an academically and professionally upward-striving, upper-middle-class German-Jewish family. The male members of the family had had doctor's degrees for many generations.

They were all doctors, lawyers, scholars, or senators in the German parliament. Several female members of the family also had doctor's degrees. The family was well-to-do financially, firmly entrenched in the formal structure of the social class, living in the creative furor of the Weimar Republic after World War I. Then I was born as the only child of the Mendel family and the last carrier of the name. A few years after my birth Hitler became chancellor of Germany.

In the first twelve years of my life I lived in a family which would not accept the changing world. The family relationships were formal. The demands upon me academically and socially were clearly outlined. I was the depository of all the background, knowledge, and hope for the future of the family. I was constantly reminded of my duties and obligations to my illustrious predecessors, of my responsibility for carrying out traditions, of being the last of the Mohicans (Mendels)' so to speak. Then came external chaos. My father who had believed himself above all such things was incarcerated in a concentration camp. My grandfather and grandmother, who had been important super-Germans, were carted off to the gas chambers. I was sent out as a refugee to England to go to school in a hostile country where suddenly I was despised for being what I was not, namely a German. I was brought up to be a German and then declared by Hitler not to be a German. I went to England because I was not a German and there was beaten up in the school yard for being a German. I came to the United States to flee from Hitler and promptly was declared an enemy alien with restricted mobility and rights. My family regrouped in Los Angeles in a German-Jewish community which pretended that it was living in Germany in 1928, not the United States of 1939. We held on to our values and attempted to live in Germany while living in wartorn United States. All property was lost, all possessions were gone, all titles had become meaningless, and yet we tried to cling to the decayed fabric and structure of the old life.

From all of this I began to understand that nothing is permanent, that nothing has real value, that all is changeable. The only value that one can depend on is one's own integrity and the ability to relate to people and time.

After returning from the American Army of World War II, I continued my schooling, went through medical school, internship and residency training, psychoanalytic training, and became a professor.

I had fulfilled the demands of my destiny. I had become a fully recognized and accredited academician, psychoanalyst, psychiatrist, and doctor. Yet, in fact, none of these was a prized possession. I had learned that they could all disappear, could all evaporate. What I prized over anything else was my personal feeling of competence, my reliance upon myself, my mobility, and most importantly my willingness to let go of acquired goods and titles and to go on to other things.

The Future

In order to understand where I am, you must know where I am going. Today I am forty-five. My boys are nearly grown up. They have left home to start their own lives in college and in the world. Many things I have enjoyed doing in the past bore me now. I do not plan to be a professor until my retirement at sixty-five. I have been a professor now for some ten years and that is about enough. I do not anticipate being an administrator much longer. It is fun to manage systems and it is good to teach people how to do things efficiently. I do it well, but I think I have had enough. I do not anticipate being a psychotherapist much longer. I took care of my first enuretic patient in the psychology clinic at Stanford in 1949. Since then I have been responsible for managing many psychotherapeutic and psychoanalytic transactions. Twenty-three years of these transactions are also enough.

Nothing should be done any longer than it is fun. At first the fun of therapy came in the mastery of the art, then the fun came in the results I achieved, then fun was to have the secondary benefits of earning high fees and much fame. Finally it is no longer fun. Then one has the choice of letting go and going on or becoming a conservator. To be conservative is doing something because I do it well and because I am successful and I try to do it as long as possible. That is not for me.

If I look at the stages of my sources of pleasure from doing psychotherapy, I can see how these have changed over the years. At the beginning it was exciting to discover the patient, to understand what was going on, and then eventually to learn not only what was happening in the patient but also what was happening in me and what was going on between us. The next stage was the pleasure in mastering and learning the techniques of intervention, of seeing how I could influence the transaction, and how I could make things happen. The next stage was one in which I was comfortable enough with my own feelings and with the mastery of the techniques to be able to really listen to the patient and to hear the many fascinating "war stories." Then after I had heard all the stories came the pleasure in the results, the ability to help people change their situations for the better, to help them become what they are and to learn what they know, and subsequently to see how their lives changed in the direction of becoming more creative, more productive, more open to fun and new experiences. In the next stage of my twenty-two years of existing as a psychotherapist, I became interested in further refinement of techniques, handling more difficult cases, doing it faster, doing it with more skill and with more finesse. I liked engaging in the acrobatics of technique, showing how good I was, how much better than anyone else, and how I could take on cases that no one else would dare handle. People came to me who had tried everything else. They were referred because I was great, famous, and successful! They paid me well. I enjoyed this for awhile and rose to the occasion by giving my best into each transaction.

But when all of these stages were past there was only one real gratification, one real pleasure which remained from the difficult, arduous task of psychotherapy. From each human contact I grew, I enlarged my horizons, I changed. Now, at this stage of my development, I do psychotherapy and psychoanalysis and engage in the helping transaction for the pleasure of the human transaction, for the fun of relating to another human being, for the delight of having another growth experience. However, I have also realized that most people who identify themselves as patients tend to lead constricted, limited lives, tend to be rather boring, and tend not to be able to give a great deal to human transactions. For this reason the time has come for me to move on to other kinds of human transaction. The expanded hearing, expanded vision, and expanded feeling which I derived from the reflective self-aware living as a psychotherapist and psychoanalyst can apply to nontherapeutic relationships and yield much more of a growth experience to me at this time. This is why psychotherapy is no longer fun and why it is time to let go and go on for me and my existence.

What then will I do with my twenty years of experience as a psychotherapist and psychoanalyst? What will I do with the skills and attitudes and knowledge I have accumulated? What will I do with my improved eyes and ears, my techniques of flowing into relationships? What will I do with my courage for intimacy? I plan to use them to explore and enjoy new relationships with many human beings in many roles. I plan to escape from the incarceration in the medical model and from the psychotherapeutic transaction into real life. I will relate to real people on a real basis and to pursue this pleasure until it is again time for me to let go and go on.

In this short sketch you can see where I have come from and where I expect to go. You have some brackets in which to set me in the present moment when I write this and when you read this. You have some basis from which to understand my attitude toward illness and health, responsibility and treatment, mental health care delivery systems and innovations as well as theory of neurosis and psychosis and treatment. These attitudes are described and worked out in my papers and books. I am not going to repeat them here. I will only give you some outline of what I think and believe now. I would remind you that I feel about ideas as I do about periods of my life. I am willing to let go and go on. What I believe today is not what I believed yesterday nor is it what I expect to believe tomorrow.

Schizophrenia

At this point in my career I have no idea what causes schizophrenia. I do not have the faintest idea how to cure it, and therefore I am in exactly the same position as everyone else. However, I do know a great deal about how to manage the patient who suffers from schizophrenia in such a way that he can live a nearly normal life with considerable effectiveness and satisfaction. I can minimize his disabilities and maximize his capacities and I can prevent him from living a life of pain, misery, and agony. A few of my colleagues know how to do the same thing. Most don't.

I believe that there is some genetic predisposition, and that there are early childhood experiences which lead to the problems which we summarize under the rubric of schizophrenia. There are also chemical changes which are identifiable and which may be related to some of the changes called schizophrenia. Most probably they are simply the result of the chronic anxiety in the physiological systems of the body. The clinical defect in the adult schizophrenic patient as I have gotten to know him consists of three factors:

First is a failure of historicity. Life's experiences, particularly the good experiences which build self-esteem, do not stick to the ribs of the schizophrenic patient. He can have a good relationship, develop a trusting transaction for many years, be loved and successful. Yet one minor event, one missed appointment, one disappointment can erase all the years of good experiences and success as though they never happened. It is as though the history which each of us lives and which makes part of our self-esteem system does not work for the schizophrenic patient. He does not have a feeling of past, present, and future. He has only the present moment of his anxiety, of horror, or pain, of facing the void. Variously this has been described by the existentialist as feelings of emptiness; by the Sullivanians as impaired self-esteem; by the behavior therapists as the schizophrenic's inability to learn from experience. The psychoanalysts have noted this defect as the schizophrenic's narcissistic attitude which makes it impossible for the patient to relate and to develop insight about relationships. The psychodynamically oriented supportive therapist talks about this defect as the "as if" personality. However, for me this difficulty in the schizophrenic existence is best described as a failure of historicity.

The second major difficulty a schizophrenic existence demonstrates is the inability of the patient to manage interpersonal relationships comfortably, successfully, and economically. Each relationship a schizophrenic patient enters seems to lead to further failure, further disaster, and further pain. Somehow he always manages to make it come out badly. He enters a relationship to get support and he gets rejected. He enters a relationship to be successful and he fails. He enters a relationship to give love and he ends up hating; he wants to get nurture and he is poisoned. He wants to fill his emptiness and he gets sucked dry. The schizophrenic patient displays a fantastic social and interpersonal clumsiness which leads consistently to terribly expensive and exhaustive attempts at supplying his needs from interpersonal transactions. This defect makes treatment extremely difficult because most of the time the patient and the therapist manage to make the transaction expensive and disastrous.

The third major defect in the schizophrenic patient's existence is his inability to manage his anxiety economically and effectively.

Usually he has a lifelong history of expending inordinate amounts of energy and activity in the process of managing his anxiety. This leads to the commonly observed clinical phenomena of pan-neurosis, free-flowing anxiety, nervous exhaustion, and physiological changes secondary to chronic anxiety states. The patient who lives a schizophrenic existence does not have the techniques or the energy to manage his anxiety effectively.

The treatment of the schizophrenic patient must address itself to these three major issues. We must take great care to give constant consultation and training to the patient to help him learn to manage his interpersonal transactions so that they do not always end in disaster. We must supply support and substitution for the patient's failure of historicity by providing an open future and an ongoing, variable support system for the rest of his life. These techniques include getting the patient off the hook when he gets in over his head in interpersonal transactions. It also includes warning him about all the complications of certain relationships and of not pushing him out of his autism more rapidly than he is able to handle the interruption of his isolation. In supportive care I teach the patient techniques to manage his anxiety. At times chemical help with his anxiety may be indicated. By formulating schizophrenia along these three observations, I have been able to develop an economical and feasible technique and theory of supportive care which allows me to provide, with minimum effort, lifelong treatment to patients with schizophrenic existences during exacerbations and remissions. I can support most of my patients with one appointment every month or two during remissions and with two or three extra appointments during exacerbations. I have described this technique and summarized it and detailed it in *The Therapeutic Management of Psychological Illness*.[1]

Expressive Psychotherapy and Psychoanalysis

These techniques of intervention are best understood as teaching-learning experiences. I see therapy as a special technique for creating an atmosphere in which the patient has the opportunity to spend leisurely time to reflect upon himself, where he is, and where he's

[1] W. M. Mendel and G. A. Green (New York: Basic Books, 1967).

going, and thus to discover alternatives to the repetition compulsion. There are two major kinds of psychotherapy. Repressive psychotherapy, which is essentially supportive, is particularly applicable for the schizophrenic patient and other psychotic people. Expressive psychotherapy, sometimes called insight psychotherapy or uncovering psychotherapy, is particularly suitable for the neurotic and the character-disordered patient. Regardless of what type of expressive psychotherapy we do, whether it is analytic, or behavior modification, or existential, or Jungian, or another humanistic approach, we essentially go through the same steps. The patient seems to go through the same stages in "getting well" in learning new attitudes, new ways of thinking, and new ways of behaving. The end point of treatment, the getting well, is when he has the tools with which to solve his problems. First always is the confrontation as the therapist holds up a mirror to the patient and says to him, "Look, as I see it these are some of the things you seem to be doing and thinking and feeling." This is a step all psychotherapies must begin with. It is also the step which is very much extended and expanded in what is called character analysis. Step two includes reflection on how the patient got to where he is now—the exploration of the events in his life which led him to the difficulty he is in now and an exploration of the attitudes, thoughts, feelings, and behavior patterns in his history. This, of course, is the step which is very much exaggerated in classical psychoanalysis and psychodynamic psychotherapy. Step three consists of recognizing that there are alternative ways of handling situations. While indeed it was true at age five or seven one could handle an overwhelmingly aggressive authority figure only by having a temper tantrum, knuckling under, or running away, when one is thirty-five or forty there are other alternatives. The patient can explore these alternatives in the psychotherapeutic transaction and in life. In the classical psychoanalytic model this exploration is done entirely within the framework of the transference. In other models it can be done as part of behavior modification techniques, as a result of insight, as a result of new experiences. Step four is to take these alternate techniques and, with the "courage to fail," try them out in life. Nobody has gotten well in the consulting room or on a couch. People need to get well in life, and that's where they must try out what they have learned about themselves and about the world. These are the four steps which are part of every expressive psychotherapeutic process. They are steps of recognizing, learning, and trying out. I think the process can be best understood in terms of learning theory.

From the patient's point of view, how does he change? First he becomes aware of what he is doing, thinking, and feeling. After he has done, thought, and felt in retrospect, he can begin to figure out what happened. Next he becomes aware of what is happening, what he is doing while it is occurring. After that he arrives at a stage of his learning where he says, "Oops, I almost did it again," but at that point he can stop himself from falling into the repetition compulsion. And then, finally, when his patterns have changed he can see how he used to do these kinds of things, have those thoughts and that set of feelings under these circumstances, but now he no longer has them. Now he can use alternate ways of viewing them.

Contrary to the views in some of my earlier work I see the future as having increasing possibilities. When I was much younger and looked at the influence of the perception of the future on psychopathology I was convinced that as we age, as we have more experiences, the future closes. Now it seems to me that I can, must, should, let go of certain functions, and each year my future seems to be more open. Each year I am more able to enjoy life, to feel better, and to be excited about all there is. This perhaps is the greatest surprise of all. I have not become blase. I have not felt that there is nothing new under the sun. Rather I feel that with each year's experience of living, with each new skill learned and with each new door open, I have improved my capacity for enjoyment and for sampling the richness of the universe in which I live. It is fascinating to me that this is even true physically. Even though I am forty-five years old I feel physically better and more able now than I did twenty years ago. I feel psychologically better and more able than I did twenty years ago. I am more efficient, more hedonistic, more effective than ever before. And each year I enjoy my relationships more.

Just as I can say to my wife "I love you and enjoy you less today than I will tomorrow," I can say about the world, the culture, and my interpersonal transactions that each day I get more from them than on the previous day.

Selected Writings

"Binswanger's Case of Ellen West." (A translation) In *Existence*. New
    York: Basic Books, 1958.
*Therapeutic Management of Psychological Illness: The Theory and Prac-
    tice of Supportive Care*. New York: Basic Books, 1967. With G. A.
    Green.
With PHILLIP SOLOMON (eds.) *The Psychiatric Consultation*. New York:
    Grune and Stratton, 1967.
(Ed.) *A Celebration of Laughter*. Los Angeles: Mara Books, 1970.
"Depression and Suicide—Treatment and Prevention." *Consultant*, 1972,
    12, 115–116.

XIII

A Psychiatrist in Spain

Juan J. Lopez-Ibor

I decided to study medicine because I always thought that in this way I would be able to draw closer to the reality of man and his mysterious being. It was when I was a second-year student in medical school that I came across the complete works of Freud. Perhaps this Spanish edition was the first translation of his works into a foreign language. The prologue contained a letter written by Freud to the translator, Lopez Ballesteros, dated May 7, 1923, in Vienna, which said: "When I was a young student, the desire to read the immortal *Don Quixote* in the language of Cervantes himself led me to learn, without teachers, the beautiful Castilian tongue. Thanks to this hobby of my youthful days I can now, in my mature age, verify the exactitude of your Spanish version of my works, the reading of which gives me great pleasure because of the extremely precise interpretation of my thought and the elegance of the style."

Translated from the Spanish by D. Tomás Monahan, Madrid.

The impact of reading Freud led me to study psychiatry after I graduated. At the medical school, while I was studying internal medicine, I was always on the lookout for books and writers which aroused a special interest in me—for example, the works of Krehl, Siebert, Weiszaker—that is, those in which the scientific-natural orientation of medicine was shown to be insufficient; I sought what was subsequently called "anthropological medicine" in Central Europe and "holistic medicine" in the United States. Although both these paths do not absolutely coincide, they are inspired by analogous motives.

At that time, the psychiatry of Central Europe enjoyed the highest reputation in Spain. When I had completed my official studies there, I went to Munich. There, in the university clinic, Kraepelin had been succeeded by Bumke who, although he came from a more flexible school of psychiatry, followed the same philosophy as his predecessor. In Munich there was also the Kraepelin-Institut, dedicated to psychiatric research, but which was mainly directed toward the somatic aspect of mental disturbances. About that time Bumke published a monograph in which he manifested his opposition to psychoanalysis. Distinct from the university there was a psychoanalytic circle presided over by von Hatinberg, and I attended the meetings regularly. Afterward, I spent some time in other clinics, both German and French. When I arrived at Kretschmer's clinic, a doctor who was one of his assistants said to me in confidence, "A new exceptional book by Freud has just been published. You ought to read it at once." This book was, in fact, *Das Unbehagen in der Kultur*. From the time I first read it, I have retained two compelling recollections: the origin of culture or civilization by means of the act of repression—"putting out the fire by means of a jet of urine"; and a metaphor I came across for the first time in Freud's writings—although it had previously been used by other German writers—"oceanic feeling" (*ozeanisches Gefühl*), which Freud said that he had never experienced.

Psychotherapeutic Practice

When I began my own psychotherapeutic practice, certain facts immediately attracted my attention. I remember one of my first cases, M. T., who was thirty when she came to consult me. By profession she was a pediatrician, as was her husband, and they practiced together. She had no children and had been a very brilliant student at the university. She consulted me because of the unbearable anxiety from which she was suffering. She did not have specific phobias, but her state of anxiety was manifested, above all, as a pan-phobia. She was afraid that something would happen to her, but she did not know what that something was.

For the purpose of psychotherapeutic treatment, she came to live in Madrid for some months, but she returned to her native city and to her profession when she was cured. In the first psychotherapeutic sessions, I endeavored to decipher the enigma of her anxiety. The spectres that haunted her were two: death and madness. She began by relating the story of her life. When she was twenty-four and had recently obtained her degree, she began to practice her profession in a hospital in the city in which she was born. At that time she had to live through a revolutionary episode that occurred prior to the Spanish Civil War. The miners in the province rose up in rebellion against the government and occupied the capital city. There were fires, armed attacks, and other acts of violence, and a continuous stream of wounded people entered the hospital where she was permanently on duty. There were many deaths and she had to certify them as deceased. The circumstances produced in her a severe and lasting state of anxiety which, however, disappeared when the situation returned to normal after about two weeks.

Another important series of anxiety-ridden memories pertained to her childhood when she was between four and six years of age. The crises of anxiety reached their peak in summer, when she went with her brothers and the rest of her family to a house in a mountain village. This house was an ancient manor which was, she said, "large, very large" and a considerable part of it was uninhabited. It also had a huge, dark garret which was full of strange noises. She recalled that she had been frequently attacked by crises of anxiety, even when she was playing with her brothers and her friends. The solitude and silence of some of their hiding places oppressed her and filled her with anxiety as well.

The detailed recounting of these and other episodes in her life required four months of therapy, at a rate of five hours a week. No sexual traumas, which could be considered as having provoked her state of anxiety, came to light. Halfway through the treatment she began to experience such an acute state of anxiety that she was compelled to change her hotel and find one closer to my office. During this period she could not stand being alone. When her husband was unable to be with her, for professional reasons, she needed the company of a different member of her family. During the last two weeks of treatment her anxiety diminished very rapidly, and at the end of the treatment she was able to take up her normal life again.

When I had finished with her, I was left with a great sense of dissatisfaction: I had not been able to see clearly *how* she had been cured. In the course of treatment I always made an effort to seek "rationalization" of the episodes of her life, past and present, as a correction against the irrational nature of anxiety. In other cases I had managed to convince myself that my psychotherapeutic work was more closely linked with the data of the conscious and unconscious life of the patient and with the manifestations of the neurosis itself. But the case of M. T. was the first in which I had found evidence of an *empty zone,* and with such a void I would not be able to grow in the understanding and interpretation of the neuroses.

Another of my early cases was that of a teacher who also suffered from an anxiety neurosis. The first day that he came to see me he told me he had an Oedipus complex. This proved to be the case. He was an only child, with all the defects incurred in the upbringing of such children. The patient was always very dependent on his parents, and especially on his mother. He was very studious and intelligent and played some sports for health reasons. He learned, for example, to play tennis by studying a book. His behavior was similar in other aspects of his life, but in reality his mother was more dependent on him than he was on her. On one occasion when he had a fit of shivering and took to his bed, his mother went to bed with him to keep him warm. In childhood he had had diphtheria and had to have a tracheotomy. When his diphtheria had been cured, his mother refused to allow the fistula, the sequel of the tracteotomy, to be closed until he was twenty, with the idea of forestalling his military service.

The patient was cured of his anxiety phase by means of psychotherapy and subsequently had a brilliant scientific career. Ten years later he again came to consult me with symptoms of anxiety and depression, which lasted for some months, succeeded by a state of hypomania, which continued with cyclothymic oscillations, very accentuated in one and another direction, and which have continued up to the present.

There has just been published the catamnesis of the Wolf-Man. This patient appeared in the consulting rooms of Freud in February 1910 and remained under analysis until July 1914. Later on Freud published "The Case of the Wolf-Man. From the History of an Infantile Neurosis." The work of Freud is extraordinarily interesting. As Gardiner states in the introduction to the book,[1] of the five famous cases published by Freud only three were really analyzed by him, and of these three only the Wolf-Man survives. The reading of his clinical history and his personal biography shows that the Wolf-Man had had cyclical depressions all his life. Gardiner says that the depressions were not, in her opinion, psychotic. But on reading his autobiography, and other commentaries contained in the book, this statement must be questioned. In a letter dated September 21, 1950, he says: "A 'tedium vitae' has taken hold of me, so that when I wake up in the morning I shudder at the thought that I must get through a 'whole day' from morning to evening."

As I have tried to describe, I found myself, at the outset of my psychotherapeutic work, in an intellectual situation similar to that raised by the case of the Wolf-Man. Anxiety, Freud said, is the key to neurosis. Anxiety has also become the key to the interpretation of the human being in certain very active currents of contemporary thought (existential philosophy, for example). I then asked myself whether both classes of anxiety are the same, equivalent, or merely analogous.

My experience with depressions taught me that the sadness of the depressives is not of the same quality as that of normal man. The melancholics, that is, the psychotic depressives, are incapable of experiencing sadness. Many depressives can make the distinction between reactive sadness which comes from the loss of a loved one and the other depression which is more profound, which comes from within, and which the phenomenologists call vital or endothymic sadness. Does not the same occur with anxiety and with similar emotive states, of which tedium itself is an example? In replying to this question, I

[1] M. Gardiner (ed.), *The Wolf-Man by the Wolf-Man: The Double Story of Freud's Most Famous Case* (New York: Basic Books, 1971).

found the way to understand that vacuum I had experienced in the case of M. T. above.

Mastery of Technique

The attitude of a psychotherapist requires a high degree of maturity. Young psychotherapists tend to be too closely bound up with problems of technique and, in general, they lack sufficient flexibility to cope with the most serious problems of psychotherapy. The fact that 60 percent of neuroses follow a phasic course and terminate spontaneously, and which some writers consider an objection to the efficacy of psychotherapy, misleads them. In the life of Freud himself it can be seen how he passed from a descriptive attitude of clinical studies to an interpretive attitude and finally to the general statement of the great problems of the human being in an attempt to develop a meta-psychology.

If all knowledge requires experience, the knowledge of the limits of the action of a man requires much more. It is precisely to contribute to this process of maturing, to avoid personal vicissitudes having an unfavorable effect on patients, to prevent the application of over-rigid theoretical moulds, that the neutrality of the psychotherapist is required. This neutrality is a working hypothesis, because the inter-subjective relationship can scarcely be neutral. What is certain is that the closer one approaches the great themes of life, such as anxiety, suffering, illness, despair, and the more one learns to cope with them as deep psychotherapy requires, the more does the maturing of the personality of the psychotherapist become accelerated.

In any event, the neutral attitude of the psychotherapist merits a detailed analysis. There is no doubt that the psychotherapist who is a tyro, or has not been forewarned, often finds himself caught up in the neurotic web and has great difficulty disentangling himself from it, more particularly if the therapeutic relationship becomes eroticized. It should not be forgotten that neurotic personalities have a pathological affective hunger and that they consequently are disposed to devour whoever allows himself to become their victim. In such cases, the psychotherapist becomes converted into an instrument in the hands of a neurotic personality. Again, this often happens even though the relationship is not erotic. Psychotherapy implies the establishment of contact but also the keeping of a distance. No psychotherapy is possible without human contact, but there can be no therapeutic action without a sufficient distance being kept. It is not possible to obtain objective knowledge of the neurotic situation if the psychotherapist immersed in it is unable to keep a certain distance from it and is therefore swept away by the strong tides that characterize it.

Since the world of illness is so varied, and since on occasion illness is found at the limits of stimulation, the case may arise of an active attitude of persistence in psychotherapy as a form of filling up life. But these cases are not, in themselves, and psychopathologically speaking, the most important. What most frequently happens is that the patient does not want to renounce certain defense mechanisms, because basically he is unable to free himself. The defense mechanisms constitute a refuge that he cannot leave except on the condition of being healthy, which implies the suppression of the advantages of the symptoms. Only when, in the process of cure, the defense mechanisms —which, in reality, are symptoms of the illness—are suppressed will it be possible to deal with the patient regarding the abandonment of still other defensive mechanisms which are not so closely linked with the illness itself. The patient does not leave his house, for example, because the first person that he meets makes him blush. The blushing can be interpreted as a defense mechanism, the same as the fact of not leaving the house. The second phenomenon, however, is a form of behavior secondary to the first. It is only the suppression of the first that will return his freedom to the patient. It is not sufficient to interpret the erythrophobia: it must disappear. The patient can make a greater or lesser effort to approximate his behavior to that of the rest of the world, and the doctor has to try to put him in a situation in which he can do so. To give him interpretations of his nonemergence from his neurotic fortress as resistance is like transferring the bad conscience of the doctor to the patient.

The inappreciable and a-logical moment that exists in transference has been duly stressed by some authors. In the process of transference, the patient exteriorizes the whole of his affective stratum only before one man, the psychotherapist. The cure comes when the patient can transfer this trusting relationship to the real world. Freud has said little on this point, not only because the exposition of this fragment of the road to cure proves to be particularly difficult, but also because

Freud knew that this fragment of the art of psychoanalysis does not permit itself to be apprehended in technical formulations. The opacity of the transferential crisis is evident, just as is the impossibility of translating it into technical schemas. It is handled like an art, just as all human contacts are handled. In the actuation of the cure, rationalization evaporates. What is it then that happens here?

The limits of the efficacy of the cure are clear. In the cases of character analysis it is not easy to indicate a natural limit, even though one holds oneself aloof from exaggerated hopes and does not propose any extreme task to the analysis. It is not possible to propose as an objective the smoothing-away of all peculiarities in favor of a schematic normalization, nor even to ask that those who have been subjected to deep analysis shall not feel any serious passion and shall not develop any internal conflict at all. Analysis must obtain the psychological conditions most favorable for the functions of the "I." When these are accomplished the task can be considered as finished. Here, "deep psychoanalysis" opens the doors to a prudent *psychogogy*. With this, Freud once again demonstrates his talent. He is not bent on going beyond the limited possibilities that the "analysis of the character" offers.

In the base of the human being, along with the negative anthropological structures there exist those which are positive. One is the necessity of keeping faith with oneself; and the other, closely linked with the first, is that of hope. Any doctor who treats incurable or doomed patients finds noteworthy the facility with which, against all logic, they cling to the minutest hope that is offered them. This form of hope does not need to take the concrete form of a new diagnosis, or considering the previous one to be slightly mistaken, or in the form of a new drug. What the patient is offered, and that to which he clings, is something vague and undefined. I have long been surprised by this same and extraordinary fact in relation to experienced doctors themselves attacked by a serious disease. Contrary to what it would be logical to suppose, they maintain their hope despite unmistakable signs of the uncontrollable advance of their malady. In reality, this is a question of a special form of hope.

In life, hope exists as the future. The very impulse to go on living, which proceeds from life itself, constitutes what we could term its biological base. The future causes the present to advance, but the future is seen, so to speak, as a populated continent. People hope to obtain this or that thing, to carry out such and such an activity, to attain a certain position. In this hope there exists a mixture of reality and fantasy, of possibilities that are attainable and others that are not. This future which is integrated in life is like a derivative of the present.

There exists another form of hope which is impossible hope: that despairing hope, unconcrete and vague, that does not come from without, that is, from the hope of the attainment of something desired, but from within, from a kind of new illumination of life. In this kind of hope it is not simply a matter of the disappearance of the symptoms of an illness, of a recuperation, although naturally this is assumed by what is hoped for. It is not a question of the disappearance of the pains, the weakness, or the symptom. It is a question of something with a wider scope whose process is amorphous, carefully unconscious, something that could be called "recovery of health." In some attempted suicides it can be seen that the person is seeking a state different from his earthly condition. In many depressives it is not so much longing for death but a longing for that other state of "existential health" that drives them to suicide. Paradoxical as the situation may seem, it is nevertheless real.

This hope is intimately related to the character of openness of the very anthropological structure of man. In the fact of its existence there is always to be found the possibility of something that does not yet exist. This is the difference between expectation and hope, between anxiety and fear. Expectation belongs to the kingdom of the concrete future, hope to the kingdom of possibility, of becoming something that has not yet been attained.

In anxiety there exists the possibility of "annulation," precisely because the being explodes into an infinity of possibilities. Annulation is to cease to be, or to be another. Vis-a-vis this "being another," this threat of alteration, there arises the principle of the fidelity of the being—that which in psychological language is called "one's self" and "the continuity of one's self" as being characteristic of the "I." Fidelity is faith. When the threat of nonbeing asserts itself, hope rises up, born of that same primordial structure. In transference we find ourselves faced with these two elements, through the personal relationship. The doctor or the psychotherapist inspires confidence. This means that, in the interior agony, the threats of anxiety will not materialize, and the being will continue to be. Hope is born, also, inspired by the presence of the doctor. The positive possibilities of the being reappear. The patient will be cleansed of guilt, from the ancestral fear linked to his phobias, from the impalpable suffering that annihilates.

Closely related to this theme is what is generally called, at times slightingly, "supportive psychotherapy." The most general example of this is what the general physician practices when he encourages a patient by giving him a pat on the back and saying a few consoling words. The psychotherapists who practice deep psychotherapy wax wroth at this attitude, as they do in general with every form of psychotherapy that may be termed "covering-up." Such practices are a form of deception, they say. The self-deception of the patient is reinforced by the deception practiced by the doctor. "All consolation is turbid," says Rilke, alluding to that lack of internal veracity that consolation embodies. Nevertheless, in consolation there is something more than this tendency to disguise reality. Consolation, in ordinary life, implies the elevation from one sphere to another, from that which has no remedy to that which has. Consolation always tries to provide man, despite the threat exercised by the infinite, with a more profound protection in the infinite. This act of freeing oneself from limiting concrete circumstances—in this case, illness—by placing one's hopes in something inconcrete is a form of belief. The step toward this belief is taken through a personal instance, that of the doctor. Such a form of belief has nothing to do with the contents of a given religious belief. This would be, in any event, a super-added action.

Supporting psychotherapy creates, to say the least, a relationship of transference which alleviates while the neurotic phase lasts, in the event that it is a phase of life which is in question. In other situations, it adds a direct moral aid that can contribute to disentangling the situational web in which the patient is enveloped.

The Ego as Therapist

The ideal of the "ego" of the psychotherapist must necessarily be linked with his own reality and must be brought up to date day after day. Each day has its own task, and taking a parallel from a great writer, we may say that he who does not have the spirit of his age has all its sufferings; but this does not refer to the age of maturity alone, but also to youth itself. The ideal is created by trying increasingly to explore one's own depths and to fulfill oneself by means of one's action on the patients.

A person recognizes himself only in encounters with others healthy or ill. Each one has his own style of life, which is slowly created through experiences which at times are favorable and at other times are marked by suffering.

For my part, I have had a very complex life, but it has permitted me to attain now a way of development much more serene than that which I was able to have in my youth. My "family romance" had scarcely any weight in my childhood and adolescence. I have always had the sensation of living life as an adventure, not on the material but on the intellectual level. At a certain moment, I created a family, which is a large one. This fact increased my impulse toward the future. The past cannot as such be changed. Only at a late stage did I come to appreciate that the past can come to be modified through my own perspective of it. This was a great discovery, commonplace in its formulation, but rich as an experience, which opened up new paths for my self-fulfillment as a psychotherapist. What is important in the past is not its facts, but the perspective which illuminates them. The past, even though traumatized and erroneous, is the source of the future. There is no doubt that a "personal demon" exists, taking this term in its Socratic sense. Socrates himself was unable to control his own demon: his failure is full of lessons for the rest of the world. The failure of the psychotherapist is pride, the *hubris* of the ancient Greeks. All of us are the playthings of destiny, and there are no supermen who can master it.

As time passes, one experiences a greater satisfaction in the exercise of psychotherapy, because one feels oneself nearer to deciphering the human enigma, although in reality one never succeeds in reaching this goal. With the passing of the years, the experience undergone is in no way tedious, but, on the contrary, interesting. Each day, when one comes to the end of one's task, one feels more enriched within, with more "human substance," one might say.

Transference occurs with great facility because the anxiety of the patient demands it. The dangers of countertransference arise when the psychotherapist feels himself insecure or subjected to some form of anxiety. A form of normal anxiety is derived from the lack of satisfaction of different aspects of life—sexual, economic, and so on. If this lack does not exist, the dangers of countertransference are less. I consider that the best means of avoiding more or less abnormal countertransferences is to have recourse to a process of sublimation in thinking and in acting. Psychotherapy always poses problems which, when one approaches them not with excessively rigid schemas but with the desire to decipher even by a fraction of an inch more the enigma of illness, of suffering, and the enigma of the human being itself, oblige one to penetrate more deeply into the life of the psychotherapist himself, thus making it possible to avoid the dangers of an abnomal countertransference.

In any event, in transference and countertransference the fact of human liberty must not be forgotten. If the patient has his liberty limited by the illness, the psychotherapist does not. If the latter surrenders his liberty, he converts himself into a plaything in the hands of the patient. His liberty is the source of his curative power, of his "knowledge of salvation."

At the present time schizophrenia is more confusing than ever because the different schools of psychiatry and psychopathology comprehend different areas of it. Bleuler introduced the word schizophrenia, thinking, and rightly so, that the dementia praecox of Kraepelin had proved to be an inadequate designation. The designation has been so successful that it is even used today in nontechnical language. (I have heard a minister of finance say that the economy of his country was suffering from schizophrenia.) The fundamental idea is that of splitting (*Spaltung*), but the splitting to which Bleuler refers is that of the psychic functions. To what has been said it may be added that Bleuler was using the model of associational psychology and was referring fundamentally to the contents of thought; but in fact splitting occurs in the psychological function itself, which is the disturbance.

Experience has shown me that the psychic functions disturbed in schizophrenia are disturbed not only by the splitting of the psychic functions (perception, thinking, feeling) but also by contamination. "Sonorous thinking," for example, is nothing more than the contamination of two functions, one of which is sensorial and the other the pure function of thinking, which is normally silent. Other examples of this nature could be given.

In any event, we find ourselves faced with a *fait accompli*. The fact is that the word schizophrenia is employed by many people to designate psychopathological pictures whose most apparent aspect is the splitting of the ego, the rupture of its unity and, in addition, the fracturing of its contact with the environment, thus creating a distance between both, as though the ego were moving in a vacuum without the capacity to establish contact with anything else. From the psychotherapeutic point of view, the clearest image is offered by schizophrenic autism. As somebody once said, the patient is like the houses of ancient Rome which have all the doors to the outside closed and have only an inner patio.

In an epoch in which the systems of communication are more advanced than ever before, it nevertheless proves to be more difficult to penetrate into the inner life of people. Perhaps something is happening in the world which reveals itself not only in the structure of the personality of the ill but also in the formation of the personality of the healthy; this empties of its contents that "internal axis" of which Seneca spoke which constitutes the real framework of the personality.

Whoever has seen schizophrenics such as those which Bleuler describes and sees them again now will note an enormous difference. Their symptomatological richness is less, having been reduced by all the therapeutic means that are available, from the pharmacological to the psychotherapeutic. However, there always remains in the patient an inner nucleus, a kind of *sanctum sanctorum*, into which it is difficult to penetrate, and if at some time one manages to do so, one has the impression of having entered into an empty place. The impression of inner solitude of which Burton speaks is undeniable.

With regard to understanding man as he is today, the problem that seems most interesting to me is that of nihilism. It is easy to understand the nihilism of the neurotic and the schizophrenic, although on many occasions its authentic roots are not discovered. What is certain is that the fundamental problem always consists in finding "the sense of life." Who ought to find it—the patient himself, or should it be suggested, in one way or another, by the psychotherapist? This second hypothesis is practically unrealizable. Any manner of vital projects can be proposed to the patient, but if they are not born from within him they will never have sufficient force to lead him to realize them for himself.

The sense of life is intimately related to the sense of history, but we may ask whether history has sense. When the history of humanity is spoken of, it is often thought that it is the creative action of man that is discovering this sense, but precisely when faced with the neurotic or the psychotic we find a certain creative incapacity. I have previously said that on many occasions anxiety has creative powers, as is demonstrated by daily experience, and especially by what has occurred in the case of many great historical personages. Aristotle must have perceived something similar when he said that genius was akin to madness. However, the inhibition, the sensation of emptiness, the tedium of the ill leads them to find life as having no sense. Can it then be affirmed, as Nietzsche did, that life has no sense? This affirmation is dangerous, since if life has no sense then the logical conclusion consists in saying that life is *absurd,* as the schools of existential philosophy hold.

Camus said that if life is absurd, its only solution is suicide. Nietzsche also affirms this. However, in his case, his own vital necessity of emerging from this closed circle leads him to think of the will to power and of the possibility of a superman. To speak of the superman is utopian, at least in the psychotherapeutic task, when one has before one a human being weakened by his neurotic disturbances and still more by his psychotic disturbances. As an evasion of this limiting situation, which is what we see every day in certain patients, Nietzsche attached himself to the idea of eternal recurrence. Anxiety is always anxiety before nothingness, felt as anxiety at the idea of death, anxiety about emptiness, anxiety about madness; in a word, anxiety is *nonbeing.* Faced with this terrible experience, the ill, for example the obsessives, cannot find any way out except that of the repetition of their acts, and in this repetition they find a support that is false but nevertheless enables them to continue living. Nietzsche's thesis attempted to make compatible the idea of history as development and progress with the idea of the historic cycles. It is curious that this same problem is found latent in the conflict that was created between Freud and Fliess. Fliess claimed to have discovered the periodicity of the vital rhythms, of which Schwoboda had already spoken in purely biological terms. The theses of Fliess were forgotten, but the thesis of Freud was not, probably because in Freud anxiety found creative ferments which constituted the justifications of his discoveries and of his psychothera-peutic action.

Selected Writings

Lecciones de Psicologia. Vol. 1. Paz Montalvo, 1956.
Discurso a los Universitarios Españoles. Rialp, 1956.
Lecciones de Psicologia. Vol. 2. Paz Montalvo, 1960.
Las Neurosis Como Enfermedades del Animo. Gredos, 1966.
Rasgos Neuroticos del Mundo Contemporaneo. Cultura Hispanica, 1964.
El Libro de la Vida Sexual. Danac, 1967.

XIV

Final Notes on the
Lives of Healers

Arthur Burton

It is not easy to generalize about the way men become psychotherapists. In this volume we have to be content with a sample of twelve.
Even so, the twelve lives are less completely depicted than one would
like. Having a psychoanalysis or a personal psychotherapy apparently
returns less of the repressed than we had formerly believed. Or possibly there is a greater reserve in professionals' talking about their
childhood in this public way than we knew. Some reluctance to deal
with psychogenesis was certainly apparent in the twelve, and this
reticence was paradoxically at odds with their often slavish interest in
the infantile genesis of their clients. And, of course, female psychotherapists play no part in this volume, an obvious deficiency on my
part. Even though at the higher reaches of psychoanalysis or psycho-

310

analytic psychotherapeutic practice, and particularly in private practice, women psychotherapists are rare, two were invited to join this
symposium, accepted the invitation, but were unable to deliver their
manuscripts by publication date. They must therefore wait for another
opportunity and, at any rate, we can make a strength out of weakness
by confining our generalizations to the vast majority of therapists who
are male.[1] Our twelve autobiographers do not at all represent therapists who are psychiatric social workers, educational counselors, marital counselors, and so on, among whom greater numbers of women
can be expected to be found. But I would insist that psychotherapy
qua psychotherapy has its own indigeneous requisites regardless of
who practices it. Our twelve may indeed be more representative than
the small sample implies.

Seven of the twelve psychotherapists in this volume are pro-
fessedly Jewish. This ratio conforms well to the frequent observation
that this particular ethnic group applies for healing membership in
much greater numbers than would be indicated by their proportion
in the population. Depending upon how psychotherapy is itself defined,
and how the sample is taken, Jews in psychotherapy can range from a
bare majority to an overwhelming one. My own expectations are that
clinical psychology, psychiatry, and psychoanalysis will become even
more heavily identified with Jewish traditions in the future.

It may be that I have in the opening chapter overstressed the
relationship between the dynamics of being a Jew and the dynamics
of doing psychotherapy. But the history of the Jews reveals that their
particular social structure and social needs led them to become healers
in the Greco-Roman, Arabic, Byzantine, Christian, and every other
culture they lived in. We might say that one does not have to be a
Jew to be a psychotherapist, but it helps. I would also guess that those
non-Jewish psychotherapists who make psychotherapy their life style
as well as profession show considerable unconscious similarity to their

---

[1] I have earlier cited the fact that the fellowship membership of
the American Psychoanalytic Association, the American Psychiatric Association, and the Division of Psychotherapy of the American Psychological Association is heavily male. For example, at the Midwinter Meeting of the Division of Psychotherapy held in Phoenix, Arizona, March 2,
1972, from which I have just returned, 90 per cent of the registrants were
male.

Jewish colleagues. Freud was always fearful that psychoanalysis would become a "Jewish science." Perhaps it has—and now Jewish and non-Jewish practitioners merge into one entity at the fundamental level of identification with the client.

Childhood

Our autobiographers disagree about whether their childhood was determinative in becoming psychotherapists. Ellis flatly comes out against it, and Rogers makes no great bones for such early ordination. Mendel, Warkentin and Burton, on the other hand, imply that their early character formation was causal in becoming healers. And English seems to ride the fence. But what is manifest is that an early and sustained physical illness is almost uniformly found in the twelve healers. English had tuberculosis; Ellis found himself with nephritis; Burton contracted bronchial asthma; Rogers had periods of undefined lassitude; Warkentin had asthmatic attacks; Steinzor developed a disease of the eye; and so it went. These illnesses usually led to long periods of quiet inaction and introspection, sometimes with a concomitant fear of death, and systematized fantasy rather than reality became the source of childhood gratification. This fits well with the current appreciation that one's life flies in the face of one's disability. In some, handicap is followed by superordinate attempts to overcome and compensate for it, along Adlerian lines, and the handicap becomes the human sensitivity and the justification for unreasonable dedication and effort. The handicapped try harder to make this a nonhandicapping world. Beds, white sheets, nurses, doctors, medication, the attention of helpful people, all help slant the ego toward the melioration process. This strange milieu then becomes the one of comfort, and if one cannot become a perpetual patient, one can at least become the doctor.

The family backgrounds are remarkable in the absence of mental illness in the progenitors. One would have expected on an actuarial basis that the immediate and distant family would have had more psychosis in it. However, my feeling is that psychosis drives people away from the psychotherapeutic field whereas neurosis brings them to it. Psychosis overpowers and quiets but neurosis activates the metaphorical search for the sources of humanity.

Our psychotherapists come from families on the move. They were busy "making it," and particularly the fathers. Of course, not making it is also subject to the rule. There is more than an average amount of mobility—intellectual and spatial—in these families and this is not to be accounted for by the European origins of many. As adults the psychotherapists themselves show little stasis and are galvanized people even though they are presumably in a passive occupation. This high activity level partly accounts for the innovative creation of our sample in the form of research projects, books, professorships, and institute memberships, as well as substantial treatment loads. It also correlates with a certain volatility revealed by them.

One would reasonably expect that as psychoanalysts or analytically oriented psychotherapists, who often have been personally analyzed by descendants or even peers of Freud, these autobiographers would report early sexual trauma in their lives. But this book is remarkably free of sex and strangely strong on logos. Are these analysts and therapists saying that the primal scene, the evolvement of pregenital character, the castration conflict, the Oedipal conflict, and similar others were unimportant in their own growth and development? Only Reuben Fine clings tenaciously to Freud's hard-won concepts and attempts—unsatisfactorily, I might add—to apply them to his genesis. As a psychotherapist myself, I would say by way of explanation that such Freudian concepts are still very much present but serve as a baseline or normative aspect, and something more than a castration complex is needed to produce a psychotherapist. These concepts seem also, clinically, to apply more readily to clients than they do to our own lives. All of this points up the fact that the sum of the erogenous zones does not add up to what a person becomes, and the self-description of a life is not indexed by its sexuality—early or late.

Psychotherapeutic Training

Very few of our autobiographers have kind words to say about their training analysis, or their personal therapy in lieu. Steinzor and Ellis are downright hostile; Burton, wistful; and Polster and English moderately worshipful and stargazing. But the "person" of the training analyst or personal therapist still shines brightly for them, perhaps in the recognition that the process was defective but the analytic per-

son tried hard and was quite human about it. All respondents feel that
their true growth has come from, and with, their clients. Much of
what they know has been self-taught; that is, our healers have great
capacity for innovative learning and process, and eschew the formal
methods available to others. In the face of this one wonders whether
the requirement of a personal analysis or personal therapy ought not
to be dropped, or at least its rational justification changed. I myself
consider it extremely important, but only in the sense that it allows the
psychotherapist to become an identified sufferer.

Therapists' Wives

It seems necessary to be married to be an authentic psychotherapist. The marriages of psychotherapists can be either very good
or very bad, with not much in between. Our autobiographers reported
their wives as having extraordinary meaning to them, almost at times
to the point of sentimental embarrassment. English, Rogers, Warkentin, Mendel, Steinzor, Polster, and others hardly see themselves apart
from their wives. Why is this?

At a workshop meeting of the Division of Psychotherapy of the
American Psychological Association,[2] at which I was present, twenty-
six therapists' wives met in an encounter group to work through their
marriages to their psychotherapist husbands. This unique group revealed that problems in their marriages are frequent and that they
personally often felt lonely. Their husbands keep clients and wives
carefully segregated and, as I have described in Chapter One, each
psychotherapist has in effect two families rather than one. But the
wives were pretty firm on the idea that they also serve as therapists to
their husbands—that they nurse them through Freudian, Rogerian,
and other stages of evolution, and the many pains which come from
being a psychotherapist as well. Many wives said they were jealous of
their husbands' clients, and even of the joy they got out of their therapeutic work.

It is evident that our twelve autobiographers are in daily touch
with their feminine side, are fundamentally related to—yes, in love
with—all women, and actually spend most of their waking and sleep-

[2] *Phoenix (Arizona) Gazette*, March 3, 1972. The group was
facilitated by Dr. Ron Fox.

ing hours with women. None of them is a member of a professional football or basketball team! The extraordinary number of female clients is certainly a part response to the welcome they receive from male psychotherapists. Attention has a way of materializing itself. But English's point is well taken: we treat female clients but we marry our wives. Our marriages endure beyond our treatment relationships; and they are, by and large, the more fulfilled side of us.

Love and Work

Each autobiographer talks of love and work. Freud was not far off in his description of love and work as the basic ingredients of mental health. And our therapists do work hard and love hard. In fact, the distinctions between love and work are often indistinguishable for them. One loves work and works at love! The happiness and well-being of the psychotherapist lie in the differential fact that he can love and work whereas his clients cannot. Becoming helped by treatment is being able to work better and to love more: that is to say, becoming more like the psychotherapist. This is perhaps one of the reasons so many of our patients want to become psychotherapists during treatment.

Management studies reveal that most people hate their work, but most healers find glory in theirs. But work and love are inseparable. Those who work unhappily also tend to love unhappily. All true creativity has this power of disestablishing time and space; and joy, in the final analysis, is the momentary freedom from temporality and death.

Luck

A most surprising finding in our study was the fact that our scientist-therapists believe they were the fortunate objects of a process called luck. This is best exemplified by Rogers who calls it luck that he consistently anticipated and preceded clinical developments which put him on the crest of every tide in his profession for three decades. English and Polster and Warkentin and Ellis similarly feel somewhat this way, without explicitly calling it luck, and most of the others genuflect in this direction as well.

Is it that we feel lucky that we are not the clients? Do we consider the profession of psychoanalysis and psychotherapy so full of demonic pitfalls that luck has to rescue us, or is luck the symbolic statement of guilt about the good thing all of us have made from the misery of our sufferers? Except in one sense I do not feel that I, personally, was lucky. I made my own breaks and consistently refused to accept failure. Some of my colleagues did accept it with even less reason than I had and fell by the wayside. Yes, I am lucky to be alive; but even here it is more a matter of genetic programing than anything the environment afforded me.

Ellis and Rogers best demonstrate careers in which, to me, luck played only a minor part. Each of these men had a finely attuned "third ear" which acted in radar fashion to bring them in harmony with the needs of society. They bet on themselves and they bet on the receptivity of the environment to their presentations. But if the bet failed to pay off, they quickly switched to another area of probability. Sex and sensitivity training are in wide demand and Ellis and Rogers are specialists in each at just the right time. Permanent failure is very rare in this group and I doubt that it could occur. Only death can call finis. If by luck one means a careful playing of the cognitive odds, then I have no objection to it. But creative men make their own luck, and modesty then leads them to ascribe their wonderful fruition to this evanescent lady. (Even then, I would not ignore the horseshoe!)

Being Crazy or Unique

Our autobiographers accept the fact—even parade it, in a sense—that they are unlike other men. This is a necessary part of their charisma; but this differentness is not only ascribed to them by others, it is a part of their own internalized image of themselves. To be "crazy" is to be inventive and innovative—to be in touch with the devil, from whom all things stem. No healer wants to be called a saint for this demeans the possibilities of his craziness.

As one reads these life stories one's head slowly wags at what often illogical and irrational people these psychotherapists are. Like Freud himself, who was a complete ass at times,[3] the child sits side by

[3] See, for example, the letters to Fliess.

side with the adult, but is apparently as necessary to the adult as the adult is to the child. Thus Steinzor's six or seven years with his lady analyst make us irritable that he didn't break it up earlier, for he obviously wanted to. And English tempting Thanatos while doing an internship with active tuberculosis, and Warkentin wanting to die because his wife spurned him from time to time, and Burton clinging to Los Angeles when the East called is all straight *mischigas*.

These examples are not the elegant and rational decisions one expects of mature psychotherapists. It was the same with great writers. Dostoevski was a fool as a gambler; F. Scott Fitzgerald a sop about high society; Henry Miller carefully kept one step ahead of any possibility of being physically heroic; and so it went. The successful Muse is a combination of cold intellectual steel and a bunch of drivel which would make even adolescents ashamed. Psychotherapy is a peculiar mixture of play and reality, of studied rationality and fantastic idiosyncrasy, of established maturity and puerile infancy, of sheer honesty and gross deception. All of this becomes critically focused in the one personality of the healer and the visible motif is often one of chaos. But do not let this fool you. In the crucible of the interpersonal relationship all faculties zero in simultaneously and the psychotherapist is there as razor sharp and authentic. He becomes for the hour almost perfectly integrated, as the needs of the client offer themselves to him. These autobiographers are sometimes funny as well as serious, and their comic aspect is just the recognition of life in its serious *and* nonserious aspects.

Future of the Therapist

I suppose that the successful outcome of a life as a healer is, as Mendel puts it, to move happily on to some nonhealing joy. One simply cannot master all the seriatim challenges of therapy and still hang in there on a constantly peaking level. Psychotherapy certainly renews itself every day, but a higher-order problem, or a higher-order person, must also be waiting in the wings to maintain the challenge. I have already said that psychotherapists find satiation difficult. To treat endlessly the same kind of people in the same way would be impossible. The many styles of current psychotherapies do not represent merely an artistry of process but the need to keep oneself immersed and motivated in continuing to do psychotherapy at all by a variety of innovated ways.

Countertransference is uniquely dissatisfaction. Being a psychotherapist requires working with the bedrock of existence and involves a perpetual philosophical questing. Irritability and dissatisfaction constantly wait at the door to be let in. Psychotherapy is not a technique but the vocation of being human. To be human one must have needs acknowledged and satisfied. I have for this reason called for an annual "satisfaction checkup" for psychotherapists everywhere.[4] Our autobiographers obviously do not reside in paradise, but they are a group of people greatly satisfied with themselves as human beings. They would do it over again in the same way.

Selection of Therapists

If one can to some extent generalize the lives of the psychoanalysts and psychotherapists self-depicted in this book, and they must be deemed successful by any known criterion, then one is left with the feeling that perhaps medical schools, graduate schools, psychoanalytic institutes, counseling centers are selecting the wrong people to train. The myths which abound in selecting people to become healers have a way of perpetuating themselves even beyond what one may find, say, in a law school. The criterion of any selection test for therapists must be not only a substantive quantum of ultimately recovered clients, but a sense of completeness and fulfillment on the part of the therapist as well. The principal distinction I find in our twelve psychotherapists is not that they have helped people in great numbers but that they have become authentic and fulfilled people themselves by so doing. They like themselves—a rare condition in these days. But I am not so sure that all of them would be admitted to formal psychoanalytic and psychotherapeutic training programs as present-day criteria go.

If I may be permitted to use the twelve lives in this book as a criterion and assume that they stand as some kind of model for future generations of psychotherapists, then the following would be among the relevant criteria for selecting candidates for healing work in psy-

---

[4] A. Burton, *Interpersonal Psychotherapy* (Englewood Cliffs, N.J.: Prentice-Hall, 1972).

chology, psychiatry, and psychoanalysis. Their absence may not necessarily result in failure of the candidate, but their presence is certainly associated with success.

(1) A psychotherapist is a person with a metaphysical hunger.

(2) A pyschotherapist idealizes his father and depreciates his mother.

(3) The psychotherapist will probably be Jewish, have Jewish origins, or have unconscious collective values similar to those represented by Judaism.

(4) Love and negative mutuality will be central to the psychotherapist's being.

(5) The psychotherapist will be comfortable with hearing confession.

(6) The psychotherapist will live closer to his unconscious but without thereby reducing his consciousness.

(7) The psychotherapist will have personally experienced depression, despair, and dissociation.

(8) The psychotherapist's family background will reveal considerable disruption and upheaval.

(9) The psychotherapist will require not one but two families.

(10) The psychotherapist will introject a therapist-ideal and will find creative meaning in the yin and yang of such idealization.

(11) The psychotherapist will be a rationalist who interprets his world as orderly, logical, and subject to cognitive rule.

(12) The psychotherapist will place a high value on talk and conversation.

(13) The psychotherapist will manifest logos but will not be institutionally religious.

(14) The psychotherapist will help society grow as well as helping his client.

(15) The psychotherapist will primally manifest (what Heidegger calls) *Sorge:* a Promethean caring for humanity and a willingness to assume the absurdities of man.

It could be said that some of these twelve have moved along innovatively with the times, and others still appear to represent the more traditional beliefs and ways of practicing psychotherapy. But are we to value one group over the other? My feeling is that Carl Rogers is Carl Rogers whether he is being client-centered, more direct with schizophrenics, or a self-effacing facilitator in an encounter group, and that it does not matter much which. The social forms by which a person plies his indigenous healing posture are almost irrelevant in his treatment outcomes. Each healer in the stages of his growth finds a platform from which he leaps into the faith of the cure, and the fact that some leap further or more often than others is not remarkable. What counts is what I have described in my fifteen personality vectors but, more than this, the summation of all of them into what I call the primal healing posture of the personality. If such sorge is present, then the healer can be expected to be motivated to heal and to offer his ego time and again in the service of the disabled. Without it formalism is apt to take over.

Training institutes are confused as to what makes a desirable candidate and whom to admit and not admit. They oscillate in their admission policies like a pennant in a gale. I want personally to say that these twelve are for me the heroes of psychotherapy, and future candidates should be accepted principally in their image. This is not vanity—it is that too—but lifetime demonstration of a clear and brilliant extension of humanism to the dehumanized. Not only that. These twelve have provided one hundredfold beyond their numbers in creative productions which have extended knowledge both generally and specifically. In this they have more than carried their weight as models. The failure of psychotherapy is that so few of us ever go beyond the client to the written word.

Psychotherapy, in my opinion, has not yet reached its zenith, and in the desperate social need of our times it is being wildly secularized. But secularization and heterodoxy have often fallen short in the past, and again and again I have found that I cannot escape the basic discoveries of Freud and Jung. Abridgement for comfort, convenience, and palatability has its limits. Perhaps we have now reached them if an encounter group or transactional group allows a client to build his resistances to insight and being rather than reduce them. A friend a long time ago said to me, and I cannot forget what he said: "Art, there are no bargains in psychotherapy; it is fruitless to look for them." I now fully agree with him.

Index

Charity and the therapist, 12–16
Chestnut Lodge: and schizophrenia, 230; Stierlin at, 132, 133–136
Childhood of psychotherapists, 312–313; Burton, 192–194, 203–204, 312; Ekstein, 263–267; Ellis, 104–108, 312; English, 78–81, 312; Fine, 222–224; Mendel, 285–286, 312; Polster, 146–151; Rogers, 29–35, 312; Steinzor, 165–167; Stierlin, 127–128; Warkentin, 244–247, 254–255, 312
Client: ideal, 24–26; learning from, 48, 94–96, 99, 135, 183–184
Co-therapy, 250
Countertransference, 318; to Ekstein, 264, 278; to Fine, 226, 227, 237–239; to Lopez-Ibor, 305–306

D

Death: deferred for psychotherapists, 22; attitude toward, of English, 101; attitude toward, of Steinzor, 185

E

Ego satiation and the psychotherapist, 21–22
EKSTEIN, R., growth and development of: childhood, 263–267; in youth movement and university years, 267–269; in psychoanalysis, 271–273; in practice, 274–275, 276; in teaching, 275–277; in philosophy, 269–271, 277–279; through wife and children, 279–280; in views on future of psychoanalysis, 280–283; in writings, 263, 272, 274–276, 277, 279, 283
ELLIS, A., growth and development of:

childhood, 104–108, 312; in student years, 108–109; in psychoanalytic training, 108–112, 313; in analysis, 110–112; in psychoanalytic practice, 112–114; in RET (rational-emotive therapy), 114–126; in group therapy, 117–118, 120–121; in combining of love and work, 122; in writings, 126
ENGLISH, O. S., 3, 18; colleagues, learning from, 88–92; and the healing encounter, 100; and patient therapy, 94–96, 99; with professional organizations, 94; self-perception of, 96–99; and sensitivity groups, 100–101; and suffering, 99–100; writings of, 97–98, 101–102
ENGLISH, O. S., growth and development of: childhood, 78–81, 312; during student years, 81–84, 317; as Commonwealth Foundation Fellow, 83–84; in psychoanalytic training, 84–87, 313; through marriage and children, 87–88, 93, 96, 98, 314, 315; in practice, 89, 91–92, 93; and developmental forces, 92–94; in attitude toward death, 101
ERIKSON, E., 63, 136, 204
Eros in psychotherapy, 199–200

F

FARSON, R., 55, 64, 66
Fathers and the psychotherapist, 17–20, 312, 319; and Burton, 192–193; and Ellis, 104–105, 115; and English, 79–80; and Polster, 46, 149; and Rogers, 29–35, 40; and Steinzor, 165–166, 169–170; and Warkentin, 247
FINE, R.: and countertransference, 237–239; and love as a universal,